# Research Methods in Nursing and Midwifery

## PATHWAYS TO EVIDENCE-BASED PRACTICE

S

**BPP**

## REFERENCE USE ONLY

### Not to be removed from the Library

# Research Methods in Nursing and Midwifery

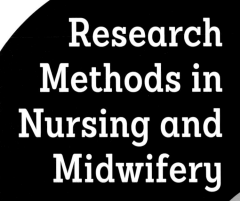

PATHWAYS TO
EVIDENCE-BASED
PRACTICE

SECOND EDITION

Edited by
SANSNEE JIROJWONG
MAREE JOHNSON
ANTHONY WELCH

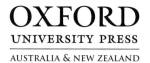

OXFORD
UNIVERSITY PRESS
AUSTRALIA & NEW ZEALAND

OXFORD
UNIVERSITY PRESS

Oxford University Press is a department of the University of Oxford.

It furthers the University's objective of excellence in research, scholarship, and education by publishing worldwide. Oxford is a registered trademark of Oxford University Press in the UK and in certain other countries.

Published in Australia by
Oxford University Press
253 Normanby Road, South Melbourne, Victoria 3205, Australia

National Library of Australia Cataloguing-in-Publication entry

Title: Research methods in nursing and midwifery / Sansnee
    Jirojwong, Maree Johnson, Anthony Welch, editors.
Edition: 2nd
ISBN  9780195528510 (paperback)
Notes: Includes index.
Subjects: Nursing—Research—Textbooks.
        Midwifery—Research—Textbooks.
Other Authors/Contributors: Jirojwong, Sansnee, editor.
                        Johnson, Maree, editor.
                        Welch, Anthony J., editor.

Dewey Number: 610.73072

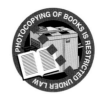
Edited by Venetia Somerset
Typeset by diacriTech, Chennai, India
Proofread by Anne Mulvaney
Indexed by Russell Brooks
Text design by Glen McClay
Printed by Markono Print Media Pte Ltd, Singapore

*To the Jirojwong family, in particular Nantaka, and the late Professor Robert MacLennan*
SANSNEE JIROJWONG

*To the courageous women in my life: Emily Condon, Pauline Johnson, Carmel Young and Judith Wilkinson*
MAREE JOHNSON

*I would like to dedicate my contributions to this book to my parents and family,*
*without whom such an achievement would not have been possible.*
ANTHONY WELCH

# CONTENTS

Below.

## 3  Introducing the Research Process    34

Maree Johnson and Cecily Hengstberger-Sims

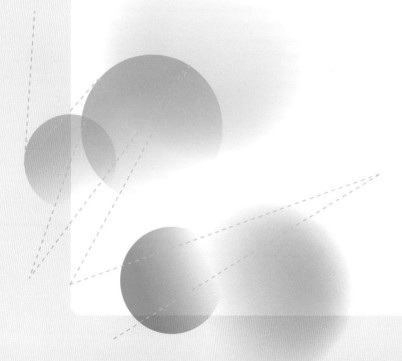

# LIST OF FIGURES

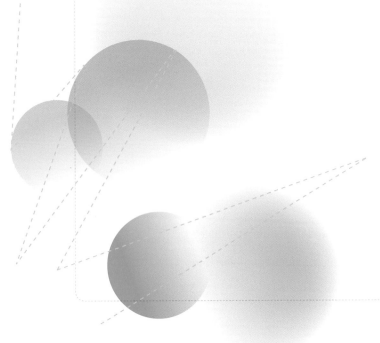

# LIST OF TABLES

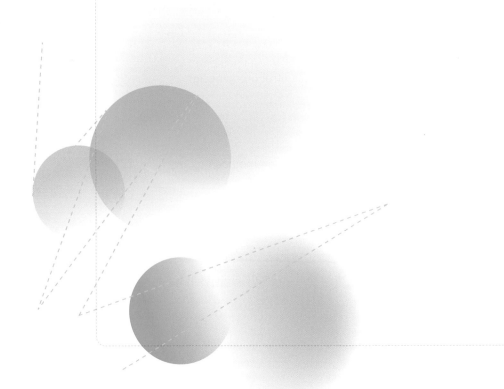

# LIST OF ABBREVIATIONS

| | | | |
|---|---|---|---|
| ABS | Australian Bureau of Statistics | MAStARI | Meta Analysis of Statistics Assessment and Review Instrument |
| ACN | Australian College of Nursing | MRSA | Methicillin-resistant Staphylococcus aureus |
| AIDS | acquired immune deficiency syndrome | NEAF | National Ethics Application Form |
| AIHW | Australian Institute of Health and Welfare | NHMRC | National Health and Medical Research Council |
| ANMAC | Australian Nursing and Midwifery Accreditation Council | OR | odds ratio |
| APA | American Psychological Association | PCA | patient controlled analgesia |
| CALD | culturally and linguistically diverse | PDA | personal digital assistant |
| CAT | critical appraisal tool | PICF | Participant Information and Consent Form |
| CATI | computer assisted telephone interviewing | PICO | Patient/Population, Intervention, Comparison, Outcome |
| CIAP | Clinical Information Access Program | PLS | Plain Language Statement |
| CINAHL | Cumulative Index to Nursing and Allied Health Literature | QARI | qualitative assessment and review instrument |
| CNC | clinical nurse consultant | QRMG | Cochrane Collaboration Qualitative Research Methods Group |
| EBMid | evidence-based midwifery | QUAL | qualitative |
| EBN | evidence-based nursing | QUAN | quantitative |
| EBP | evidence-based practice | RCT | randomised controlled trial |
| ED | emergency department | RN/M | Registered nurse/midwife |
| EMS | extended midwifery services | RR | relative risk |
| GDM | gestational diabetes | SAB | surfactants, allantoin and benzalkonium chloride |
| GP | general practitioner | SARS | Severe Acute Respiratory Syndrome |
| HAPI | Health and Psychosocial Instruments (database) | SD | standard deviation |
| HIV | human immunodeficiency virus | VAS | visual analogue scale |
| HREC | human research ethics committee | WHO | World Health Organization |
| IQR | inter-quartile range | WMD | weighted mean difference |
| JBI | Joanna Briggs Institute | | |

# ABOUT THE EDITORS

**Sansnee Jirojwong** (PhD) received a PhD at the University of Melbourne and taught nursing and midwifery students at undergraduate and postgraduate levels. She undertook research projects in Thailand, Brunei Darussalam and Australia. Sansnee's projects have focused on the health of disadvantaged groups such as migrants and rural people. She has worked with local communities and disadvantaged groups to increase the accessibility of health and social services. One of her projects used the participatory communication concept as a framework to develop health education resources for Vietnamese-born pregnant women who have gestational diabetes. The resources based on this project received the Commendation New South Wales Multicultural Health Communication Award. Sansnee's research articles are published in international refereed journals and conference proceedings. In 2012, this research textbook was shortlisted for the Australian Educational Publishing Awards. Sansnee now lives in Thailand, her birth country, where she is assisting junior researchers undertaking their research projects.

**Maree Johnson** (RN, PhD Epidemiology & Population Health) is a Clinical Professor with the School of Nursing and Midwifery, University of Western Sydney, with 30 years' experience in nursing and health research. As Director of the Centre for Applied Nursing Research (a joint facility of the University of Western Sydney and Sydney Western Sydney Local Health District) she has assisted academics and clinicians to successfully complete research projects (Honours, Master's and PhDs). Her expertise includes the use of complex sampling procedures, conducting national surveys, instrument design and testing, clinical trials, and grounded theory and ethnographic studies in qualitative research. Other aspects of her current role include undertaking systematic reviews and developing clinical guidelines for health professionals. Professor Johnson has published in national and international refereed journals in nursing and health and has a contemporary understanding of the learning requirements of undergraduate and postgraduate research students.

**Anthony Welch** (PhD) is an Associate Professor of Mental Health Nursing at the School of Nursing and Midwifery CQUniversity Australia. Anthony is the Head of Program for the Master of Mental Health Nursing and Discipline Head of Mental Health Nursing. Anthony has extensive experience in supervision of higher degrees by research candidates in the areas of suicide prevention, resilience, recovery, compassion and caring in healthcare delivery, depression, men's health and spirituality. His research expertise is in qualitative research methods. Anthony continues to act as a consultant to a number of universities in South East Asia in relation to research supervision and the application of qualitative research findings to clinical practice.

# ABOUT THE CONTRIBUTORS

**Petra Gertraud Buettner** (PhD) Associate Professor Buettner completed her PhD with the Technical University and the Free University of Berlin, Germany. Since 1995 she has worked at James Cook University. Her research interests include design and analysis of epidemiological studies. She has authored more than 200 research publications in peer-reviewed journals and book chapters. Her book *Epidemiology* was published by Oxford University Press.

**Monika Buhrer-Skinner** (DrPH) completed her DrPH in 2011. Since 2003 she has worked at James Cook University as lecturer and taught quantitative research methodology to undergraduate and postgraduate health science students. Her main research interests include sexual and reproductive health, especially Chlamydia trachomatis infection, which was also the subject of her doctoral project.

**Sungwon Chang** (PhD) has extensive experience in quantitative data analysis. Sungwon has had a number of collaborative research projects within health services and clinical research. She has recently received a Chancellor Post-Doctoral Research Fellow from the University of Technology Sydney. Her areas of research interest include exploring a range of measures in clinical trials.

**Keri Chater** (PhD) completed her nursing degree in 1980 and received a doctoral degree at La Trobe University. She has worked in acute care, aged care and community sectors as well as lecturing at RMIT. Her areas of specialty include nursing ethics. She has extensive experience in aged care research and currently is a member of the Western Health Ethics Committee where she reviews research applications.

**Ritin Fernandez** (PhD) is Professor of Nursing at the School of Nursing, Midwifery and Indigenous Health, University of Wollongong and St George Hospital and the Director of the Centre for Evidence Based Initiatives in Health Care, a collaborating Centre of the Joanna Briggs Institute. Her teaching and research interests include evidence-based practice and randomised controlled trials. Ritin has published over 100 peer-reviewed journal articles.

**Rhonda Griffiths** AM. (RN; RM; B.Ed(Nursing); MSc(Hons); Dr.PH.) Professor Griffiths is Dean of the School of Nursing and Midwifery at University of Western Sydney. Rhonda is an experienced administrator, researcher and educator and has held senior positions in public health services and universities. She was appointed as a Member in the General Division of the Order of Australia (AM) 'for service to public health, particularly through contributions to diabetes research and education, and to the nursing profession'. She was also recognised with the award of Honorary Life Member of the Australian Diabetes Educators Association and the Sir Kempton Maddox Award for her contributions to Diabetes Australia and to people with diabetes. Rhonda completed her first research project in 1988 and since then has been awarded research grants of AU$4 million. She has published 150 peer-reviewed journal articles and book chapters and over 200 peer-reviewed and invited conference presentations.

**Cecily Hengstberger-Sims** (PhD) is an Associate Professor at the School of Nursing and Midwifery, University of Western Sydney. Cecily has successfully supervised a number of Honours and research higher degree students. She retains an active interest in evidence-based practice and nursing research and her research interests include effective team communication and innovative teaching.

**Jackie Lea** (MN) is a registered nurse, lecturer and clinical coordinator in the School of Health, University of New England. Jackie teaches clinical nursing practice at undergraduate and postgraduate levels. Her research interests include new graduate nurses, rural nursing practice and retention issues in nursing. She has published widely in refereed journals and has presented papers at conferences and workshops.

**Janice Lewis** (DBA) is the Program Leader for Health Policy and Management courses in the School of Public Health, Curtin University, Western Australia, where she teaches health services management and qualitative research methodology at postgraduate level. Her interests are health policy and qualitative research methods. She has also developed a research methodologies unit for Open Universities Australia, which combines both qualitative and quantitative methodologies.

**Phillip Maude** (PhD) is an Associate Professor at Royal Melbourne Institute of Technology University and the Director of Research Programs and a coordinator of mental health/addictions programs. Phil's research interests include practice development and cognitive behavioural interventions. He has supervised PhD students who use diverse research methods and engaged them in using research evidence to improve clinical practice.

**Reinhold Muller** (PhD) is the Principal Epidemiologist/Biostatistician at the School of Public Health and Tropical Medicine, James Cook University. As principal investigator, Associate Professor Muller has been conducting, analysing and publishing a number of epidemiological studies including nursing, rehabilitation and cardiology. He teaches quantitative research methodology. He has more than 250 articles in international peer-reviewed journals and three textbooks on evidence-based quantitative research methodology.

**Penny Paliadelis** (PhD) is Dean at the School of Health Sciences, University of Ballarat. Her research interests include the broad area of rural nursing practices as well as the organisational culture of healthcare systems. She has a reputation for encouraging and supporting scholarly and research collaborations within and across health disciplines, in partnership with clinical colleagues.

**Glenda Parmenter** (PhD) is a registered nurse and lecturer at the School of Health, University of New England. Her clinical background focused on aged care nursing and community-based palliative care. Her research interests concern the social lives of rural nursing home residents and professional development of nurses in rural areas. She has published a book chapter and journal articles and presented her work at conferences.

**Karen Pepper** (MA Hons) has lectured on research methodology and data analysis for the health and behavioural sciences at the University of Sydney and the University of Wollongong. Her research interests include investigating the relationship between psychological factors and health, with an emphasis on the application of statistical analysis to health and behavioural research.

**Jamie Ranse** (MCritCareNurs) is an Assistant Professor in Nursing at the University of Canberra. His research interests are in disaster and mass gathering health. His projects have been supported by competitive research grants. His work is published in peer-reviewed journals. Jamie is completing a PhD at the Flinders University.

**Jan Taylor** (PhD) is a midwife and Associate Professor in the Faculty of Health, University of Canberra. Jan teaches in the Bachelor of Midwifery as well as supervising higher degree research students. She is particularly interested in survey research and her research interests revolve around women's experiences following birth.

**Jane Warland** (PhD) is a Senior Lecturer in Nursing and Midwifery, University of South Australia. She completed her PhD at the University of Adelaide. Jane's research interests include population health, mental health and maternity. She uses qualitative, quantitative and mixed methods in her projects and has had more than 30 articles published in peer-reviewed journals.

**Lisa Whitehead** (PhD) is an Associate Professor at the Centre for Postgraduate Nursing Studies, University of Otago, Christchurch and director of the strategy to enhance research in nursing and allied health. Dr Whitehead's community health practices and research focus on developing self-management of long-term conditions to allow people to remain in their own homes.

# ACKNOWLEDGMENTS

This book could not have been completed without the support of many people. The University of Western Sydney—School of Nursing and Midwifery provides support through their library and office resources. The reviewers of the first edition of the book provided critical comments that were useful to its revision. Ideas and opinions from many readers of the first edition are valuable for the updating.

Sansnee Jirojwong would like to acknowledge the late Professor Robert MacLennan, an experienced researcher and epidemiologist, who provided encouragement as the book was going through an early stage of the revision. His support will be remembered. Nantaka Jirojwong has quietly made sure that no disruption occurred while Sansnee was carrying out her tasks and responsibilities as senior editor and a contributor to several chapters. Special thanks to her.

Maree Johnson would like to thank Sansnee for her vision and Tony for his support during this revision. She thanks both for making a life-time dream become a reality.

Anthony Welch would like to acknowledge his companion and friend Stephen Gellion for his continuing support and encouragement over the years as he has ventured down the path of his professional pursuits and personal aspirations. To his sisters and brothers who have been an ongoing source of pride and love. A special thanks to his beautiful Old English Sheepdog Pierre who on many occasions corralled him in his office and maintained the watch to prevent any disruptions or distractions throughout the process of working with Sansnee and Maree on this book.

We also would like to thank Debra James and Shari Serjeant at Oxford University Press for their patience and understanding of our situations as university academics, researchers and laypersons. Their collegiality is much appreciated by all of us. We value the input from all OUP staff during the process of book conception to print. We appreciate the important contributions by all contributors, who have been so marvellous in responding to our emails, requests and explanations. They have shared their research experiences in their individual chapters.

The authors and publisher are grateful to the copyright holders for granting permission to use the various figures, examples (or modifications of them) and data in this book. Every effort has been made to trace the original source of the material reproduced in this book. Where the attempt has been unsuccessful, the authors and publisher would be pleased to hear from the copyright holder concerned to rectify any omission.

# INTRODUCTION

## Sansnee Jirojwong and Anthony Welch

In 1971, Professor A. L. Cochrane published *Effectiveness and Efficiency: Random Reflections on Health Services*, a seminal book about the need to evaluate medical and social services on the basis of scientific evidence rather than on tradition, clinical opinion, expert or anecdotal observation. He called for the assessment of disease treatment, screening, diagnosis, midwifery and social work. The book has had a profound influence, not only on medicine but also on other healthcare disciplines such as public health, pharmacy, nursing and midwifery.

About antenatal care, he wrote: 'This service is basically a multiple screening procedure, which, by some curious chance, has escaped the critical assessment to which most screening procedures have been subjected in the last few years and there seems no reason why the same approach that has proved so useful elsewhere should not be used here.' He went on to say, 'Much more doubtful is the therapeutic use of iron and vitamins…My general impression is that the emotive atmosphere should be removed and the subject treated like any other medical activity' (p. 66).

Over the past 40 years, especially since the 1990s, evidence-based practice has been adopted worldwide as an important principle in healthcare. Despite Cochrane's achievement, much still needs to be evaluated.

Over more than seven decades, the professions of nursing and midwifery have made considerable advances in the development of discipline-specific knowledge and clinical expertise. Such advances can be attributed to the application of new information to clinical practice. This has led to quality improvement in all areas of professional practice in nursing and midwifery. The generation of new knowledge has not occurred in isolation but as a result of applying a systematic and rigorous approach to the search for answers to issues arising in everyday professional practice. Research is the process of questioning and searching for answers to a problem or issue of concern.

Within contemporary nursing and midwifery practice there are few clinicians, educators and students who fail to perceive that learning about research is relevant to their practice. They acknowledge the benefits of research but still see it as something 'out there' to be accessed if needed but not viewed as part of professional practice.

We read the results of research published in the press or listen to discussions about research findings on the radio. They can also appear as short messages flashing on internet websites. Healthcare consumers who are searching for information from these media to improve their health may use these findings. As healthcare professionals, we need to be able to read and decide whether the results are credible, whether they are to be used by healthcare consumers or not. This means we need to understand the concept of research process and research methodology.

Evidence-based practice depends on a careful recording of evidence, such as is widely carried out in healthcare. For example, What is the evidence for deciding to have a flu vaccination? can be asked when you suggest to a patient to increase their immunity against flu. Evidence is also based on the synthesis of research results. People who take on the task of generating or creating the evidence need to be able to identify and differentiate the evidence from 'good' projects from that resulting from 'not so good' projects.

Different kinds of knowledge can be generated by different pathways. Researchers can generate knowledge by conducting research and collecting data from participants in the field or in clinical areas. They can have data retrieved from records kept by hospitals, long-term care settings or community health organisations. Knowledge can be also generated by analysing and synthesising the results of a number of research studies. This research textbook is written in order to demonstrate that research is a process and there is a pathway that readers and researchers can follow.

Many health issues are complex. Clinicians often ask why such issues are occurring. There may be so many questions to ask about a particular health issue that it will be difficult for clinicians to answer all of them at once. Many questions may be answered by the findings of quantitative research; let us think, for example, about a warm sponging and rest as ways to reduce body temperature. Many others can be answered by qualitative research; let us think about having elders included as important persons who can link healthcare workers and Indigenous patients in some communities so that the care can be increasingly accepted or adopted by the patients.

# GUIDED TOUR

**Part openers** introduce and follow the characters of Ann and Bob as they embark on a research project, drawing out the main issues discussed in the following chapters.

**PART 1**

## GETTING STARTED IN RESEARCH

Ann and Bob are registered nurses working in a busy emergency department (ED) of a large referral hospital. They observe that many patients who present with chest pain are discharged after a few hours of observation. However, it is also observed that half of these patients repeatedly re-present to the ED. Ann and Bob would like to explore why this group of patients continue to re-present to ED and what additional services can be provided after discharge to help them manage their condition better and therefore reduce the rate of re-presentations. Ann and Bob are aware that a number of research publications are available, including systematic reviews and guidelines for pain management, and so they decide to review what is known about pain management before deciding how to go about researching this issue. As this is their first project, Ann and Bob want to ensure that the project will be conducted to the best of their ability—in a systematic and rigorous manner. As the hospital has links with a local university Ann and Bob decide first to consult experienced researchers for direction and guidance. The decision to undertake this project sets them on the path of research.

Chapter 1 gives important information about beginning the research journey: the processes involved in starting your first piece of research, for example identifying a researchable question, and working with experienced researchers as mentors. Chapter 2 briefly explains what evidence-based practice is and where to locate the evidence from various sources. It is important to note that we focus on the review of research publications, though readers should be aware that other sources of evidence can be used, such as expert opinions. Chapter 3 introduces the reader to the processes involved in developing a research proposal: s...
literature to...
for the prop...

Under...
directly fro...
health-rela...
information...
confidence,...
drawn up. C...
research cr...
potential fo...

After r...
information...
study. The p...
this early st...

**CHAPTER 1**

## THE IMPORTANCE OF RESEARCH IN NURSING AND MIDWIFERY

Sansnee Jirojwong and Anthony Welch

### CHAPTER LEARNING OBJECTIVES

After reading this chapter you will be able to:
- recognise the importance of research and evidence-based practice in nursing and midwifery
- differentiate major philosophical approaches in the conduct of research and their use in nursing and midwifery services
- understand developments in nursing and midwifery research in the context of society, politics and history
- understand the links between nursing and midwifery services, education and research
- recognise the importance of nursing research and its contribution as part of interdisciplinary research and healthcare services

**KEY TERMS**

**Chapter openers** introduce the key terms and objectives that students will explore throughout the chapter.

---

**CHAPTER 3** INTRODUCING THE RESEARCH PROCESS

How much literature should be considered in the literature search? For some topics with extensive literature, such as HIV, researchers may choose to do a random selection of literature. A general guide for topics with extensive literature is to ensure coverage within the past five years; for more obscure topics you may need to search literature dating back to the 1960s when databases commenced.

### TIPS AND SKILLS

**LITERATURE COVERAGE**

The question of how do you know whether you have searched the literature thoroughly enough can be answered within the searching itself.

When researchers find and gain access to an article and all relevant materials referred to in that article, they are described as covering most of the literature. Clearly, it is impossible to cover every article. It is covering contemporary debates or methods adequately that is at issue.

#### Synthesis of the existing knowledge

Synthesis is a difficult task and is achieved by reading the literature, segmenting the literature into similar aspects of the topic and then logically ordering both the overall direction of the review and the aspects to be covered in the topic. Where identified, studies that support or refute the premises of your study should be emphasised. This allows the researcher to progressively develop an argument on how your study provides knowledge that fills the gap in existing knowledge. Remember, synthesis does not mean that every study you have read should be included, but only essential works.

The literature review is a critical review of the literature; some material will be omitted while other material will be shaped into a set of similar and dissimilar aspects of the topic. Synthesis is where the nurse/midwife researcher presents a thorough understanding of the material that focuses on key issues and includes several studies that support or refute these key issues. Synthesis is not the mere presentation of every study, case by case. If there are many studies to be presented, often a table that defines the chronological order of the related studies is presented, perhaps as an appendix. The literature review section of the proposal represents the end point of synthesis and critical reflection on the material examined (Raw 2011).

The literature review is often summarised in two paragraphs that revise the key aspects covered and reiterate the problem being addressed by the study (Falk 2006). Readers should see Chapter 14 for a detailed discussion on the literature review. Researchers often use wording like 'this study uniquely contributes to knowledge in the area of...' or 'this study examines for the first time key issues of...'

### THINKING DEEPLY

**Literature review**

Having identified your topic area, decide how you will locate literature to further inform your study. What key terms will you use to locate appropriate and relevant literature? What literature search engines are available and what search parameters will you use? How do you plan to organise and synthesise the literature you retrieve?

**Thinking deeply** boxes encourage further discussion and critical reflection of a topic and take students beyond a basic level of understanding.

**Margin notes** illustrate key terms and concepts, which are in bold throughout the text.

**Tips and skills** provide guidance on key aspects of the research process.

**Implications for evidence-based practice** boxes bring to light the key issues from the chapter and highlight the implications for evidence-based practice in nursing and midwifery.

**Summaries** at the end of each chapter help students identify the most important issues covered in the chapter.

**Practice exercises** help students apply their learning and stimulate critical thinking.

**Further reading** and **weblinks** provide valuable resource materials encouraging students to extend their knowledge further.

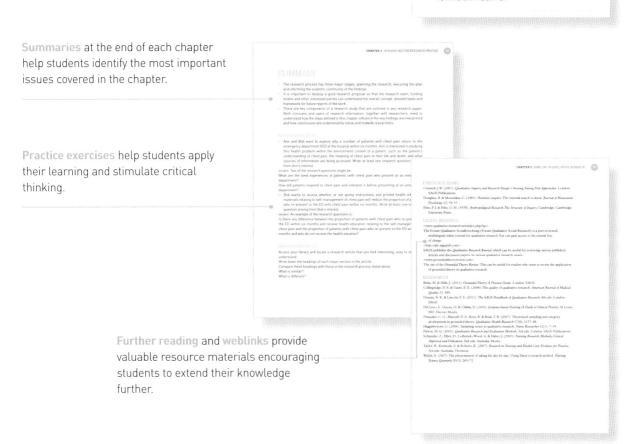

# PATHWAYS TO
# EVIDENCE-BASED PRACTICE

------------------------------------------------

## RESEARCH PATHWAY

Getting started:

» Selecting a topic of interest, or a problem area
» Defining the scope of the research topic or problem—literature review
» Defining the research question, or outline the aim and/or hypothesis—feasibility and ethical considerations

Deciding on the best research approach to answering the research question or hypothesis:

» Selecting the approach—the type of data required to answer the research question or hypothesis: quantitative/qualitative/mixed method
» Design—ensuring the design is consistent with the research question or hypothesis
» Sampling—making sure that the sampling process and the type of sampling procedures reflect the aim or purpose of the study
» Setting—being clear about where the proposed study will take place
» Data collection—choosing appropriate method/s for collecting data
» Analysis of procedures/processes—making sure that the analysis procedures/processes are consistent with the original aim and design of the study

Interpreting and applying the findings to the practice setting:

» Interpreting the data—this activity will differ between quantitative/qualitative/mixed method
» Presenting the findings/writing up a report or a research paper

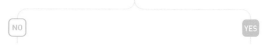

**GETTING STARTED**

**Asking questions:**

» Why do you think this should be explored/investigated?

» Can you gain access to people?

» What exactly do you want to know?

**Is this a suitable area for investigation?**
Questions to consider below:

» Is it feasible? (time, money, experiences of team or mentor)

» Is there any ethical issue/s which you need to consider?

» Can the ethnical issue/s be addressed?

NO                                                          YES

» Review the issue and may have          » Further define the research question, aim
   to look at the problem again             of the research project and/or hypothesis

» Go back to the 'Asking                          » Will this research question be answered
   questions'                                             by a specific qualitative, quantitative or
                                               mixed method design?

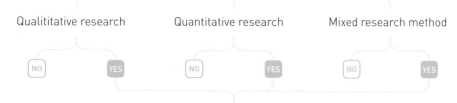

Qualititative research          Quantitative research          Mixed research method

NO     YES               NO     YES               NO     YES

» Do literature review

» Define the scope of the research question/problem

» Outline and revise the research question/problem—aim and/or hypothesis

» **What is the lived experience of patients who present to ED with chest pain?**

Qualitative research

» Select the research design?
  *See Chapter 6 Qualitative Research Design*
» What type of data is to be collected?
  *See Chapter 6 Qualitative Research Design and*
  *Chapter 7 Data Collection: Qualitative Research*
» What data collection approaches and processes will be used? For example face to face interview, focus group interview, oberservation, document search
  *See Chapter 5 Sampling in Qualitative Research and*
  *Chapter 7 Data Collection: Qualitative Research*

Data analysis
Qualitative research

» Is the analysis process descriptive, interpretive, critical or theory building?
» What processes will be used? Thematic analysis, content analysis, coding (using manual or computer programs)
  *See Chapter 7 Data Collection: Qualitative Research and Chapter 8*
  *Qualitative Data Analysis*

» Interpreting and presenting the findings

» What are the characteristics (age, gender, social support) of
  patients who present to ED with chest pain?
» Will patients with self management tools have fewer
  presentations to ED than patients who do not?

Quantitative research

» Select research design
  *See Chapter 10 Quantitative Research Design*
» What is the sample?
  *See Chapter 9 Sampling in Quantitative Research*
» What is the study setting?
  *See Chapter 4 Ethical and Legal Considerations in Research*
» How will data be collected?
  *See Chapter 11 Data  Collection: Quantitative Research*

Data analysis
Quantitative data

» What are the types or scales of the data?
» Is it a nominal, an ordinal or a continuous scale?
» Will the research question and the data be answered by
  univariate, bivariate or multivariate analysis?
  *See Chapter 12 Quantitative Data Analysis*

» Interpreting and presenting the findings

» What is the meaning for patients attending an ED who experience chest pain?
» What factors influence the decision of patients with chest pain to attend an ED?

Mixed research method
» Outline the research questions, aims and/or hypothesis
» There will be at least two research questions involved

Selecting the methods

» Recheck again whether both qualitative and quantitative research is needed for the study:

NO
go back to a single research method

YES
see Chapter 13 Mixed Methods Research

» What is the primary focus of the research? Is it to be answered by both qualitative research and quantitative research?
» Does the qualitative or quantitative component have a complementary or unique contribution to the study?
» Are the qualitative and quantitative components of equal or unequal importance in the study?
» In what order does the research question need to be answered? or the data collected? Nested, parallel, sequential?

Select research design:
» What is the sample?
» What is the study setting?
» How will data be collected?
   *See relevant chapters both quantitative and qualitative research*

Data analysis both qualitative and quantitative data
*See relevant chapters both quantitative and qualitative research*

» Interpreting and presenting the findings

**Interpreting and presenting the findings**
» **Qualitative, quantitative, mixed research methods**

» Have the research questions been answered? OR
Has the hypothesis been tested? Is it statistically significant or
non-significant?

» How will the qualitative data be analysed and presented as
part of the study?

» Have the findings been compared and contrasted with findings from other
studies?

» Are there conditions and factors that may affect the findings that have
been identified?

» Are there other studies required for further investigation?

» What are the implications for patients, clinicians, educators, managers
and other healthcare professionals?

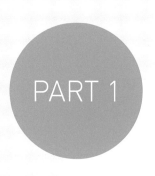

# PART 1

# GETTING STARTED
# IN RESEARCH

Ann and Bob are registered nurses working in a busy emergency department (ED) of a large referral hospital. They observe that many patients who present with chest pain are discharged after a few hours of observation. However, it is also observed that half of these patients repeatedly re-present to the ED. Ann and Bob would like to explore why this group of patients continue to re-present to ED and what additional services can be provided after discharge to help them manage their condition better and therefore reduce the rate of re-presentations. Ann and Bob are aware that a number of research publications are available, including systematic reviews and guidelines for pain management, and so they decide to review what is known about pain management before deciding how to go about researching this issue. As this is their first project, Ann and Bob want to ensure that the project will be conducted to the best of their ability—in a systematic and rigorous manner. As the hospital has links with a local university Ann and Bob decide first to consult experienced researchers for direction and guidance. The decision to undertake this project sets them on the path of research.

Chapter 1 gives important information about beginning the research journey: the processes involved in starting your first piece of research, for example identifying a researchable question, and working with experienced researchers as mentors. Chapter 2 briefly explains what evidence-based practice is and where to locate the evidence from various sources. It is important to note that we focus on the review of research publications, though readers should be aware that other sources of evidence can be used, such as expert opinions. Chapter 3 introduces the reader to the processes involved in developing a research proposal: selecting the topic, developing a researchable question, reviewing the research literature to identify what is already known about the topic, establishing aims and objectives for the project, and exploring an appropriate research design.

Undertaking research in health means that information, that is, data, is obtained either directly from individual participants or from health records of individuals held by health or health-related organisations. It is not uncommon for researchers to have access to sensitive information about people. To ensure that such information is treated with respect, and in confidence, legal and ethical regulations and guidelines for conducting research have been drawn up. Chapter 4 discusses what the researcher needs to consider in order to achieve research credibility. Issues addressed in this chapter include confidentiality, privacy, benefits, potential for harm and how to obtain ethics approval.

After reading the four chapters of Part 1, Ann, Bob and you the reader, will have enough information to get started in putting together ideas about the actual focus of the intended study. The pathway shown in the front of the book summarises the major steps involved at this early stage of the research journey.

CHAPTER 1

# THE IMPORTANCE OF RESEARCH IN NURSING AND MIDWIFERY

Sansnee Jirojwong and Anthony Welch

## CHAPTER LEARNING OBJECTIVES

After reading this chapter you will be able to:

- recognise the importance of research and evidence-based practice in nursing and midwifery
- differentiate major philosophical approaches in the conduct of research and their use in nursing and midwifery services
- understand developments in nursing and midwifery research in the context of society, politics and history
- understand the links between nursing and midwifery services, education and research
- recognise the importance of nursing research and its contribution as part of interdisciplinary research and healthcare services.

### KEY TERMS

quantitative
 research
phenomenon
inductive approach
deductive approach
paradigm
theory
positivist
naturalist
model

## Introduction

There are various ways by which we as human beings come to know and understand our everyday world. Over the centuries different forms of knowledge have been developed and valued by individuals and societies. As a young child we come to value the knowledge of our parents. We go to them for information and for guidance. As we move into our teens we begin to question what they know and start to seek out our own way of understanding our world and what is important to us. At high school and university we enrol in different subjects to acquire particular forms of knowledge for our future career pathway such as nursing, teaching, architecture or psychology. Within your nursing program you study different subject areas to gain particular forms of knowledge: science, to understand the molecular world of the cell; biology, to learn about the workings of the human body; psychology, to understand human behaviour and the way people think and interact; and research, to learn how to determine what is the most appropriate form of knowledge or the best evidence on which to make clinical decisions, for example about aseptic technique, pain management, caring for a person with a mental illness and their family, or deciding whether breastfeeding or bottle feeding is best for a mother and her new baby.

Over the past six decades scientific knowledge and technology have expanded. The health of populations has improved significantly, with an increase in life expectancy and a reduction of morbidity and mortality from infectious diseases (Beaglehole & Bonita 2004). Changes to nursing and midwifery services, education and research have occurred in many developed and developing countries such as the USA, UK, Australia, New Zealand, Thailand, Indonesia and Malaysia.

In Australia, nurses and midwives achieved formal recognition as healthcare professionals in the early 1980s. This was the result of political, social and professional forces such as scientific discoveries, the use of technologies in medicine and public health services, the expansion of Australian universities, the increasing number of nursing and midwifery leaders with postgraduate qualifications in education, and the requirement of undergraduate education preparation for beginning nurse clinicians (Greenwood 2000). Nursing and midwifery education is now located in the tertiary education sector. Knowledge of the practice of nursing and midwifery has expanded as the professions have become increasingly cognisant of the need for clinical practice to be underpinned by research. Clinical practice informed by research is increasingly demanded by the general public, who expect practising nurses and midwives to provide care that is evidence-based (International Council of Nurses 2006; Nursing and Midwifery Board of Australia 2010).

The professions of nursing and midwifery will experience ongoing changes in response to an increasingly ageing population, rising healthcare costs and the use of technology in the healthcare sector. The shift towards empowering health consumers to be active participants in managing their health, and the increasing expectation of the consumer to self-manage, challenges nurses and midwives to be responsive and adaptable to these trends.

In this chapter, the importance of nursing and midwifery research and evidence-based practice is emphasised. The identification of existing and emerging challenges in nursing and midwifery are discussed from the perspectives of two major philosophical approaches, positivism and naturalism. Both approaches will be described in the context of nursing and midwifery research. The future of research in nursing and midwifery and of evidence-based practice will be presented in the context of ongoing changes in Australian social, political and professional environments.

## The place of research in generating knowledge

Let us reflect on how health knowledge has been generated in traditional societies. People observed that certain behaviours would have certain outcomes. Women who were carers would encourage sick people to rest and drink plenty of fluid because they saw that the recovery process was faster when the sick attempted to do something rather than do nothing. The use of trial and error as an approach to problem-solving was the most common means of identifying what worked and what did not. Communities and individuals depended on cultural beliefs, social customs, traditional healers and acknowledged experts as the main sources of knowledge for decisions about health and quality of life. Over time, trial and error has been replaced with a more effective way of generating knowledge and applying it systematically.

As nurses and midwives, we have improved our practices as new knowledge of what is more effective has become available through research and questioning the relevance of convention, custom and tradition, through the opinion of experts, through observations and through the experience of trial and error in contemporary healthcare delivery (Burns & Grove 2009). Examples are early ambulation among post-operative patients, and the use of pets in providing emotional support for residents in long-term care. Planned investigations help consumers of research—nurses, midwives, researchers and educators—to apply research results to their work environment. The result has been improved practice.

We all use research results in one form or another. For example, clinical guidelines based on the synthesis of research results are used in our daily working life. We care for patients and their families who vary in their knowledge of their illness and their ability to manage it. As health professionals it is our business to ensure that our patients have the most up-to-date and appropriate knowledge with which to make informed decisions about their care and management. To be effective in improving health outcomes for patients and their families, we need knowledge that is evidence-based. As nurses and midwives, we also need to be competent in evaluating the strengths and weaknesses of research studies, and the applicability of their findings to our work environment.

## The importance of evidence-based nursing and midwifery practices

As mentioned earlier, health professionals such as nurses and midwives use different sources of information for the delivery of services. In the 1960s Archie Cochrane found that much of clinical practice in health services lacked evidence of effectiveness, resulting in wastage of healthcare resources and sub-optimal outcomes. Cochrane was a strong advocate of randomised controlled trials (RCTs) (Cochrane 1972; Cochrane Collaboration 2010). In 1976 the first systematic review of controlled trials in perinatal medicine commenced in the UK. The Cochrane Centre opened in Oxford in 1992 with registration of the Pregnancy and Childbirth Group and its Subfertility Group. In 1993 at a conference in New York, the concept of the Cochrane Collaboration was presented by the New York Academy of Sciences. Since that time there has been rapid and extensive adoption of the concept. By August 2013 there were more than

5600 completed Cochrane reviews and 2300 protocols (see the approach used for this research in Chapter 15), which are available to healthcare workers and consumers.

Sackett and his colleagues (1996), pioneers of the Cochrane Collaboration and the Centre for Review and Dissemination, defined evidence-based medicine as 'a conscientious, explicit and judicious use of current best evidence in the decision-making about the care of individual patients' (p. 2). In 2000, the definition was expanded further to include patient values and clinical expertise. The evidence needs to be generated by systematic investigation. Patients' illness condition, rights and preferences are considered when making clinical decisions about their treatment. Clinicians use their personal expertise and the best available evidence in the delivery of care. The definition of evidence-based medicine is also applied to evidence-based nursing (EBN) and midwifery (EBMid) (see Chapters 2 and 15).

Since the early 1990s evidence-based nursing and midwifery practices have been actively promoted by York University and McMaster University (Craig & Smyth 2007). Over these two decades, there has been a growth of publications of EBN and EBMid practices by different organisations including the International Council of Nurses, the Australian Nursing and Midwifery Council, and the Joanna Briggs Institute (JBI) (see Greenwood 2000; Usher & Fitzgerald 2008). These publications are as brief as a one-page summary or as long as a comprehensive document of more than 40 pages. The length and format of these publications accommodate the needs of consumers who may wish to access such evidence.

## TIPS AND SKILLS

Antiretroviral treatment (ART) improves the health and prolongs the lives of persons with HIV. Long-term ART treatment is crucial for the health and well-being of individuals and reducing the risk of HIV transmission. The World Health Organization recommends that the ART treatment needs to be initiated in hospitals with maintenance in peripheral health facilities such as community-based organisations or home-based services (WHO 2013).

**Quantitative research:** A systematic investigation with a rigorous and controlled design, using precise measurements and obtaining quantifiable information to answer a research question.

Levels of evidence are classified according to the validity and reliability of research (NHMRC 2009). Comprehensive criteria used to assess the quality of **quantitative research** have been well developed (see Chapter 15). Analysis and synthesis of experimental research are considered to be level I evidence. It should be noted that the Australian National Health and Medical Research Council (NHMRC) does not allocate any level to the opinions of experts (see Table 1.1).

**Table 1.1** Levels of evidence according to the type of intervention

| Level | Intervention |
|---|---|
| I | A systematic review of Level II studies |
| II | A randomised controlled trial |
| III-1 | A pseudo-randomised controlled trial (i.e. alternate allocation of some other method) |

| III-2 | A comparative study with concurrent controls:<br>• Non-randomised, experimental trial<br>• Cohort study<br>• Case-control study<br>• Interrupted time series with a control group |
|-------|---|
| III-3 | A comparative study without concurrent controls:<br>• Historical control study<br>• Two or more single-arm studies<br>• Interrupted time series without a parallel control group |
| IV | Case studies with either post-test or pre-test/post-test outcomes |

Source: NHMRC 2009

However, Polit and Beck (2010, p. 37) have included levels V, VI and VII:

- Level V: Systematic review of descriptive, qualitative or physiologic studies
- Level VI: Single descriptive, qualitative or physiological study
- Level VII: Opinions of authorities or expert committees.

Compared to quantitative research, qualitative research has been classified at levels V and VI evidence, based on qualitative evaluation of reliability and validity. Currently the Cochrane Qualitative Research Methods Group is calling for researchers to register their evaluation evidence from the perspective of qualitative research. Resources for conducting qualitative syntheses are also made available by various organisations through the Cochrane Collaboration website (2013).

## The purposes of research

What is research? We do research because we are curious and interested in solving problems. 'Research is a systematic investigation which aims to discover new knowledge or to validate and refine existing knowledge' (Burns & Grove 2009, p. 2). The professions of nursing and midwifery are committed to generating new knowledge that informs their practice and validates best practice for healthcare delivery.

Nurses and midwives are in a good position to generate research questions because they provide direct and continuous care to individuals, families and communities. New knowledge can be generated through our observations. For example, a nurse in Sydney was the first to observe an increase in congenital malformations in newborn children of mothers who had been treated with thalidomide during pregnancy. Subsequent investigations confirmed that this was a worldwide **phenomenon** (McBride 1962; Smithells & Newman 2009).

**Phenomenon:** Any observable thing or occurrence that is worth noting; plural, phenomena.

Nursing and midwifery care vary across a broad range of contexts from health promotion, illness prevention, acute and chronic care settings and school health, to terminally ill persons who are receiving palliative care at home or in a hospice. Our clients can also be a community, such as people in rural and remote areas or disadvantaged people.

Like other professionals, nurses and midwives need to be aware of new knowledge about emerging trends and innovations in healthcare delivery that are informed by research. It is quite common to find a single issue investigated by many researchers. Of these, few projects may have findings that corroborate each other, while the findings of other projects may contradict each other. The question that needs to be asked is, which study gives the most credible findings and provides the best outcomes that we can use? The process used to critically analyse a large number of research studies concerned with exploring the same issue is called a systematic review (Cochrane Collaboration 2010; Craig & Smyth 2007; see Chapter 15).

Knowledge development is an ongoing process. It occurs in response to a continual advance in technology and the changing healthcare needs of clients and society. As part of a multidisciplinary healthcare team, it is important to be aware that knowledge in nursing and midwifery can be improved or confirmed through the synthesis of knowledge from research into other health disciplines.

## THINKING DEEPLY

### Patient information

Nurses observe that a few post-operative patients require pain relief medication more than other patients. They start talking to patients in order to understand why. One possibility is patients' fear of surgery and the post-operative situation. The nurses know that fear can be reduced by providing patients and their family with knowledge about the operation and what is to be expected post-operatively.

To investigate the problem, two approaches to research can be used: quantitative research and qualitative research. The choice of approach depends on the philosophical orientation of the nurses and the question to be answered. Aspects of both approaches are often used to explore the same problem. Qualitative research is based on enquiry into human quality of life and human action and therefore should consider all circumstances in which that quality of life and action of the individual and family occur. What is important is researcher commitment to explore these phenomena (Law 2007; Rée & Urmson 2004). Open-ended questions (qualitative) provide an opportunity to explore a broad sweep of questions such as, what does it mean to care for another who is in pain? The knowledge generated from such a study can provide information that can be tested by quantitative research strategies. Both approaches are legitimate means by which new knowledge can be generated (Law 2007; Thompson 2003).

Quantitative and qualitative research have arisen from worldviews on how knowledge can be generated. Characteristics of both research methods are summarised in Table 1.2. The philosophical approach of quantitative research is that knowledge is good, that it accumulates through time and that it builds on previous knowledge. If the knowledge is true, it needs to stand the scrutiny of time or be tested in different environments and groups of people. An event cannot occur without preceding events, so it has to occur as the result of previous events. A particular event needs to be precisely observed or measured without any interference from other events. The hypotheses about the occurrence of an event can be tested in different environments and different groups of people. Hypotheses can never be proved absolutely because no event in the world can be proved, since there could be alternative hypotheses not considered (Susser 1986).

## THINKING DEEPLY

### Systematic research

People in European countries always see white swans. It would be incorrect to state that 'All swans are white' as there are black swans in Australia. A better way to make such a statement is, 'Not all swans are white' and test this statement in different locations. Researchers or testers can falsify their statement and have more and more confidence that a swan is likely to be white. When they come across a black swan, then the statement is accepted as true.

This indicates that researchers are unable to check an event that occurs all over the world. The best they can propose is to 'falsify' that the event is not true.

You can apply this situation to many health issues. For example, we may assume that patients with terminal illness may want to know the prognosis so they can plan their life or activities. This may not be true in certain cultures as there may be a cultural belief that the psychological health of patients with terminal illness should be maintained by not letting them know about imminent death. This knowledge will not be confirmed if no systematic investigations or research are conducted among different cultural groups.

## Implications for evidence-based practice

### QUANTITATIVE RESEARCH—THE CONCEPT

Based on observations described in Thinking deeply on p. 8, a team of nurses plan to assess the influence of fear and social support on some patients' perceived pain so that their care can be improved. If they can provide evidence that fear has more impact on the level of pain than social support, interventions can be made in order to reduce fear before the operation. If social support has more impact, supporters of patients may need to be included in the pre-operative care so that their support can be enhanced, potentially reducing the patients' pain. The literature provides information that fear, social support and pain can be investigated and measured. Based on the team's philosophical approach, quantitative research is likely to be used.

The use of quantitative research to explore human behaviours has been criticised because it includes phenomena that have been predetermined by researchers and separated from their overall context, and because the control applied in quantitative research does not allow the voice of participants to be heard. Nurse and midwife researchers who want to focus on human experience and ways by which humans come to understand and interpret their everyday world therefore prefer a qualitative research approach to enquiry. Qualitative research generates information that produces understanding of the human condition in all its manifestations.

More than 40 terms are used to explain qualitative research. Among them are research frameworks or designs (ethnography, phenomenology, grounded theory), theoretical perspectives (naturalist, constructivist, humanistic) and methods (interviewing, observation, document analyses) (Goodrick 2010). Chapter 6 discusses various qualitative research designs and theoretical perspectives. Readers are advised to seek detailed information from advanced qualitative research textbooks.

The foundation of qualitative research is the philosophical stance that reality is constructed by individuals as part of their everyday experience of living. Lincoln and Guba (1985) support such a notion by suggesting that a constructed reality 'fosters the idea that there are multiple realities…and [therefore] there is more than one way to know something and that knowledge is context bound' (Streubert & Carpenter 1995, p. 9). In the context of research, 'ideas and knowledge belong to participants (agents) rather than the researcher (spectator)' (Flew 1971, p. 258). The characteristics of qualitative research as shown in Table 1.2 reflect the nature of the research paradigm.

Note that the term 'naturalistic' has a range of meanings. It may mean that data collection is conducted in a natural setting where participants feel comfortable about providing information on their experiences devoid of any control by the researcher. It is holistic in that the context of the experience is captured. The results of qualitative studies can generate hypotheses that can form the basis of both qualitative and quantitative studies.

## Implications for evidence-based practice

### QUALITATIVE RESEARCH—THE CONCEPT

Based on the scenario in Thinking deeply, the team of nurses discuss the problem and find out that their patients are from several social and demographic backgrounds. Their responses to pain also vary. Long-term illness and previous use of analgesics appear to affect patients' perceived level of pain. The team concludes that the experience of pain from the perspectives of their patients needs to be explored. They expect that the results of their research will help to provide care that meets the needs of an individual patient.

**Table 1.2**  Major characteristics of qualitative and quantitative research

| Characteristic | Qualitative research | Quantitative research |
|---|---|---|
| Philosophical approaches to knowledge development | Naturalistic, interpretive, humanistic, metaphysical | Logical positivism |
| Focus | Broad, subjective, holistic | Concise, objective, reductionist |
| Reasoning | Dialectic, inductive | Logistical, deductive |
| Basis of knowing | Meaning, discovery, understanding | Cause-and-effect relationship |
| Theoretical orientation | Generates theory | Tests theory |
| Researcher involvement | Shared interpretation, subjective | Control, objective |
| Methods of measurement | Unstructured | Structured |

| Data | Words | Numbers |
|------|-------|---------|
| Analysis | Interpretive | Statistical analysis |
| Findings | Understanding of phenomena | Generalisation |

Source: Adapted from Burns & Grove 1997

## Inductive and deductive reasoning in research

**Inductive** and **deductive** reasoning are applied in human reason and enquiry (Thompson 2003). Inductive reasoning works from 'a set of specific facts to a general conclusion. Specific phenomena are observed and a general statement is later formed' (Burns & Grove 1997, p. 6). Inductive reasoning is applied in qualitative research.

In contrast, deductive reasoning begins from a general premise with logical consequence to a specific conclusion. If the premise is false, generally the conclusion is also false. Deductive reasoning is used in quantitative research. The hypothesis testing and probability used in quantitative research have been developed from the argument that true understanding can be achieved by testing whether a premise is false. If the premise can be tested and is shown to be not false, it remains as probable but is never confirmed. Therefore, it is more accurate to use deductive reasoning to observe the falsifiability of a premise (Susser 1986). Table 1.3 gives a schematic representation of differences between inductive and deductive reasoning.

**Inductive approach:** The method of moving from the specific to the general: from empirical data to theory generation.

**Deductive approach:** A method of moving from the general to the specific: from the macro to the micro.

**Table 1.3** Examples of inductive and deductive reasoning

|  | Inductive reasoning | Deductive reasoning |
|--|---------------------|---------------------|
| Characteristic | From specific to general | From general to specific |
| Example | Specific: Bleeding during pregnancy is stressful to pregnant women. Having high blood sugar during pregnancy is stressful to pregnant women. General: All symptoms during pregnancy are stressful to pregnant women. | General: All humans are mortal. Specific: John and Mary are human. Therefore, John and Mary are mortal. |

The hypothesis to be tested in quantitative research (see Chapters 10 and 12) is stated as, 'No relationship between two variables (null hypothesis)'. If it is proved that this null hypothesis is false, the relationship between both variables is probable. In other words, an alternative hypothesis which stated that 'There is a relationship' is likely to be valid, given a good study design, lack of bias, appropriate sample and adequate sample size.

Two examples of hypotheses used in quantitative research are:

- *Null hypothesis*: There is no relationship between healthcare workers' perceived risk of infection and their hand-washing.
- *Alternative hypothesis*: There is a relationship between healthcare workers' perceived risk of infection and their hand-washing.

Quantitative research is considered a scientific approach. Original hypotheses may result from observations, intuitions and human imagination. Observations and subsequent systematic investigations can provide information that refutes traditionally held beliefs such as stress causing peptic ulcer (Marshall & Warren 1984; Marshall et al. 1988) and shoes causing a higher prevalence of Hallux valgus in women (MacLennan 1966). Possible hypotheses may be proposed and considered so that the most likely hypothesis can be formally investigated to explain a phenomenon (Thompson 2003). Demonstrating that a hypothesis is false may lead to the generation of another hypothesis.

One requirement of the knowledge generated from scientific investigations is that it needs to be scrutinised. New knowledge may refute or support currently held knowledge. Acceptance of new knowledge by others in the profession may take years, as in the research by Marshall and Warren (1984). Traditional beliefs held by medical practitioners were that stress and acidity caused peptic ulcer. An alkali was one of the treatments. Marshall and Warren reported research results that bacteria cause peptic ulcer, which challenged standard clinical practice and greatly reduced the cost of treatment.

## Paradigms for nursing and midwifery research

**Paradigm:** In the research context, paradigm has come to mean the commitments, beliefs and values, methods and outlooks shared across a research discipline.

A **paradigm** is the thought pattern in a scientific discipline or the **theory** of knowledge (Flew 1971). Historically, knowledge was gained through observations and trial and error. An individual who accumulated knowledge or expertise on particular issues was another source. The truth of this knowledge could be tested.

Since the late 19th century, technologies and scientific enquiries have been used to improve the health of populations. This improvement was gained through scientific methods such as laboratory experiments and field trials. This theory of generating knowledge is referred to as the **positivist** paradigm (see Table 1.2) and it underpins quantitative research.

**Theory:** A set of interrelated assumptions put forward to describe or explain a given phenomenon.

The application of a positivist approach to research, especially in the area of human behaviour, was criticised for its apparent inability to explore human experience from a holistic perspective. The limitations of the positivist paradigm to conduct research in this complex area of human existence have led to the development of another research paradigm, the '**naturalist paradigm**'.

**Positivist:** Someone who believes in the concepts of an objective reality and the notion of determinism.

Qualitative research methods are still evolving and need to be consolidated. However, researchers such as Kleinman (1980) and Leininger (1988), pioneers in using qualitative research in health, proposed conceptual frameworks that have been used in many nursing and midwifery research studies (Fawcett 2002).

Recently the combination of qualitative and quantitative approaches, referred to as a mixed methods approach to research, has been applied to many disciplines, including nursing and midwifery. Understanding the principles behind this approach is necessary because it is not a simple matter of combining quantitative and qualitative approaches in a study. Chapter 13 explains mixed methods research in detail.

**Naturalist paradigm:** The exploration of phenomena as they occur in their natural setting.

## The role of theory in nursing and midwifery research

**Model:** A structure or framework designed to symbolise a concept or phenomenon.

Increasing death and illness due to chronic diseases, the increasing cost of technology in healthcare, and the shift towards a holistic view of the aetiology of illness have led to the development of **models** and theories to explain individual health and illness in families and communities. The development of such theories in nursing and midwifery has a similar history. The Nightingale theory, which emphasised cleanliness in individuals and environments (Geison 1995), was developed at a time when infectious diseases were the leading causes of death. Poor nutrition, environment and public health infrastructure were discovered to be major contributing factors to illness and death.

The growth of current nursing theories began in the early 1980s, initially in the USA and the UK. Professionalism and nursing education at tertiary level were major factors leading to the development of nursing theories. More than 27 theories have been proposed, falling into four classes: philosophy, grand theory, middle-range nursing theory and micro theory (Marriner-Tomey 1994; Marriner-Tomey & Alligood 2006) (Table 1.4). As research and evidence-based practices grow, new knowledge is being generated. New theories such as Trans-cultural Dynamics in Nursing and Cultural Safety theory have been developed and tested, while some theories such as the Behavioural System by Johnson have been found to have limited use. Some theories such as the Cultural Care Theory and the Pender Health Promotion Model have been reviewed and revised as the result of their use in research projects. Readers who are interested in learning more about nursing theories are recommended to read other sources that focus on these matters (see Further reading).

**Table 1.4** Examples of theories and research using some of these theories

| Major levels of nursing and midwifery theories or models | Examples of theories or models |
| --- | --- |
| Philosophy of nursing | F. Nightingale, *Modern Nursing*<br>E. Wiedenbach, *The Helping Art of Clinical Nursing*<br>V. Henderson, *Definition of Nursing*<br>L. Hall, *Core, Care and Cure Model*<br>J. Watson, *Philosophy and Science of Caring*<br>P. Benner, *From Novice to Expert—Excellence and Power in Clinical Nursing Practice* |
| Grand theory | D. E. Orem, *Self-Care Deficit Theory of Nursing*<br>M. R. Rogers, *Unitary Human Beings*<br>C. Roy, *Adaptation Model*<br>B. Neuman, *System Theory*<br>I. King, *Theory of Goal Attainment* |
| Middle-range theory | I. J. Orlando, *Nursing Process Theory*<br>R. T. Mercer, *Maternal Role Attainment*<br>K. E. Bernard, *Parent-Child Interaction Model*<br>M. Leininger, *Cultural Care Theory*<br>N. J. Pender, *The Health Promotion Model* |
| Micro theory | Stress-Strain-Coping Theory<br>Pain Gate Theory |

Sources: Greenwood 2000; Marriner-Tomey 1994

## What is the purpose of theory for research and evidence-based practice?

In the early 1970s recognition of nursing and midwifery as health professions in North America and the UK led to changes in education, research and practice. Nurses, midwives and other health professionals clearly indicated their need to have a body of knowledge relevant to their specific disciplines. The educational backgrounds of leaders have also influenced the development of theories. Early theories were originally used as philosophical frameworks of educational programs in tertiary education institutions (Gruending 1985; Tompkins 2001; Walsh 1998). These theories included Philosophy and Science of Caring, From Novice to Expert—Excellence, Power in Clinical Nursing Practice, and Humanbecoming, each of which has been used in educational and clinical practice research. Research projects have been conducted to evaluate the application of selected elements of theories to the world of clinical practice. These theories are still evolving. Some of the theories have proved useful in their application to clinical practice, while others have had limited success (see also Greenwood 2000).

While educators and researchers have focused on the conduct of primary research, many practising nurses and midwives have questioned the relevance or applicability of research in light of the complex and ongoing changes occurring in clinical environments. The application of research is influenced by socio-cultural and political backgrounds and contexts of healthcare systems, communities, clinicians and clients. At an individual level, barriers to using research include lack of time, lack of interest, and inability to access or understand research publications (Usher & Fitzgerald 2008).

The implementation of research in a specific location or organisation depends on the development of professional relationships between researchers and clinicians. Many strategies have been established to link researchers and clinicians in research endeavours. Some of these include in-service training programs, creation of research positions in health organisations, and joint appointments between universities and hospitals.

The emergence of the evidence-based practice movement and the establishment of organisations such as the Cochrane Systematic Review Groups, the Joanna Briggs Institute and the Evidence-Based Nursing Institute at York University have facilitated the translation of research findings to the actual points of care by practising nurses and midwives. These organisations have devoted resources to reviewing and summarising the findings of research publications that identify best practice outcomes (see also Chapter 15). Many journals, for example *Australian Journal of Advanced Nursing*, *Journal of Advanced Nursing* and *Advance in Nursing Sciences*, have also published results of systematic reviews of research publications. Organisations such as the International Council of Nurses and the World Health Organization Nursing and Midwifery program (WHO 2002) also provide evidence-based information for nurses and midwives.

Qualitative research has become increasingly accepted as a philosophical approach to knowledge development. Meta-synthesis has been developed to identify evidence from the results of such research. However, ongoing assessments are needed of the translation of the evidence to actual care in clinical areas. Healthcare systems, healthcare professions, and social and cultural characteristics of clients are major factors that can influence the applicability of evidence. Details of the systematic review including meta-analysis and meta-synthesis can be found in Chapter 15.

## TIPS AND SKILLS

Saunders and Griest (2009) plan to reduce the social, recreational and non-military occupational noise exposure among veterans in the USA. They use the Health Belief Model and the Health Promotion Model of Pender as frameworks to develop a multimedia hearing loss prevention program. This program aims at preventing the progression of hearing loss. Their target groups are likely to be those who have different levels of hearing loss at the beginning of the program.

## The future use of nursing and midwifery theories and frameworks in research

Changes in societies will influence the advancement of theories and frameworks in research and evidence-based practices. An ageing population, increased healthcare costs, the high expectation placed on healthcare services and the empowerment of healthcare consumers are some factors to which nurses and midwives must respond. Health information is now widely available to consumers through the internet and many commercial publications. Increased understanding of genetics and its use in screening and the provision of care has the potential to impact significantly on future healthcare. Healthcare personnel also have to increase their evidence-based knowledge so that credible, valid and effective care is provided. All of these factors will influence the use of theories and frameworks in nursing and midwifery research.

## Implications for evidence-based practice

**CARING FOR THE ELDERLY**

Elderly people become constipated more often than younger people. This is related to lack of mobility, no roughage in their diet such as vegetables or fruit, and inadequate fluid intake. One of the guidelines developed by the Joanna Briggs Institute focused on caring for elderly people who are at risk of constipation. The guideline recommended that 'For persons unable to walk or who are restricted to bed or otherwise incapacitated, exercises such as low trunk rotation, pelvic tilt and single left lifts are advised' (JBI 2008, p. 1).

Use your own words to explain why this guideline generates nursing knowledge based on research studies.

**MENTORING**

Maria is a third-year nursing student who has her clinical placement at a medical ward. She is mentored by Yvonne, a registered nurse. Maria observes that Yvonne has drawn up heparin in advance before checking the prescriptions of her patients. Yvonne explains that it is a routine that medical patients receive heparin to reduce the chance of deep vein thrombosis. Does Yvonne use the results of research correctly? Why/Why not?

Comments: There are at least two major issues relating to the use (or incorrect use) of research findings by Yvonne. The first is that not all patients have equal risk of having deep vein thrombosis. The second is that Yvonne is not complying with the rules of medication administration. She is introducing a health risk to patients because of her practice.

## Developments in Australian nursing and midwifery research

As professions, nursing and midwifery have made significant advances in Australia and New Zealand over the past four decades. The evolution of these advances is integral to contemporary nursing and midwifery practice, research and education. The relocation of nursing education from the vocational and hospital sectors to universities has been instrumental in achieving recognition of nursing and midwifery as professions. Nursing and midwifery education in Australia and New Zealand is underpinned by a strong focus on research and evidence-based practice.

Acknowledgment of the importance of research to advancing clinical practice and the increasing interest in nurses and midwives engaging in research is evidenced by the number of research journals and research institutes now in existence, and the number of universities offering undergraduate and postgraduate studies in nursing and midwifery.

The Joanna Briggs Institute has reviewed and issued more than 57 nursing and midwifery best practice publications (JBI 2010). There are more than 30 nursing schools/departments/faculties that offer undergraduate and postgraduate programs (Hobsons 2009), and more than six refereed journals that publish both quantitative and qualitative research findings. In the Australian and the New Zealand tertiary education sectors, there is a demand on student places for higher degrees by research. The collaboration between education and practice sectors in the development of clinical guidelines has been a significant advancement in the provision of quality patient care.

## Looking ahead: Research and its application in nursing and midwifery care

Nurses and midwives are parts of a healthcare team. Their roles and responsibilities in contributing to community health are well recognised. Support has been provided by the Australian Federal Government, which has allowed nurse practitioners and midwives to access Medicare benefits and PBS prescribing (Medicare Australia 2010).

Increasing control of local healthcare services requires nurses and midwives to be responsive to local needs and to be accountable for their services. For this, research-based knowledge and evidence-based practice are required.

The social and demographic characteristics of healthcare consumers are continually changing. The proportion of aged persons from culturally and linguistically diverse (CALD) backgrounds will increase faster than the aged population from Anglo-Saxon backgrounds (Aged and Community Services Australia 2008; Australian Institute of Health and Welfare 2007). Varying healthcare needs of different population groups such as the disadvantaged Indigenous, long-term unemployed and homeless people must be met. Socially and culturally appropriate care is needed. The complexity of the healthcare workforce, the high turnover rate and the lack of healthcare workers in certain locations will continue to be problems. Research leading to evidence-based practice and the provision of quality holistic healthcare seem the only solutions.

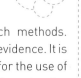

### Implications for evidence-based practice

Not all health issues can be investigated by quantitative research methods. Descriptive research and qualitative research can also provide quality evidence. It is important that researchers and research users are aware of reasons for the use of a particular research design. Systematic reviews such as meta-analysis and meta-synthesis are used to evaluate the results of quantitative and qualitative research. Different sources ranging from refereed journals, professional organisations and healthcare organisations provide many evidence-based practices and practice guidelines. Nurses and midwives need to gain access to information applicable to their practices.

In Australia and New Zealand evidence-based nursing and midwifery have great potential because of their contributions in the educational and healthcare sectors. It is important that they continue to be responsive and proactive to emerging health issues in society.

# SUMMARY

This chapter has discussed important key points which include:

- Significant advances in nursing and midwifery over more than six decades.
- Both the professions of nursing and midwifery have provided leadership in the development of policy and advancement of global healthcare practices. These advancements can be attributed to developments in nursing and midwifery education, research and practice.
- Theory development informing practice and paradigm shifts in philosophical beliefs have been influential in determining what constitutes professional practice.
- The increasing complexity of the healthcare needs of individuals, families and communities have been key elements influencing the changing patterns of professional practice.
- One of the main challenges for nursing and midwifery is to recognise the importance of research evidence as an integral component of professional practice.

## PRACTICE EXERCISE 1.1

a  Based on your personal experiences, list three major changes in Australian nursing and midwifery professions. To what extent have education and research influenced these changes?

b  You may come across a health issue that can lead to a research question. Reflect on your personal view of this issue. What will be the research approach you use: quantitative, qualitative or mixed methods? Why?

## PRACTICE EXERCISE 1.2

Write a few sentences on your opinion of the following conversations over dinner among friends:

Jane: Nurses have to have knowledge in both health sciences and the arts. They also have to develop the knowledge of their own disciplines because they can't keep on borrowing knowledge from other disciplines. Their patients also want to know more and start asking questions about their care.

Peter: I won't argue about that. But nurses mainly use their skills during their day-to-day work. Very little of their work needs any scientific knowledge.

Jane: If you are sick, do you want to receive care from a nurse who has both knowledge and skills or a nurse who has very good skills?

Peter: You got me!

## PRACTICE EXERCISE 1.3

a  In Australia, a number of Vietnamese pregnant women with gestational diabetes are admitted to a hospital to have their blood sugar controlled. The rate is approximately 11%, which is three times higher than the rate in Australian-born women (3.5%) (AIHW: Thow & Waters 2005). Midwives at a maternity unit observe that Vietnamese women tend to eat very little and appear very concerned when insulin is given.

The midwives would like to know how the women interpret their illness and the impact of lifestyle modification and use of insulin on their own health and the baby's health. Is qualitative research or quantitative research suitable to gain answers for the research questions? Explain.

b   Despite strict procedures used to administer medication to patients by nurses, medication errors still occur. At a medical unit, there are at least four reports of medication error. The clinical nurse manager observes that the errors tend to happen between 3 a.m. and 7.30 a.m. and involve at least a casual or agency nurse. Does this observation warrant research? If yes, does it require a lot of money to conduct the research?

## FURTHER READING

Chang, E. & Daly, J. (eds) (2007). *Transitions in Nursing: Preparing for Professional Practice*. Sydney: Elsevier Churchill Livingstone.

Greenwood, J. (2000). *Nursing Theory in Australia: Development and Application*. Sydney: Pearson Education.

## USEFUL WEBSITES

International Council of Nurses (ICN): <www.icn.ch>

You can find current nursing issues at this international organisation website. The ICN has also organised a major congress every four years when the global development of the nursing profession is shared among more than 5000 participants.

World Health Organization, Nursing and Midwifery program: <www.who.int/hrh/nursing_midwifery/en>

This WHO website contains core information about nursing and midwifery professions. It focuses on the service delivery in poorly resourced countries.

Selected list of qualitative research journals: <www.slu.edu/organizations/qrc/QRjournals.html>

This website can be used as a source to locate qualitative research on a topic that interests you. The following website gives more specific journals that present research results using quantitative and qualitative research designs.

*Journal of Research in Nursing*: <www.jrn.sagepub.com>

## REFERENCES

Aged and Community Services Australia. (2008). *Fact sheet 1: An Ageing Australia*. <www.agedcare.org.au/PUBLICATIONS-&-RESOURCES/General-pdfs-images/ACSA%20Fact%20Sheet%201%20 2008-%20An%20Ageing%20Australia.pdf>.

Australian Institute of Health and Welfare (AIHW). (2007). *Older Australians at a Glance*. Canberra: AIHW.

Beaglehole, R. & Bonita, R. (2004). *Public Health at the Crossroads: Achievements and Prospects*. Cambridge: Cambridge University Press.

Burns, N. & Grove, S. K. (1997). *The Practice of Nursing Research: Conduct, Critique, and Utilization*. Philadelphia: W. B. Saunders.

Burns, N. & Grove, S. K. (2009). *The Practice of Nursing Research: Appraisal, Synthesis, and Generation of Evidence*. St Louis, MI: Saunders Elsevier.

Cochrane, A. L. (1972). *Effectiveness and Efficiency: Random Reflections on Health Services*. London: Nuffield Provincial Hospitals Trust.

Cochrane Collaboration. (2010). History. <www.cochrane.org/about-us/history>.

Cochrane Collaboration. (2013). *Resources for Conducting Qualitative Syntheses*. <http://cqim.cochrane.org/resources-conducting-qualitative-syntheses>.

Craig, J. V. & Smyth, R. L. (2007). *Evidence-based Practice Manual for Nurses*. Edinburgh: Churchill Livingstone.

Fawcett, J. (2002). The nurse theorists: 21st-century updates—Madeleine M. Leininger. *Nursing Science Quarterly* 15(2), 131–6.

Flew, A. (1971). *Introduction to Western Philosophy: Ideas and Argument from Plato to Sartre*. London: Thames & Hudson.

Geison, G. L. (1995). *The Private Science of Louis Pasteur*. Princeton, NJ: Princeton University Press.

Goodrick, D. (2010). Qualitative research: Design analysis and representation. Workshop note, Australian Consortium for Social and Political Research Incorporated (ACSPRI) Summer program. Victoria: ACSPRI (manuscript).

Greenwood, J. (2000). *Nursing Theory in Australia: Development and Application*. Sydney: Harper Educational Publisher.

Gruending, D. L. (1985). Nursing theory: A vehicle of professionalization? *Journal of Advanced Nursing* 10(6), 553–8.

Hobsons. (2009). *The Good Universities Guide to Education, Training and Career Pathways*. Melbourne: Hobsons.

International Council of Nurses. (2006). *The ICN Code of Ethics for Nurses*. <www.icn.ch/images/stories/documents/about/icncode_english.pdf>.

JBI (Joanna Briggs Institute). (2008). Management of constipation in older adults. *Best Practice* 12(7), 1–4.

JBI. (2010). The Joanna Briggs Institute. Best Practice series. <www.joannabriggs.edu.au/pubs/best_practice.php>.

Kleinman, A. (1980). *Patients and Healers in the Context of Culture: An Exploration of the Borderland Between Anthropology, Medicine, and Psychiatry*. Berkeley, CA: University of California Press.

Law, S. (2007). *Philosophy*. London: Dorling Kindersley.

Leininger, M. M. (1988). Leininger's theory of nursing: Cultural care diversity and universality. *Nursing Science Quarterly* 1(4), 152–60.

Lincoln, Y. S. & Guba, E. G. (1985). *Naturalistic Inquiry*. Beverly Hills, CA: SAGE.

MacLennan, R. (1966). Prevalence of hallux valgus in a neolithic New Guinea population. *Lancet* 1(7452), 1398–400.

Marriner-Tomey, A. (ed.) (1994). *Nursing Theorists and Their Work*. St Louis, MO: Mosby.

Marriner-Tomey, A. & Alligood, M. R. (eds) (2006). *Nursing Theorists and Their Work*. St Louis, MO: Mosby.

Marshall, B. J. & Warren, J. R. (1984). Unidentified curved bacilli in the stomach of patients with gastritis and peptic ulceration. *Lancet* 1(8390), 1311–15.

Marshall, B. J., Goodwin, C. S., Warren, J. R., Murray, R., Blincow, E. D., Blackbourn, S. J., Phillips, M., Waters, T. E. & Sanderson, C. R. (1988). Prospective double-blind trial of duodenal ulcer relapse after eradication of Campylobacter pylori. *Lancet* 2(8626–27), 1437–42.

McBride, W. G. (1962). Thalidomide and congenital abnormalities (letter), *Lancet* 2, 1358.

Medicare Australia. (2010). *Nurse practitioner and midwives*. <www.medicareaustralia.gov.au/provider/other-healthcare/nurse-midwives.jsp>.

NHMRC (National Health and Medical Research Council). (2009). *NHMRC Levels of Evidence and Grades for Recommendations for Developers of Guidelines*. <www.nhmrc.gov.au/_files_nhmrc/file/publications/synopses/cp30.pdf>.

Nursing and Midwifery Board of Australia. (2010). Competency standards. <www.nursingmidwiferyboard.gov.au/Codes-and-Guidelines.aspx>.

Polit, D. F. & Beck, C. T. (eds) (2010). *Essentials of Nursing Research: Appraising Evidence for Nursing Practice*. Philadelphia: Wolters Kluwer.

Rée, J. & Urmson, J. O. (2004). *The Concise Encyclopaedia of Western Philosophy and Philosophers*. London: Routledge.

Sackett, D. L., Rosenberg, W. M. C., Gray, J. A. M., Haynes, R. B. & Richardson, W. S. (1996). Evidence based medicine: What it is and what it isn't. *British Medical Journal* 312, 71.

Saunders, G. H. & Griest, S. E. (2009). Hearing loss in veterans and the need for hearing loss prevention programs. *Noise Health* 11(42), 14–21.

Smithells, R. W. & Newman, C. G. H. (2009). The Thalidomide Story. <www.thalidomide.org.uk/Thalidomide.aspx>.

Streubert, H. J. & Carpenter, D. R. (1995). *Qualitative Research in Nursing*. Philadelphia: J. B. Lippincott Company.

Susser, M. (1986). The logic of Sir Karl Popper and the practice of epidemiology. *American Journal of Epidemiology* 124(5), 711–18.

Thompson, M. (2003). *Teach Yourself Philosophy of Science*. Abingdon: Bookprint Ltd.

Thow, A. M. & Waters, A. M. (2005). *Diabetes in Culturally and Linguistically Diverse Australians: Identification of Communities at High Risk*. AIHW cat. no. CVD 30. Canberra: Australian Institute of Health and Welfare.

Tompkins, C. (2001). Nursing education for the twenty-first century. In E. Rideout (ed.), *Transforming Nursing Education through Problem-Based Learning*. Sudbury, MA: Jones & Bartlett, pp. 1–20.

Usher, K. & Fitzgerald, M. (2008). Introduction to nursing research. In S. Borbasi, D. Jackson & R. W. Langford (eds), *Navigating the Maze of Nursing Research: An Interactive Learning Adventure*. Sydney: Elsevier.

Walsh, M. (1998). What is the basis for nursing practice? In *Models and Critical Pathways in Clinical Nursing*. London: Baillèire Tindall, pp. 1–25.

WHO (World Health Organization). (2002). *The Nursing and Midwifery Programme at WHO: What Nursing and Midwifery Services Mean to Health*. <www.who.int/hrh/nursing_midwifery/leaflet.pdf>.

WHO. (2013). HIV/AIDS, 9.4.3 Decentralizing HIV treatment and care. <www.who.int/hiv/pub/guidelines/arv2013/operational/servicedelivery/en/index5.html>.

CHAPTER 2

# EVIDENCE-BASED PRACTICE FOR NURSES AND MIDWIVES

Maree Johnson and Ritin Fernandez

## KEY TERMS

evidence-based
  practice
Archie Cochrane
clinical guidelines

## CHAPTER LEARNING OBJECTIVES

By the end of this chapter you will be able to:

- define evidence-based practice
- identify the key concepts in evidence-based practice
- understand why evidence-based nursing practice is essential for good patient care
- describe the critical skills a registered nurse or midwife needs for evidence-based practice
- understand the fundamental skill of evidence-based practice in a critical review of research
- describe ways that nurses develop evidence.

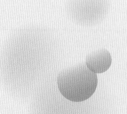

# Introduction

Nurses and midwives are increasingly involved in key decision-making about patient care along with their medical and allied health colleagues (Mantzoukas 2008). Nurses therefore have to use the best available evidence from scientific research in their clinical judgments and decisions. In 1998 DiCenso, Cullum and Ciliska made a plea to the profession in their statement that 'each nurse must care enough about her[/his] own practice to want to make sure it is based on the best possible information' (Kitson et al. 1966). This challenge still remains. In this chapter we will introduce readers to practical ways in which nurses and midwives can find the best evidence on which to base their practices.

**Evidence-based practice** (EBP) is a systematic approach using the best available evidence from research, along with patient preferences and clinical experience, when making clinical decisions (Sackett et al. 2000; Titler & Adam 2010). This represents a substantial paradigm shift from tradition-based practice for nurses and other health professionals (Rycroft-Malone et al. 2013). You have probably heard nurses say 'But we've always done it this way', representing tradition-based practice.

The goal of EBP is to eliminate ineffective or even harmful practices in favour of those that have demonstrated better health outcomes. The pioneer of EBP was **Archie Cochrane**, who suggested that the available resources should be used judiciously to provide healthcare which has been shown in properly designed evaluations (randomised controlled trials) to be effective (Cochrane 1999). Later he stated, 'It is surely a great criticism of our profession that we have not organised a critical summary, by specialty or subspecialty, adapted periodically, of all relevant randomised controlled trials' (Cochrane 1979, p. 1). The foundations laid by Archie Cochrane were built upon by Sackett and colleagues, who identified evidence-based medicine as 'the conscientious, explicit, and judicious use of current best evidence in making decisions about the care of individual patients' (Sackett et al. 1996, p. 71).

**Evidence-based practice:** A process that requires the practitioner to identify knowledge gaps, find research evidence to address knowledge gaps, and determine the relevance of the evidence to a particular client's situation.

**Archie Cochrane:** A pioneer and advocate of evidence-based practice.

## THINKING DEEPLY

Consider this clinical situation:

Mary Freidsen, a registered nurse working in the cardiology unit, has just come to your orthopaedic unit, and noted that you are changing your intravenous (IV) therapy cannulae too frequently. Mary says to you: 'We only change our cannulas when there are signs of infection, not every 72 hours. Haven't you seen the research?' You check the ward policy and note that it still says 72 hours. Mary gives you a copy of a large Australian study (Rickard et al. 2012) that has convincing evidence of no clinical benefit in changing peripheral IVs every 72 hours. How do you decide what to do?

Although it would seem that you might want to just change your practice in a case like this, you would need to follow a series of steps to consider the evidence carefully. EBP is underpinned by the procedures of review of the literature and collating the results of many rigorously conducted studies to inform guidelines or policies. So in this case, one study alone may not be sufficient evidence. For example, the study may not be conducted in an appropriate manner, or the results may not apply to your setting. Therefore it may be that you should not be changing practice. If the nurse or midwife is to act on the evidence or research available, they will require a set of skills to be learnt and regularly used.

## Skills required for evidence-based practice

Evidence-based practice is an active process and involves six major steps: identifying a gap in the knowledge; formulating a precise clinical question; retrieving the most relevant and best evidence; appraising the evidence for its reliability, validity and applicability; integrating the evidence along with clinical judgment and patient preferences; and assessing the outcome of the evidence implementation (Finotto et al. 2013).

1  *Identifying a gap in the knowledge* Identifying a gap between evidence and practice is the first step in EBP (Kitson & Straus 2010).
2  *Formulating a precise clinical question* The clinical question should be clear and precise and should focus on outcomes that are important in practice (Kloda & Bartlett 2013). Chapter 15 will outline how to develop a precise clinical question.
3  *Retrieving the best and most relevant evidence* This involves methodically searching the medical, nursing and allied health databases to acquire the most relevant evidence (Cullum et al. 2008).
4  *Appraising the evidence for its reliability, validity and applicability* The ability to critically appraise research reports is a fundamental skill for evidence-based practice. For a nurse or midwife to be able to do this competently requires an extensive knowledge of how research is conducted. The content of this textbook will provide information about these key aspects of research reports, and Chapter 14 will outline how to critically appraise a research report.
5  *Integrating the evidence along with clinical judgment and patient preferences* This step often results in **clinical guidelines** or recommendations for practice.
6  *Assessing the outcome of the evidence implementation* Nurses are slowly changing their practice based on evidence. However, they rarely evaluate the effects of the practice change. It is important for nurses to assess the effect of the practice change as it will provide evidence if the particular treatment has worked (Taylor 2013).

**Clinical guidelines:**
Recommendations for practice based on the best available evidence.

## Why evidence-based practice?

Contemporary leaders in practice change continue to support nursing and midwifery practice being based on the best available evidence. But why is this so? Using an evidence-based approach in nursing has numerous advantages (Bellamy et al. 2013; Gerrish et al. 2012). These include:

- better outcomes for patients
- greater autonomy and professional credibility for nurses
- auditable research bases for clinical guidelines
- demonstrated value of what nurses do
- providing nurses with better opportunities to deliver cost-effective care.

Although the evidence-based practice movement has been in progress for nearly two decades, patients are still not receiving the best treatment based on the available research evidence.

A recent Australian study by the National Stroke Foundation (2010) found that although its Clinical Guidelines for Acute Stroke Management had existed since 2007, the Guidelines' recommendations were not fully implemented in Acute Stroke Units throughout Australia (Hill et al. 2009). A trial by Middleton and colleagues (2011) further demonstrated the importance of these guidelines because they showed there were improved patient outcomes within 90 days for patients in Acute Stroke Units who were in the trial. This trial was a nurse-led implementation of multidisciplinary guidelines. Further implementation of these guidelines (National Stroke Foundation 2010) is under way. As can be seen, however, seven years (in 2014) have passed and these guidelines are still not fully implemented in practice.

## TIPS AND SKILLS

Locating existing clinical guidelines through internet search engines will often deliver both the guidelines and the systematic reviews on which they are based, and their authors will make recommendations about the potential application in practice.

## Do nurses participate in evidence-based practice?

Despite the obvious benefits of evidence-based practice, studies show that in nursing, medicine and allied health, research results are not always applied to practice. The literature indicates that a 10- to 15-year gap exists between the discovery of innovations and the implementation of these in clinical practice (Bostrom & Wise 1994). An example is a systematic review of randomised controlled trials that demonstrated the effectiveness of thrombolytic therapy for the treatment of myocardial infarction; only 13 years later was this treatment established as the norm (Antman et al. 1992).

Nurses' and midwives' uptake of best practice is generally reported as being slow (Ross 2010). In a recent study conducted with 546 acute-care nurses, positive beliefs towards EBP did not necessarily result in EBP activities (Thorsteinsson & Sveinsdóttir 2013). Key behaviours of nurses or midwives that demonstrate engagement in EPB were defined in a five-year longitudinal study of nurses (n = 2234) (Rudman et al. 2012). Only '10% of nurses appraised research reports' while '80% used information sources other than databases to search for knowledge', and this pattern remained stable over the five-year period (Rudman et al. 2012, p. 1494). The study, although conducted in Sweden, may reflect similar patterns of behaviour in Australasian nurses and midwives. This study did articulate specific behaviours that could be considered the critical skills required of an evidence-based nurse or midwife. To be able act on the evidence or research available, the nurse or midwife will need to learn critical skills and use them regularly.

## TIPS AND SKILLS

Evidence-based clinicians are nurses or midwives who:

- regularly form clinical questions that lead them to search current research
- use databases to search for knowledge on a clinical problem
- appraise the research available
- contribute to change by implementing knowledge
- participate in evaluating whether clinical practice reflects current knowledge.

## Working together works well in EBP

Most reviews of clinical practice are conducted by groups of nurses (Fernandez et al. 2012; Jefferies et al. 2010) and midwives (Sandall et al. 2013) or a multidisciplinary team

(Jefferies et al. 2011). Here are some examples of systematic reviews or a collection of the research studies (see Chapter 15 for further explanations) undertaken by either a single discipline or a multidisciplinary team. Later in this chapter, Practice exercise 2.1 provides a link to a video presentation of how teams work together to conduct a systematic review or develop the evidence.

## Nutritional systematic review (multidisciplinary)

This review was conducted in collaboration with clinicians, consumers and dietitians to develop a policy defining how nurses could support their patients' nutritional care (Jefferies et al. 2011). The evidence obtained from 40 studies was developed into standards that assisted nurses in supporting the oral nutrition of their patients. These included a focused mealtime, management of mealtime environments, management of staff mealtimes and a designated nutrition support nurse in each clinical area to monitor and evaluate the implementation of the policy.

## Models of care in nursing systematic review

This review, conducted by nurses, investigated the effect of the various models of nursing care delivery using the diverse levels of nurses on patient and nursing outcomes. Results from the 14 studies included in the review indicated that the team nursing model of care resulted in significantly decreased incidence of medication errors and adverse intravenous outcomes, as well as lower pain scores among patients. However, this model had no effect on the incidence of falls (Fernandez et al. 2012). Wards that used a hybrid model of care showed significant improvement in quality of care, but no difference in the incidence of pressure areas or infection rates.

## Midwife-led continuity models versus other models of care for childbearing women

This systematic review, conducted by midwives and published in the Cochrane library, included 13 trials involving 16 242 pregnant and postpartum women (Sandall et al. 2013). The results indicated that women who had a midwife as their main carer throughout pregnancy and birth were about 23% less likely to have a premature baby than women whose care was shared between different obstetricians, general practitioners and midwives. Midwife-led continuity of care was also associated with a lower risk of foetal loss before 24 weeks' gestation and reduced likelihood of labour interventions such as episiotomies or use of forceps.

All these reviews used an approach that brought together nurses or midwives across several hospitals or countries to work with a specialised team to review the evidence, synthesise the evidence, and provide direction as to the strength of the evidence.

### Implications for evidence-based practice

Nurses and midwives need to gain knowledge and develop skills required to provide evidence-based practice. Individuals working as a team in a supportive environment can facilitate the ongoing improvement of care via the EBP. Clients also play an important role in reaching the satisfactory outcomes of health services.

# Where do you find the evidence?

Many research organisations have assisted in making evidence available to clinicians to improve patient care. Advances in technology have led to the development of databases that provide a repository of research evidence easily accessible to healthcare workers. Following is a list of selected organisations. Please also see Chapter 15 for information on other organisations.

## The Cochrane Collaboration

The Cochrane Collaboration is an international not-for-profit and independent organisation, dedicated to making up-to-date, accurate information about the effects of healthcare readily available worldwide. It produces and disseminates systematic reviews of healthcare interventions and promotes the search for evidence in the form of clinical trials and other studies of interventions. You can gain information through <www.cochrane.org>.

## The Joanna Briggs Institute

The Joanna Briggs Institute was founded on the premise that an evidence base for nursing practice was essential, but that it was important to also develop strategies for the effective dissemination and implementation of that information in practice. The staff of JBI have helped to make evidence available by providing clearly presented summaries of research findings called 'Best Practice Information Sheets' in simple language which can be used by nurses at the point of care. Information can be accessed through <www.joannabriggs.org>.

## Clinical Evidence

Clinical Evidence describes the best available evidence from systematic reviews, RCTs and observational studies when appropriate for assessing the benefits and harms of treatments. Its website is <www.clinicalevidence.bmj.com>.

## Essential Evidence

Essential Evidence is a one-stop reference that includes evidence-based answers to clinical questions concerning symptoms, diseases and treatment. The information is available via <www.essentialevidenceplus.com>.

## UpToDate

UpToDate is an evidence-based, peer-reviewed information resource available via the web, desktop/laptop computer and PDA/mobile device. For more information, see UpToDate at <www.uptodate.com>.

## PubMed

PubMed comprises more than 22 million citations for biomedical articles from MEDLINE and life science journals. Citations may include links to full-text articles from PubMed Central or publisher websites. Free access to PubMed is at <www.ncbi.nlm.nih.gov/pubmed>.

## Barriers to EBP

Nurses face a real challenge when translating best evidence into clinical practice. Research studies from Australia and internationally (Breimaier et al. 2011; McInerney & Suleman 2010; Shepperd et al. 2013; Solomons & Spross 2011) have identified a number of obstacles to the implementation of evidence-based practice:

1   large volumes of publications (Jones et al. 2007)
2   insufficient research evidence on which to base practice (McInerney & Suleman 2010; Shepperd et al. 2013)
3   contradictory findings in research reports (Shepperd et al. 2013)
4   nurses may not be convinced of the usefulness of good scientific research for their practice (Rolfe et al. 2008)
5   nurses do not have the time to keep up to date with the research literature (Majid et al. 2011)
6   many nurses do not have the ability to search the literature (Younger 2010) or to evaluate the quality of research reports so that only valid and reliable evidence is applied to practice (Gerrish et al. 2012)
7   many nurses do not have the skills to interpret research findings (Majid et al. 2011)
8   inability to understand statistical terms, and inadequate understanding of the jargon used in research articles (Majid et al. 2011)
9   limited access to evidence-based literature provided by healthcare organisations (McInerney & Suleman 2010)
10  healthcare organisations do not provide resources such as access to information technology to implement evidence-based practice (Majid et al. 2011)
11  organisation culture that does not provide a supportive environment and value evidence-based practice (Gerrish et al. 2012)
12  limited authority or power given to nurses to change practice based on research findings (Heckenberry et al. 2006)
13  shortages of experienced nursing staff (Gerrish et al. 2012).

Although these barriers are substantial, some enlightened organisations such as South Western Sydney Local Health District are developing strong cultures within their nursing and midwifery communities that are leading national and international change in the profession.

## Developing an evidence-based profession

Extensive national and international efforts are in progress to develop nursing as an evidence-based profession. Within Australia key professional bodies such as the Australian Nursing and Midwifery Council and later the Australian Nursing and Midwifery Accreditation Council (ANMAC) have stipulated that nurses practise within an evidence-based framework and the current Nursing and Midwifery Board of Australia specifically mandates standards and competencies for nurses relating to EBP as shown in Box 2.1.

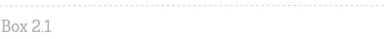

Box 2.1

**STANDARDS AND COMPETENCIES FOR NURSES RELATING TO EBP BY THE NURSING AND MIDWIFERY BOARD OF AUSTRALIA**

3  Practice within an evidence-based framework:

3.1  Identifies the relevance of research to improving individual/group health outcomes.

3.2  Uses best available evidence, nursing expertise and respect for the values and beliefs of individuals/groups in the provision of nursing care:

Uses relevant literature and research findings to improve current practice

Participates in review of policies, procedures and guidelines based on relevant research

Identifies and disseminates relevant changes in practice or new information to colleagues

Recognises that judgements and decisions are aspects of nursing care, and

Recognises that nursing expertise varies with education experience and context of practices

3.3  Demonstrates analytical skills in access and evaluating health information and research evidence.

Source: National Competency Standards for the Registered Nurse 2006; The Nursing and Midwifery Board of Australia (National Board). <www.nursingmidwiferyboard.gov.au/ Codes-Guidelines-Statements/Codes-Guidelines.aspx#competencystandards>

The inclusion of EBP in undergraduate nursing courses has provided student nurses with skills so that they can critically appraise the literature as competently as they can measure a patient's heart rate.

Many health institutions have also developed their own repository of databases to ensure that nurses have access to the best research evidence to incorporate into clinical decision-making. For example, the NSW Health Department has developed the Clinical Information Access Program (CIAP) which consists of Medline, CINAHL, Embase, Cochrane Library and other databases. The CIAP is readily available on the internet for employees of NSW Health. They can gain access to many databases that are invaluable for evidence-based practice. Other opportunities have been created by universities and healthcare institutions to teach nurses EBP skills. For example, librarians are an essential resource for evidence-based practice and they provide training in efficient advanced searching strategies to locate high-quality research evidence.

# SUMMARY

- An evidence-based practice approach to nursing and midwifery is essential to ensure that patients receive the best possible care based on the strongest evidence available.
- The essential skill of EBP is appraising the literature or conducting a critical review of a research study.
- Specific skills can be learnt to demonstrate competence in evidence-based practice as required by registering authorities.
- Repositories exist for nurses and midwives to find existing reviews or guidelines relating to their practice.
- Using evidence in practice remains an ideal for all registered nurses and midwives, and the transition to all nurses using evidence may take some time.

### PRACTICE EXERCISE 2.1

Take 10 minutes to find out how a systematic review is undertaken within the Cochrane Collaboration. Members of the team speak about their experiences.
Please copy or click on this URL
<www.cochrane.org/multimedia/video/introduction-collaboration> (6 minutes).

### PRACTICE EXERCISE 2.2

This exercise demonstrates how to access systematic reviews through podcasts from the Cochrane Library.

Nurses are often faced with managing children with acute gastroenteritis. The following podcast describes the best evidence in relation to managing an acute episode in children. Listen to the podcast, then review the evidence and consider how this affects your current practice.

Treatment of acute gastroenteritis in children: an overview of systematic reviews of interventions commonly used in developed countries:

<www.cochrane.org/podcasts/evidence-based-child-health/treatment-acute-gastroenteritis-children-overview-systematic-rev>

Click on the play button and listen to an overview of the review. View the review also by clicking on the review icon.

A comparison of oral hydration, antiemetics and intravenous therapy and probiotics is considered.

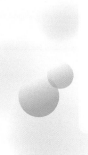

## FURTHER READING

Beyea, S. C. & Slattery, M. J. (2013). Historical perspectives on evidence-based nursing. *Nursing Science Quarterly* 26(2), 152–5.

Barker, A. L., Kamar, J., Tyndall, T. J., White, L., Hutchinson, A., Klopfer, N. & Weller, C. (2013). Implementation of pressure ulcer prevention best practice recommendations in acute care: An observational study. *International Wound Journal* 10(3), 313–20.

Centrella-Nigro, A. M. & Flynn, D. (2012). Teaching evidence-based practice using a mock trial. *Journal of Continuing Education in Nursing* 43(12), 566–70.

## USEFUL WEBSITES

Listen to an online tutorial explaining evidence-based practice: <www.youtube.com/watch?v=me7BDrpiLd4>

View the evidence-based argument as a short discussion which outlines some of the current debates surrounding evidence-based practice: <www.youtube.com/watch?v=xQyQqZ5tLoo>

View the humorous application of the evidence relating to checking the location of patients' nasogastric tubes in nursing: <www.youtube.com/watch?v=Q7ODSQrjB88>

## REFERENCES

Antman, E. M., Lau, J., Kupelnick, B., Mosteller, F. & Chalmers, T. C. (1992). A comparison of results of meta-analyses of randomized control trials and recommendations of clinical experts: Treatments for myocardial infarction. *Journal of the American Medical Association* 268(2), 240–8.

Bellamy, J. L., Mullen, E. J., Satterfield, J. M., Newhouse, R. P., Ferguson, M., Brownson, R. C. & Spring, B. (2013). Implementing evidence-based practice education in social work: A transdisciplinary approach. *Research on Social Work Practice* 23(4), 426–6.

Bostrom, J. & Wise, L. (1994). Closing the gap between research and practice. *Journal of Nursing Administration* 24(5), 22–7.

Breimaier, H. E., Halfens, R. J. & Lohrmann, C. (2011). Nurses' wishes, knowledge, attitudes and perceived barriers on implementing research findings into practice among graduate nurses in Austria. *Journal of Clinical Nursing* 20(11–12), 1740–56.

Cochrane, A. L. (1979). *1931–1971: A Critical Review, with Particular Reference to the Medical Profession.* London: Office of Health Economics.

Cochrane, A. L. (1999). *Effectiveness and Efficiency. Random Reflections on Health Services.* London: Royal Society of Medicine Press.

Cullum, N., Ciliska, D., Haynes, R. B. & Marks, S. (2008). *Evidence-based Nursing: An Introduction.* Blackwell Pub./BMJ Journals/RCN Pub.

Fernandez, R., Johnson, M., Tran, D. T. & Miranda, C. (2012). Models of care in nursing: A systematic review. *International Journal of Evidence-Based Healthcare* 10(4), 324–37.

Finotto, S., Carpanoni, M., Turroni, E. C., Camellini, R. & Mecugni, D. (2013). Teaching evidence-based practice: Developing a curriculum model to foster evidence-based practice in undergraduate student nurses. *Nurse Education in Practice* 13(5), 459–65.

Gerrish, K., Nolan, M., McDonnell, A., Tod, A., Kirshbaum, M. & Guillaume, L. (2012). Factors influencing advanced practice nurses' ability to promote evidence-based practice among frontline nurses. *Worldviews on Evidence-Based Nursing* 9(1), 30–9.

Heckenberry, M., Wilson, D. & Barrera, P. (2006). Implementing evidence-based nursing practice in a pediatric hospital. *Pediatric Nursing* 32(4), 371.

Hill, K., Middleton, S., O'Brien, E. & Lalor, F. (2009). Implementing clinical guidelines for acute stroke management: Do nurses have a lead role? *Australian Journal of Advanced Nursing* 26(3), 53–8.

Jefferies, D., Johnson, M., Griffiths, R., Arthurs, K., Beard, D., Chen, T., Edgetton-Winn, M., Hecimovic, T., Hughes, M., Linten, K., Maddox, J., McCaul, D., Robson, K., Scott, S. & Zarkos T. (2010). Engaging clinicians in evidence based policy development: The case of nursing documentation. *Contemporary Nurse* 35(2), 254–64.

Jefferies, D., Johnson, M. & Ravens, J. (2011). Nurturing and nourishing: The nurses' role in nutritional care. *Journal of Clinical Nursing* 20(3–4), 317–30.

Jones, T. H., Hanney, S. & Buxton, M. J. (2007). The information sources and journals consulted or read by UK paediatricians to inform their clinical practice and those which they consider important: A questionnaire survey. *BMC Pediatrics* 7(1), 1.

Kitson, A. & Straus, S. E. (2010). The knowledge-to-action cycle: Identifying the gaps. *CMAJ* 182(2), E73–77.

Kitson, A., Ahmed, L. B., Harvey, G., Seers, K. & Thompson, D. R. (1966). From research to practice: One organizational model for promoting research-based practice. *Journal of Advanced Nursing* 23(3), 430–40.

Kloda, L. A. & Bartlett, J. C. (2013). Formulating answerable questions: Question negotiation in evidence-based practice 1, 2. *Journal of the Canadian Health Libraries Association* 34(02), 55–60.

Majid, S., Foo, S., Luyt, B., Zhang, X., Theng, Y. L., Chang, Y. K. & Mokhtar, I. A. (2011). Adopting evidence-based practice in clinical decision making: Nurses' perceptions, knowledge, and barriers. *Journal of the Canadian Health Libraries Association* 99(3), 229–36.

Mantzoukas, S. (2008). A review of evidence-based practice, nursing research and reflection: Levelling the hierarchy. *Journal of Clinical Nursing* 17(2), 214–23.

McInerney, P. & Suleman, F. (2010). Exploring knowledge, attitudes, and barriers toward the use of evidence-based practice amongst academic health care practitioners in their teaching in a South African university: A pilot study. *Worldviews on Evidence-Based Nursing* 7(2), 90–7.

Middleton, S., McElduff, P., Ward, J., Grimshaw, J. M., Dale, S., D'Este, C., Drury, P., Griffiths, R., Cheung, N. W., Quinn, C., Evans, M., Cadilhac, D., Levi, C. & QASC Trialists Group. (2011). Implementation of evidence-based treatment protocols to manage fever, hyperglycaemia, and swallowing dysfunction in acute stroke (QASC): A cluster randomised controlled trial. *Lancet* 378(9804), 1699–706.

National Stroke Foundation. (2010). Clinical Guidelines for Acute Stroke Management.<http://strokefoundation.com.au/site/media/clinical_guidelines_stroke_managment_2010_interactive.pdf>.

Rickard, C. M., Webster, J., Wallis, M. C., Marsh, N., McGrail, M. R., French, V., Foster, L., Gallagher, P., Gowardman, J. R., Zhang, L., McClymont, A. & Whitby, M. (2012). Routine versus clinically indicated replacement of peripheral intravenous catheters: A randomised controlled equivalence trial. *Lancet* 380(9847), 1066–74.

Rolfe, G., Segrott, J. & Jordan, S. U. E. (2008). Tensions and contradictions in nurses' perspectives of evidence-based practice. *Journal of Nursing Management* 16(4), 440–51.

Ross, J. (2010). Information literacy for evidence-based practice in perianesthesia nurses: Readiness for evidence-based practice. *Journal of Perianesthesia Nursing* 25(2), 64–70.

Rudman, A., Gustavsson, P., Ehrenberg, A., Boström, A.-M. & Wallin, L. (2012). Registered nurses' evidence-based practice: A longitudinal study of the first five years after graduation. *International Journal of Nursing Studies* 49(12), 1494–504.

Rycroft-Malone, J., Seers, K., Chandler, J., Hawkes, C. A., Crichton, N., Allen, C., Bullock, I. & Strunin, L. (2013). The role of evidence, context, and facilitation in an implementation trial: Implications for the development of the PARIHS framework. *Implementation Science* 8(1), 28.

Sackett, D. L., Rosenberg, W., Gray, J. A. M., Haynes, R. B. & Richardson, W. S. (1996). Evidence based medicine: What it is and what it isn't. *British Medical Journal* 312, 71–2.

Sackett, D. L., Straus, S. E., Richardson, W. S., Rosenberg, W. & Haynes, R. B. (2000). *Evidence-based Medicine: How to Practice and Teach EBM*. Edinburgh: Churchill Livingstone.

Sandall, J., Soltani, H., Gates, S., Shennan, A. & Devane, D. (2013). Midwife-led continuity models versus other models of care for childbearing women. *Cochrane Database Systematic Review* 8, CD004667.

Shepperd, S., Adams, R., Hill, A., Garner, S. & Dopson, S. (2013). Challenges to using evidence from systematic reviews to stop ineffective practice: An interview study. *Journal of Health Services Research & Policy* 18(3), 160–6.

Solomons, N. M. & Spross, J. A. (2011). Evidence-based practice barriers and facilitators from a continuous quality improvement perspective: An integrative review. *Journal of Nursing Management* 19(1), 109–20.

Taylor, R. (2013). *The Essentials of Nursing and Healthcare Research*. London: SAGE.

Thorsteinsson, H. S. & Sveinsdóttir, H. (2013). Readiness for and predictors of evidence-based practice of acute-care nurses: A cross-sectional postal survey. *Scandinavian Journal of Caring Sciences*. <www.unboundmedicine.com/medline/citation/24111971/Readiness_for_and_predictors_of_evidence_based_practice_of_acute_care_nurses:_a_cross_sectional_postal_survey>

Titler, M. & Adam, S. (2010). Developing an evidence-based practice. In G. Lobiondo-Wood & J. Haber (eds), *Nursing Research. Methods and Critical Appraisal for Evidence-based Practice*, 7th edn. USA: Mosby-Elsevier, pp. 385–436.

Younger, P. (2010). Internet-based information-seeking behaviour amongst doctors and nurses: A short review of the literature. *Health Information and Libraries Journal* 27(1), 2–10.

CHAPTER 3

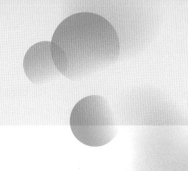

# INTRODUCING THE RESEARCH PROCESS

Maree Johnson and Cecily Hengstberger-Sims

## KEY TERMS

research question
hypothesis
problem statement
method
population
variable
dependent variable
independent
 variable
research design
research proposal
 plan

## CHAPTER LEARNING OBJECTIVES

By the end of this chapter you will be able to:

- define the steps in the research process
- discuss the essential features of a research proposal
- develop and present a logical argument to support a research problem
- demonstrate awareness of the differences between aims, research questions and hypotheses
- appraise the feasibility and ethical aspects of a research problem
- outline aspects of budgeting and timelines.

# Introduction

As student nurses or midwives, when we first learnt to give an injection in our nursing courses we were given a set of discrete tasks that we followed. The order of the tasks was defined, and we could not do the second task unless the first was completed. With practice, we gained confidence and knew the order of the tasks, and could complete the entire process safely and competently.

Giving an injection is a practical skill, and the conduct of nursing research and the research process is similar. Readers and novice researchers should first understand all the steps, learn how to complete each step and how to carry out these steps in a logical order to completion. With practice, understanding or doing, research can become very manageable. Research has a unique language and its own set of terms, which will require some attention before they are grasped. Continue to revise the key terms throughout this chapter as often as you wish. Research is a subject that requires ongoing reading to remain conversant with the contemporary changes in methods; it is a subject of lifelong learning.

In this chapter, we introduce readers to the key steps and the overall plan for research. By exploring key aspects of the research process, you will become familiar with the language and logical order of research. Subsequent chapters will provide more detail on each of the steps in the process.

The research process is a complex series of sequential activities that are carried out to allow nurses and midwives to develop new knowledge and skills for nursing and midwifery practice, management or education. The research process consists of 13 major steps in three main stages: planning the research, executing the research plan, and informing the scientific and clinical community.

- Stage 1—Planning the research
  - Select a suitable research problem and topic.
  - Review and synthesise the existing literature and topic.
  - Identify a frame of reference and define terms.
  - Develop aims, objectives, **research questions** and **hypotheses**.
  - Choose the appropriate methods (design, sampling, data collection and analysis) to answer the research questions and hypotheses posed.
  - Consider feasibility and ethical issues.
  - Finalise the research proposal or plan (budget, timeline, dissemination strategies, research team profile).
- Stage 2—Executing the research plan
  - Obtain ethical approval.
  - Obtain funding (optional).
  - Collect the data.
  - Analyse the data.
- Stage 3—Informing the scientific and clinical nursing and midwifery community of the research results
  - Write up the study findings.
  - Disseminate the findings.

The focus of this chapter is on Stage 1 of the process.

**Research question:** The question being asked by the research—the issue it sets out to explore.

**Hypothesis:** A statement about the relationship between two or more variables (factors or characteristics in a study).

# Planning the research

The research proposal, plan or protocol is the initial plan developed by the researcher to explain the research process to be undertaken to other team members, funding bodies and interested parties such as ethics committees. The proposal 'forces the investigator to create, define, and refine the research project…[This] time to fully conceptualise and synthesise the proposal will enhance the investigator's ability to conduct a better study and will provide the framework for future reports of the work' (Inouye & Fiellin 2005, p. 274). A proposal that is perceived as meeting a 'good' standard is described by Harper (2007, p. 15) as one that answers the following questions:

- What is this research trying to find out: what questions is it trying to answer?
- How will the proposed research answer these questions?
- Why is this research worth doing?

The research proposal required for service managers, ethics committees, funding bodies or other health professional reviewers can have slightly differing components to be completed by the researchers (Harper 2007). We present here the most common format (see Box 3.1) of the proposal and strongly advise researchers to read the specific instructions for the particular committee or persons requiring the proposal (Harper 2007; Martin & Fleming 2010). As Endacott (2008) notes, the research plan or proposal must 'convince others that the work is necessary, soundly constructed and expects to generate outcomes worthy of pursuing' (p. 212).

## Box 3.1

**KEY COMPONENTS OF A PROPOSAL**

- Synopsis (often in layperson's language)
- Problem
  - Aim of the study
  - Background (introduction/literature review/definition of terms/frame of reference)
- Aim/specific objectives
  - Hypotheses/research questions
- Methods
- Design
- Sample and setting
- Data collection tools
- Data collection procedures
- Analysis procedures
- Ethical considerations
- Timeframe
- Budget
- Funding sources
- Dissemination strategies
- References
- Profile of researchers or research team

## Implications for evidence-based practice

**RESEARCHING THE COST: BENEFIT RATIO**

Alison Thompson, Clinical Nurse Consultant (CNC) for Ambulatory Care, had visited the Clinical Nursing Research Unit at Raymond House Hospital. Alison was seeking advice from the Senior Research Fellow for Nursing and Midwifery Research. Alison said that she had been changing the intravenous cannulae for community clients receiving antibiotic therapy every 72 hours or when required, while other services were changing them every 48 hours or when required. Alison believed there was no difference in the patient outcomes and wanted to compare the two approaches as she thought there were considerable benefits for the patients and cost savings for the health service.

# Step 1: Select the topic and research problem

The first step in any research study is to select the topic. There are many approaches to this. Clinicians often identify topics from problems experienced during their clinical practice, as in the case study above. Occasionally new technologies or health policies may prompt nurses and midwives to explore the merit of new treatments or policies within their practice. Other authors suggest that even casual conversations with patients and their families can be a rich source of research topics (Ayres 2007; Pierce 2009). For experienced nurse and midwifery researchers, national health priorities may influence the selection of topics because these topics are likely to be funded. Vivar and associates (2007) define the topic as 'what specific situations have been observed that require a research question to be answered' (p. 71).

## Shaping the research topic into a manageable research problem

Shaping the research topic is a process whereby a broad research topic is narrowed into a researchable question (Houser 2008).

The word 'problem' is often used to reflect the focus of the study similar to the topic. The problem is often presented in a research proposal in terms of the issue or the impact or scale of the problem. In a study of coping styles of pregnant adolescents, the problem is presented in the introduction in terms of the rate of pregnancy in adolescent populations in Australia and other countries (Myors et al. 2001). The problem should be presented in a manner that engages the reader, or convinces the reader that the study is important because of the nature of the problem (Francis et al. 1979; Martin & Fleming 2010; Pierce 2009).

However, a **problem statement** is considerably more precise and is used to describe what the situation is that requires changing or understanding and how the study will address this situation or problem (Francis et al. 1979). Similarly, Houser (2008) defines the problem statement as a 'declaration of disparity; the difference (gap) between what is known and what needs to be known about a topic' (p. 113). For example, a problem statement may be as follows:

> There is considerable research comparing intermittent versus continuous nasogastric feeding of patients undergoing gastro-intestinal surgery. However, there is little research comparing these feeding methods in patients experiencing facial surgery. This study will use a randomised clinical trial to compare the benefits of intermittent versus continuous nasogastric feeding in patients undergoing facial surgery.

**Problem statement:** Describes what the situation is that requires changing or understanding and how the study will address this situation or problem.

The problem could be understood as feeding in patients undergoing facial surgery; the problem statement is a series of related statements positioning the research within existing knowledge.

Reviewing the literature or exploring the background to the problem will help shape the research problem. Aspects such as the definition of terms, limiting the scope of study for sampling, defining how the methods might influence the problem or directing which outcomes are likely, are all important components of shaping the problem (Vivar et al. 2007).

## .THINKING DEEPLY

**Getting started: Identifying the research problem**

Reflect on a recent clinical experience where you encountered an issue or problem with patient care. In a brief paragraph, write down what you thought the problem or issue was and how this problem might be resolved or what you wanted to understand more clearly. Review your statement. Does it clearly identify the issue/problem? Does it identify and express what you want to do about it?

## Step 2: Review and synthesise the literature

The purpose of undertaking the literature review is, first, to collect all the recent literature on the topic area. A comprehensive review of viewpoints, debates, methods, findings or areas for further research is the focus of the review; seminal literature can also be used. Second, the researcher should synthesise the literature and develop an argument reflecting the omissions or 'gaps' in the literature (Abrams 2012; Endacott 2008). The researcher needs to read the literature and to comprehend, summarise and synthesise it (Foster 2013).

The literature should be read in a systematic manner. You may find it helpful to place readings from authors with similar viewpoints together or similar methods together, or sources that focus on instruments or measurement tools. Synthesis, or the bringing together of like-minded positions, or similar or dissimilar methods or findings, should be carried out before writing the literature review.

A suitable database or table can be invaluable to both the novice and advanced researcher when managing volumes of papers or monographs. Once the scope of the aspects to be discussed is identified, the researcher can develop a logical order to the presentation in the literature, such as from general to specific issues (Pierce 2009). In Figure 3.1, for example, articles related to similar positions or methods can be located together when writing the material and important differences in the works noted for the literature review (see p. 40). The use of the spreadsheet is to organise material logically before putting down what is similar and what is contrasting literature. This gives researchers a balanced presentation of the material examined and allows them to position their own study in relation to the existing material, in other words to begin shaping their argument. Chapter 14 presents a thorough discussion on searching through databases, the scope of literature to be examined, and sorting the literature.

As Hamilton and Clare (2004) point out, it is important to decide on a 'line of argument or discussion to be taken to support or enhance the research [that] introduces the literature at strategic points to support that argument…[and] establishes the "case" for the research' (p. 9).

How much literature should be considered in the literature search? For some topics with extensive literature, such as HIV, researchers may choose to do a random selection of literature. A general guide for topics with extensive literature is to ensure coverage within the past five years; for more obscure topics you may need to search literature dating back to the 1960s when databases commenced.

## TIPS AND SKILLS

### LITERATURE COVERAGE

The question of how do you know whether you have searched the literature thoroughly enough can be answered within the searching itself.

When researchers find and gain access to an article and all relevant materials referred to in that article, they are described as covering most of the literature. Clearly, it is impossible to cover every article. It is covering contemporary debates or methods adequately that is at issue.

## Synthesis of the existing knowledge

Synthesis is a difficult task and is achieved by reading the literature, segmenting the literature into similar aspects of the topic and then logically ordering both the overall direction of the review and the aspects to be covered in the topic. Where identified, studies that support or refute the premises of your study should be emphasised. This allows the researcher to progressively develop an argument on how your study provides knowledge that fills the gap in existing knowledge. Remember, synthesis does not mean that every study you have read should be included, but only essential works.

The literature review is a critical review of the literature; some material will be omitted while other material will be shaped into a set of similar and dissimilar aspects of the topic. Synthesis is where the nurse/midwife researcher presents a thorough understanding of the material that focuses on key issues and includes several studies that support or refute these key issues. Synthesis is not the mere presentation of every study, case by case. If there are many studies to be presented, often a table that defines the chronological order of the related studies is presented, perhaps as an appendix. The literature review section of the proposal represents the end point of synthesis and critical reflection on the material examined (Rew 2011).

In a proposal, the literature review is often summarised in two paragraphs that revise the key aspects covered and reiterate the problem being addressed by the study (Falk 2006). Readers should see Chapter 14 for a detailed discussion on the literature review. Researchers often use wording like 'this study uniquely contributes to knowledge in the area of…' or 'this study examines for the first time key issues of…'

## THINKING DEEPLY

### Literature review

Having identified your topic area, decide how you will locate literature to further inform your study. What key terms will you use to locate appropriate and relevant literature? What literature search engines are available and what search parameters will you use? How do you plan to organise and synthesise the literature you retrieve?

### HOW TO WRITE A GOOD ARGUMENT

a   Describe the previous research in the area.

b   Identify the gaps in knowledge.

c   Explain how the proposed research addresses the gap.

d   Summarise some studies and give specific details of the studies that relate most to your study (Abrams 2012; Schmelzer 2006).

## Other aspects of managing the literature

There are many bibliographic software packages available. Useful websites at the end of this chapter includes several products the reader can explore.

One example is EndNote. This computer software can be used to locate references by exporting the reference details directly from library search engines; it also allows for material to be inserted as an electronic file directly within the reference listing. Figure 3.1 demonstrates a computer screen capture of an EndNote library relating to patient safety.

Considerable time and energy is saved by the use of bibliographic software. These packages include embedding the reference directly in the text when writing the literature review and locating the article with the reference in the library. The ability to alter the reference format from American Psychological Association (APA) or Harvard or other forms (depending on the requirements of journals or other parties) will save time (see an example shown in Figure 3.1).

Librarians advise novice nurse researchers to have only one bibliographic library and sort or search files by keywords or author's name.

Figure 3.1    Endnote library relating to patient safety

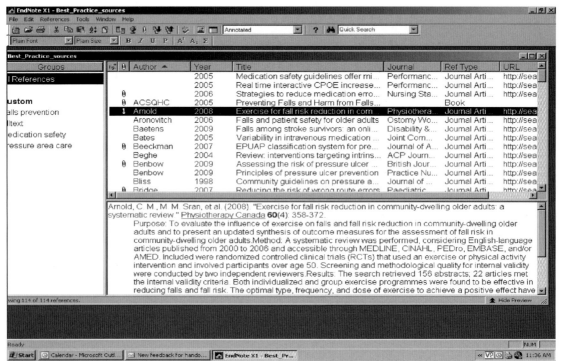

# Step 3: Identify a frame of reference and/or define the terms

The frame of reference or the way the researcher understands aspects of a study can inform the research aims, **methods** and interpretation of the data.

Not all studies will use or require a conceptual framework or a set of related general concepts (Proctor et al. 2012). In nursing and midwifery research, a conceptual or theoretical framework or established theory 'provides the structure to guide the development of the study' (Engberg & Bliss 2005, p. 157).

In some cases, the researcher is studying the theory or its components or relationships in a specific group of patients or clinical settings (Engberg & Bliss 2005). Theories in nursing, psychology, social sciences or biology have all been applied to nursing and midwifery research.

We advise the reader to review Chapter 1 on the use of theory in nursing and midwifery research. In theory-testing research, the research aims, questions or hypotheses test the relationships between components of the theory as defined by the theory or conceptual framework (Engberg & Bliss 2005). The following example emphasises the use of a theoretical framework that influenced the design of an instrument to measure nurses' self-concept.

Contemporary self-concept research has established that self-concept is a multidimensional construct (Craven et al. 2003; Marsh & Perry 2005), particularly when related to adult **populations** (Marsh & Ayotte 2003). When studying self-concept in an adult population such as registered nurses, it would be expected that multiple dimensions of self-concept will be related to behavioural outcomes, such as job satisfaction (Cowin et al. 2008).

Throughout the literature review, it is important to identify any key terms. In the example above, the term 'self-concept' can mean many things to many readers. However, for the purposes of the study, Marsh and Perry (2005) defined self-concept as 'a person's self-perceptions that are formed through experience with and interpretations of one's environment' (p. 72).

All terms should be defined in clear language and these should appear early in a research proposal to avoid misinterpretation by the readers. Definitions can be obtained from existing literature such as dictionaries, books of synonyms and technical glossaries (Francis et al. 1979) or from other research studies. The form of the definition taken by the researcher is often referred to as the 'operational definition' (Francis et al. 1979; Polit & Beck 2010). The following example demonstrates the operational definition for the biological measure of heat gain:

> Heat gain (°C) refers to the number of degrees of temperature the subject had to gain to reach 36°C (i.e., 36°C minus arrival temperature at recovery). (Clevenger 1994)

Operational definitions are also portrayed as the way the construct (abstract interpretation) is measured within the study: 'Depression, as measured by the Edinburgh Post-natal Depression scale' (Cox et al. 1987).

Having reviewed the literature and developed the argument in support of the study to be undertaken, the researcher presents a case for the significance of the study and then refines the research question further to form aims or specific objectives, hypotheses or research questions.

**Method:** The prescribed systematic procedures and protocols involved in carrying out a research project.

**Population:** A clearly defined grouping of people, animals or objects that can be identified by specific characteristics or properties useful to research.

**TIPS AND SKILLS**

The term 'research question' is often used in a broad or general sense and means the broad topic of the research; 'question' here is roughly equivalent to 'problem' or 'matter', as in 'the question of fever management in children'. For example, 'refining the research question' means that the researcher reduces the topic or aspects of the topic to a more precise definition of the problem that is to be researched. Specific research questions are a set of questions to be answered by the data that will be collected by the researcher. This is often confusing to novice researchers. Research questions are not the questions the researchers will ask in a survey or at an interview.

## Step 4: Develop aims, objectives, research questions and hypotheses

Research studies, whether undertaken by quantitative (using numbers) or qualitative (using text) methods, all have research aims or purposes (Martin & Fleming 2010). A research aim is a general statement about the research: 'The aim of this study is to compare differing warming procedures for post-surgical patients' or 'The aim of this study is to explore how carers experience living with partners with chronic heart disease'. Specific objectives are clear statements of what is to be achieved by the study, or they provide detail on what is expected as outcomes (Parahoo 2006). Examples of specific objectives may include describing the characteristics of carers, outlining the procedures used in techniques that use warmed blankets, or developing an education program for nurses using technology-based warming devices.

Research questions and hypotheses are the most precise statements of a research proposal. Polit and Beck (2010) define research questions as 'specific queries researchers want to answer in addressing the research problem' (p. 46). They qualify this statement by noting that when researchers can make 'specific predictions about answers to research questions [they] pose hypotheses that are tested empirically'.

Hypotheses are statements about the relationship between two **variables**: **independent variable** and **dependent variable** (factors in a study). In some cases, there can be independent variables or factors that cause change in the dependent variables and outcome factors (Polit & Beck 2010).

Research questions are used in both quantitative and qualitative research, although the use of a hypothesis is preferred when testing relationships or examining differences in interventions (Martin & Fleming 2010; Pierce 2009).

What are the characteristics of a 'good' research question?

Research questions and hypotheses should have the following components: the participants, the clinical context, the phenomenon of concern (if applicable in qualitative studies), intervention (if applicable in quantitative studies), comparison group (if applicable in quantitative studies) and outcomes (if applicable in quantitative studies).

In a qualitative study the aim/purpose and the research question appear very similar. For example:

> The purpose of this research was to explore the strategies used by women to manage fatigue in the first six months following childbirth (Taylor & Johnson 2010, p. 369). The research questions written for this study were:

> How do women manage fatigue? How do the strategies change over time? (Taylor & Johnson 2010, p. 369).

**Variable:** A characteristic or factor that will vary within a study (e.g. age, blood pressure, depression scores).

**Independent variable:** The variable expected to cause or influence the dependent variable. In an experimental study, researchers manipulate this independent variable.

**Dependent variable:** The outcome variable that is thought to depend on or be caused by another variable, the independent variable.

Hypotheses are generally not used in qualitative research and many qualitative researchers believe that only research aims or objectives should be used.

## Specific types of hypotheses

For quantitative research, depending on what is known about a research topic and question, hypotheses may take the form of a directional, non-directional or null hypothesis.

A directional hypothesis is by far the most common. The researcher reviews the literature and then develops the hypothesis based on those findings, often concluding that a new intervention of X will result in improved patient outcomes, for example reduced time to wound healing, reduced depression, reduced readmission rates. The hypothesis predicts that there is a direction of the change either increasing or decreasing the dependent or outcome measure (Houser 2008; Nieswiadomy 2002, 2008, 2012; Polit & Beck 2012).

Houser (2008) defines the directional hypothesis as 'a one-sided statement of the research question that is interested in only one direction of change' (p. 126). An example would be:

> Mild (35.5–36.0°C) or moderate (34.5–35.4°C) hypothermic patients who have undergone surgery for greater than 20 minutes, and who received Bair-Hugger™ warming, will achieve normothermia in less time (increased rewarming rate) than hypothermic patients receiving only warmed cotton blankets. (Stevens et al. 2000, p. 270)

A non-directional hypothesis is likely when the literature suggests that there will be a change in the dependent variable or outcome measure, but there is no clear direction as to whether outcomes will improve or deteriorate. In this situation a non-directional hypothesis is posed. Houser (2008) defines a non-directional hypothesis as 'a two-sided statement of the research question that is interested in change in any direction' (p. 126). For example,

> There is a relationship between mothers' first birthing methods and their satisfaction with subsequent birthing methods.

A null hypothesis is posed when the literature and the researcher believe there will be no difference between the groups receiving the intervention. This is relevant when there is a change in interventions in a clinical context where there is little harm evident, such as childbirth. Houser defines a null hypothesis as 'a statement of the research question that declares no difference between the groups' (p. 126).

Some researchers also distinguish between simple and complex hypotheses. A simple hypothesis includes one independent variable (factor or intervention being manipulated) and one dependent variable (factor or outcome of the study). Complex hypotheses include more than one independent variable and/or one or more dependent variables.

## •THINKING DEEPLY

You have identified your problem or issue, reviewed the literature and should now have a clearer picture. It is time for you to draft the purpose of the study and identify your research questions. If your study seeks to test or compare, you should also write appropriate research hypotheses.

# Step 5: Choose appropriate methods to address the research questions or hypotheses

**Research design:** The overall plan for answering a research question, including an appropriate detailed plan for enhancing the integrity of the study.

In this section the researcher defines the **research design** and overall methodology or approach. Every method has strengths and weaknesses and your study will fall into general areas. 'Your choice should be based upon careful consideration of how appropriate each available methodology fits your purpose [aim], and the feasibility of each method depending on the limits of your time and resources' (Francis et al. 1979).

Choosing the best or most appropriate design is a challenging task and is largely reliant on the research questions or hypotheses posed and the type of data (numbers or text) that are to be collected. Method includes the design of the study, the sample and setting, the data collection instrument or tools, data collection procedures and analysis approaches. The choice of qualitative or quantitative approaches can be made with a thorough understanding of the range of designs, sampling, data collection procedures and tools available in both these paradigms (see Chapters 6 and 10 on design, Chapters 5 and 9 on sampling, Chapters 7 and 11 on data collection and Chapters 8 and 12 on data analysis).

In general terms, qualitative research is frequently used when little is known about a topic, when factors cannot be easily defined or 'theories are not available to explain behaviour' (Vivar et al. 2007, p. 64), and the data collected is usually text. Qualitative research examines the human experience and is concerned with description and understanding. Quantitative research is appropriate when there is measurable information and defined relationships or there is prediction between variables, and the data collected is usually numeric (Martin & Fleming 2010; Pierce 2009; Vivar et al. 2007).

Other considerations when choosing a method may relate to the researcher's method of choice; for example, a Master's student may have quantitative skills and is seeking to develop qualitative research skills in their doctorate.

Some data collection methods such as face-to-face interviews may be more in keeping with the philosophical position of the researcher. In some rare cases, there may be only a small number of cases with a specific research condition and so quantitative methods may not be possible or suitable.

**THINKING DEEPLY**

Using your research questions and/or hypotheses, begin to determine what type of study design you will use. Provide a rationale supporting your choice of design—why is this the most appropriate method for your study?

# Step 6: Defining the significance and outcomes of the research

One of the most important aspects of any proposal is outlining the significance or likely outcomes or products from the study. This is the 'So what?' aspect of the study (Nieswiadomy 2008, p. 78).

The significance statement emphasises the importance of your study 'as distinct from any and all other studies that might address the same topic' (Francis et al. 1979, p. 25). Your study may address or inform key state or national policies, use innovative methods or instruments/technology, affect specific healthcare groups or clinicians, test theories in differing settings or samples, or provide knowledge for health consumers, nurse managers, educators or others. Often the social and economic benefits of research are set out in this section. Falk (2006) states that 'the significance of the grant should clearly point out why the problem addressed is important and how scientific knowledge will be advanced by the proposed study' (p. 511). As far as possible, the study's outcomes should be specifically defined.

## Scope and limitations

Outlining the scope and limitations of a research study can be just as important as identifying the topic. Containing the study allows it to become more manageable or allows a more precise comparison study than would otherwise be possible. For example, a study may be proposed to examine all older people receiving oral medications. Some older people take two medications per day while others may be prescribed 12 doses per day and may be more vulnerable to adverse events.

The researcher can define or contain the scope of the study as older people, living in the community, receiving 12 medication doses or more per day. Hence the study, or more particularly in this case the sample and setting, is constrained. Similar constraints may be applied to methods, instruments or other methods used to collect data, and indeed, analysis procedures. Disclosure of the scope and limitations of the study allows others to determine whether the study has been thoroughly considered by the researcher.

## Step 7: Consider the feasibility and ethical issues

How can novice nurse researchers evaluate whether the research question or problem they have selected is an important one that is feasible and ethical? One approach is to apply the FINER (an acrostic) model to the question as proposed by Houser (2008, p. 122):

- Feasible: Adequate subjects, technical expertise, time and money are available; the scope is narrow enough for the study.
- Interesting: The question is interesting to the investigator.
- Novel: The study confirms or refutes previous findings or provides new findings.
- Ethical: The study cannot cause unacceptable risk to participants and does not invade privacy.
- Relevant: The question is relevant to scientific knowledge, clinical and health policy, or further research directions.

Nurses and midwives can apply this model to their research questions and problems in order to clarify the issues of appraisal of a research problem inclusive of feasibility and ethical considerations. Other authors also identify that a systematic approach that considers several aspects of the proposal can assist in gaining approval or funding (Proctor et al. 2012). A comprehensive discussion on the issues of concern relating to ethics is presented in Chapter 4.

## Step 8: Finalise the research proposal plan
### Budget

Estimating the budget required to conduct a project is an important task of the lead researcher (Harrison 2012; Singh et al. 2005). There are two major categories of grants available: project funding or researcher development support (Inouye & Fiellin 2005).

**Research proposal plan:** The initial plan developed by the researcher to explain the research process to be undertaken.

For project funding there are several major components of a budget: personnel, consultants or technical/support staff, supplies, equipment, services, computer hardware and software, survey formatting and printing, postage, photocopying, travel, incentives/ compensations for subjects and other support technology such as telephones, mobiles and faxes (Bliss 2005).

Personnel may include research assistants with Master's degrees, or post-doctoral qualifications as required by the project. Personnel often reflect the major cost of the budget and the cost is determined by how many supporting research officers are needed, the hourly rate and the number of weeks they will be required. Consultants are often budgeted on an hourly rate and can be used for statistical support, design, analysis of data or occasionally to collect data. Specialised equipment required for the study or consumables such as dressings should always be precisely costed within the budget.

As a guide, small studies such as a qualitative study of 20 people would be expected to cost around $20 000 to $60 000, while large studies such as multicentre trials may cost from $500 000 to $1 million or more. Research projects should always be properly funded.

There are various funding sources to be considered, such as external grants (e.g. Australian Research Council or NHMRC grants), internal grants (small funding provided by the university or the health service) or in-kind funding (such as health staff allocated to data collection for a short period, or facilities such as office space, equipment, computers). The budget and funding body are selected depending on the level of funding being sought and the priorities of the funding bodies.

**Table 3.1**    Research budget

| Item | Description | Cost |
| --- | --- | --- |
| Salary | Clinical Nurse Educator (engaged in research) with a Master's qualification in nursing or a related discipline | $7718 for 170 hours ($45.40 per hour: base rate with on-costs for superannuation and casual allowances) data collection and entry/ data analysis/report writing/ assistance with coaching and education material preparation |
| Administration | Workshop materials (photocopying/printing and binding) × 100 workbooks | $500 |
| Research materials | NVivo 8 software for data analysis | $800 |
| Miscellaneous | Transcription services for two focus groups of one hour duration | $360 |
| Miscellaneous | Use of telephone/fax and other services | $600 |
| Equipment | Digital recorder (popular brand) | $500 |
| Total | | $10 398 |

Justification of the budget is important. Each item identified in the study will need to have an explicit and clearly related role in the potential completion of the study and this should be made immediately apparent to potential funding bodies. Inclusion of budget items that are unrealistic, poorly justified or unrelated may threaten the possibility of securing funding.

## Timeframe

A timetable of the specific tasks to be completed throughout the process informs the reviewers and the study team of the required time in which to complete tasks (Martin & Fleming 2010).

Realistic timelines are always recommended. All the tasks described in this chapter would usually appear in the timeline: finalising the literature and proposal, ethics approval, development of data collection instruments (survey or interview schedule), recruitment of participants, data collection, data analysis, and writing up or reporting on the study. Most of these tasks require between one and six months each. Be generous with your time allocations as in some cases you will be required to comply with them or give reasons for any non-adherence. Table 3.2 suggests a timeframe for a simple survey research study.

**Table 3.2**  Timeframe for tasks in a simple research study

| Date | Activity |
| --- | --- |
| January–March | Finalise literature review and proposal |
| March–May | Secure ethics clearance and approval |
| May–June | Identify potential survey recipients<br>Finalise print survey instrument and prepare for mail dissemination |
| July | Commence data collection with dissemination of mail survey<br>Develop code for data entry |
| August–September | Data entry of returned survey responses |
| September–November | Analysis of data responses |
| November–December | Write up findings and identify potential sources for dissemination of findings (journals/conferences) |
| January–February | Finalise written report and send to funding authorities/ethics committee and identified prospective disseminators of study results |

### THINKING DEEPLY

Now it is time to consider the implications for your proposed study. What sort of resources do you need to conduct and complete the study? What costs are involved? What are the specific stages of the research proposal? How long will you allow for each stage?

## Dissemination of findings

As noted at the start of this chapter, informing the scientific and clinical nursing and midwifery community of the research findings is the final and very important part of the process (Pierce 2009). Nurses and midwives can present their findings to their local community, or at national or international conferences. Unfortunately, conference proceedings are not widely available to the international research community and researchers should always strive to publish their research in national or international refereed journals.

A thorough discussion is provided in Chapter 16 on the procedures to follow when presenting a paper at a conference or publishing a paper.

When writing a proposal, the nurse researcher is required to detail when and where papers from this study will be presented for review by the scientific community. Many funding bodies request substantial detail on this topic and some may judge the proposal on the ability of the study to be published in high-ranking academic journals.

## Writing the synopsis

Finally, the synopsis is a summary of key aspects of a research proposal or plan. The synopsis is the final section of the proposal to be written but appears first in the proposal or may appear separate from the main proposal. Aspects of the plan are included briefly: the problem, aim, method or methodology, and likely outcomes of the research. Many funding bodies and ethics committees require that this section be written in plain English or layperson's language; in other words, don't use complex health terms.

The length of this section is between 150 and 250 words and often the most difficult to write.

# SUMMARY

- The research process has three major stages: planning the research, executing the plan and informing the scientific community of the findings.
- It is important to develop a good research proposal so that the research team, funding bodies and other interested parties can understand the overall concept, detailed tasks and framework for future reports of the work.
- There are key components of a research study that are outlined in any research paper. Both clinicians and users of research information, together with researchers, need to understand how the steps defined in this chapter influence the way findings are interpreted and how conclusions are understood by nurse and midwife researchers.

## PRACTICE EXERCISE 3.1

a  Ann and Bob want to explore why a number of patients with chest pain return to the emergency department (ED) at the hospital within six months. Ann is interested in studying this health problem within the environment context of a patient, such as the patient's understanding of chest pain, the meaning of chest pain to their life and death, and what sources of information are being accessed. Write at least one research question arising from Ann's interest.

ANSWER: Two of the research questions might be:

What are the lived experiences of patients with chest pain who present at an emergency department?

How did patients respond to chest pain and interpret it before presenting at an emergency department?

b  Bob wants to assess whether or not giving instructions and printed health education materials relating to self-management of chest pain will reduce the proportion of patients who re-present to the ED with chest pain within six months. Write at least one research question arising from Bob's interest.

ANSWER: An example of the research questions is:

Is there any difference between the proportion of patients with chest pain who re-present to the ED within six months and receive health education relating to the self-management of chest pain and the proportion of patients with chest pain who re-present to the ED within six months and who do not receive the health eduation?

## PRACTICE EXERCISE 3.2

Access your library and locate a research article that you find interesting, easy to read and understand.

Write down the headings of each major section in the article.

Compare these headings with those in the research process listed above.

What is similar?

What is different?

PRACTICE EXERCISE 3.3

Access your library and locate a simple research article that you find interesting, easy to read and understand. This may be the same one used in the previous exercise.

Read the article and locate the following:

- Research aim or purpose.
- Research question(s) and/or hypothesis(es).

Are the hypotheses directional, non-directional or null, and why? Note that sometimes only the aim is presented, particularly in descriptive studies.

# APPENDIX 3.1
# EXAMPLE OF A QUANTITATIVE RESEARCH PROPOSAL

**Title**: Outcomes with home follow-up visit after postpartum hospital discharge.
**Researchers**: Dr Sansnee Jirojwong, Ms Barbara Ritchie, Ms Erin Russell, Ms Sandra Walker.

## AIMS AND OBJECTIVES

The major aim of this comparative study is to identify the health outcomes of home follow-up visits provided by midwives to women after the birth of their infants.

Specific objectives are to:

- describe and compare characteristics of mothers who receive home follow-up visits and those who do not
- assess the relationship between the home follow-up visits and mothers' physical health outcomes
- assess the relationship between the home follow-up visits and mothers' psychological health outcomes
- assess the relationship between the home follow-up visits and mothers' satisfaction with healthcare after discharge
- assess the relationship between the home follow-up visits and infants' physical health outcomes
- assess the relationship between the home follow-up visits and breastfeeding
- describe mothers' comments relating to home follow-up visits and other early postpartum care.

## EXPECTED OUTCOMES

This study will include all postpartum women who meet the study criteria and give birth at Hospital ABC. It will identify characteristics of postpartum women who receive home follow-up visits and those who do not. The difference in maternal and infants' health outcomes between these two groups of women will be evaluated. The results of this study will help strengthen or broaden existing home follow-up visits provided to postpartum women by midwives. Health information given to women may be formalised in a systematic approach. A booklet containing essential information which can be used widely can be developed. A summary of methods of assessing current health education provided to early discharge patients including postpartum women can be developed.

## BACKGROUND AND SIGNIFICANCE

### Background

The introduction of casemix and diagnostic-related groups (DRG) in Australia has reduced the average length of hospital stay of patients admitted for treatments and procedures. This casemix and DRG has been used as a tool to compare hospital performance, provide a basis for funding and charging for hospital services, and aid interpretation of other aspects of care such as cost and quality (AIHW 1996). Patients affected by the DRG systems also include postpartum women who have normal births and births with complications. The length of postpartum stay in hospital among mothers has decreased over the decade. Annual Australian Institute of Health and Welfare (AIHW) reports (1994, 1996, 1999) showed that the average duration of postnatal hospital stay was reduced from 5.3 days in 1991 to 4.1 days in 1997. The figures include all postpartum women regardless of the types of birth, maternal medical and obstetric complications, neonatal morbidity and specific hospital policies of early discharge. Queensland and New South Wales have a relatively shorter stay on average (4.0 days) than other states. The latest data show that in Queensland public-insured postpartum women stay in hospitals for a shorter period (3.2 days) compared with private-insured women (5.4 days) (AIHW 1999).

In order to prevent and detect complications early among postpartum women and their infants, many hospitals and community health centres have introduced home follow-up services by midwives. There is a variation of practices from one locality to another relating to the number of visits, time of initial and subsequent visits after the hospital discharge and the range of protocol of services. However, the services generally include physical, psychological and social assessment, health education and anticipatory guidance (Ghilarducci & McCool 1993; Grullon & Grimes 1997; Williams & Cooper 1993). If required, women or their infants are referred to other health professionals such as social workers or paediatricians for appropriate care.

### Studies of home follow-up visits after postpartum discharge and its outcomes

Studies in many countries including the United Kingdom, the United States, Canada and Australia have assessed the outcomes of home follow-up visits after postpartum discharge (Carty & Bradley 1990; Frank-Hanssen et al. 1999; Ghilarducci & McCool 1993; Johnson et al. 1999; Lieu et al. 2000). Comparing the results of one study with others is problematic due to the difference in outcome measures, study designs, period between hospital discharge and data collection, protocol and content of home visit, and types of healthcare providers (Frank-Hanssen et al. 1999; Johnson et al. 1999; Lieu et al. 2000). For example, Johnson et al. assess the success or continuation of breastfeeding, while Lieu et al. assessed a number of mothers' and infants' outcomes including newborn hospitalisation, newborn urgent clinic visit, maternal re-hospitalisation and maternal postpartum depression. Only women who had vaginal births were included in the study by Meikle et al. (1998), while Armstrong et al. (1999) included high-risk women in their study.

In the 1980s and 1990s many studies were conducted to evaluate the maternal and infants' health outcomes of postpartum women who were discharged early with home follow-up visit compared with women who had a longer hospital stay (Armstrong et al. 1999; Brooten et al. 1994; Brumfield et al. 1996; Carty & Bradley 1990; Serwint et al. 1991). The results of these have supported the provision of home visits to postpartum women; particularly first-time mothers, single mothers and mothers who intend to breastfeed their infants. A wide range of outcomes have been measured including maternal depression (Carty & Bradley 1990), satisfaction with care, and the reduction of readmission (Brooten et al. 1994). Another common and consistent outcome derived from these studies is that mothers who received the home visit were more likely to be satisfied with the postpartum care (Brooten et al. 1994) or to be confident to seek help from healthcare providers (Ghilarducci & McCool 1993) than women who did not receive the home visit. However, these studies were conducted in major hospitals. Women who lived in rural and remote areas were not included in the studies.

### Social support during postpartum period

During the early postpartum period, women may receive support from many sources including their partners, family members, friends, general practitioners, paediatricians and midwives (Jirojwong 1995). As mentioned earlier, midwives provide a range of support such as information and psychological support during the home follow-up visits. The women's supporters may also provide similar types of help as midwives, particularly to those who do not have any home visits. This important factor has not been taken into account in many studies which assess the outcomes of home follow-up visits (Carty & Bradley 1990; Frank-Hanssen et al. 1999; Ghilarducci & McCool 1993; Johnson et al. 1999; Lieu et al. 2000). It also should be noted that outcomes of social support assessed by researchers were similar to outcomes of home follow-up visits by midwives.

### Hospital ABC and home follow-up visits

Hospital ABC is a major hospital which serves the population in a large geographical area that includes Central Queensland, Central Highlands and Central West Queensland. Publicly insured and privately insured women can receive care during all stages of their perinatal period. After the birth of their child, a home follow-up visit or extended midwifery services (EMS) are offered to postpartum women who meet the criteria of being women who live in Town XYZ and nearby geographical area and are willing to have a midwife visit their homes. Approximately 90% of women who meet the criteria receive at least one home visit. Other women, who are not eligible to receive the EMS services, may or may not receive home follow-up visits depending on the policies of the hospital located nearest to them.

No systematic investigation was conducted to assess a range of potential outcomes of EMS, although the hospital EMS was initiated in 1991. Despite anecdotal data of beneficial effects to the health of both the women and their infants, only one systematic evaluation has been conducted to assess the continuation of breastfeeding between women who have a home visit and women who do not. Preliminary results indicate no difference in breastfeeding between two groups (Personal communication 2000). The lack of EMS effects can be explained by the women's intention to breastfeed before their child is born. This clearly indicated the need to demonstrate the beneficial effects of healthcare resources provided to women in the community.

This study aims to assess the EMS outcomes by comparing the difference of health measures among women who receive the EMS and those who do not. The results of this study will help strengthen or broaden the existing services. Similar services such as access to healthcare personnel by telephone may be initiated or formalised for postpartum women who live in rural and remote communities. A referral system between hospital ABC and smaller healthcare organisations may be established as a result of this project.

Two major aspects of social support will be included in this study: sources of support and types of support. The sources of support include significant individuals who help a postpartum woman in various ways. The types of support can be categorised as emotional, material, information and appraisal supports (Cronenwett 1985a,b; Weiss 1974). These support persons can be included in health education sessions provided to women early in their pregnancy.

## METHODOLOGY AND TIMING

A prospective study will be conducted at Hospital ABC. All postpartum women will be invited to participate in the study. If a woman is younger than 18 years old, permission will be sought from her parents or guardian.

Informed consent will be sought from all women regarding access to their hospital records and willingness to be contacted again following discharge. The objectives of the study, namely potential benefits to women, will be explained to them. They can refuse to participate in the study at this time and will be informed that their refusal will not have any effect on the EMS services. Ethical clearance is being sought from Central Queensland Health District and from Central Queensland University.

### Sample selection and sample size

There are approximately 90 births per month at the study hospital (Queensland Health 1999). Based on information from a study previously conducted at the hospital, it is anticipated that 15% will decline to participate in the study. Data collection will be categorised in two stages. Over a period of six months, a total of 450 women are to be included in the first stage of the study. The second stage will comprise two groups of women: a sample of women who have home visits (an EMS group, 90 women) and a sample of those who do not (a non-EMS group, 90 women). As far as possible, the two groups will be of similar age and parity. Other variables which may influence outcomes will not be matched but will be included in analyses. Information from hospital records and the initial interviews will be used for selecting women for the second stage of the study.

### Data collection

All women: Information relating to obstetrics and socio-demographic characteristics of all participants will be based on hospital records. The first stage will include all participants, limited descriptive data on the recipient, and number of home follow-up visits. Demographic and obstetrics history will also be collected. These will be followed up by telephone interviews two weeks after hospital discharge. The following information will be gathered from the telephone interview: physical health, psychological health and overall satisfaction with postpartum care.

EMS and non-EMS groups: Outcomes of women with home follow-up visits will be compared with women without the visits. The following data will be gathered by telephone interviews, two weeks after their hospital discharge: sources of support (healthcare personnel including midwives, family members, non-family members), types of support provided to women and their infants (emotional, material, information, appraise support), overall satisfaction with the support, knowledge of available health resources during the early postpartum period, breastfeeding and postpartum check-up.

## Variables and their measurements

Measurements used by four studies will be modified to design data collection tools: Jirojwong (1995); Jirojwong and Skolnik (1990); Lieu et al. (2000); Serwint et al. (1991). The study variables and measurement are as follows:

- Independent variables: home follow-up visits (no visit, 1–2 visits, 3 or more visits)
- Dependent variables: physical health (selected items of SF-36, emergency visit or re-hospitalisation of mother or infant)
- Psychological health (postpartum depression measure and feeling confidence in maternal roles)
- Knowledge (information relating to healthcare resources)
- Overall satisfaction with postpartum care
- Breastfeeding
- Postpartum check-up.

  Other variables (confounding variables) are: obstetrics factors (number of antenatal clinic attendances and obstetric abnormalities); socio-demographic factors (age, types of healthcare insurance, education level, occupation of main income earner); and sources and types of social support during the postpartum period.

## Data analyses

Quantitative data will be analysed using the SPSS program. Number percentage, range and mode will be used to analyse and present descriptive data. In order to assess group differences, a chi-square test for categorical variables and the student t-test or the Wilcoxon rank-sum test for continuous variables will be used. Multivariate logistic regression analyses adjusted for any confounding variables will be used in the final analyses in order to assess the group differences in outcome variables.

## Research timeline

Personal in-depth interview (1–2 months): The design questionnaire will be validated by personal in-depth interviews among 10 postpartum women. The researchers will explore factors included in the questionnaire and their applicability. If required, the questionnaire will be modified.

Pilot study (1–2 months): When the questionnaire is completed, it will be used in a pilot study among 20 postpartum women. Differences between the information gained from personal interviews and telephone interviews will be explored. The extent of variation between two data collection methods will be assessed using the correlation coefficient. When applicable, records will be used as a principal source to validate the data collected from the women.

- *Sample recruitment* (6 months) with additional follow-up of the second stage data collection period (2 months)
- *Data analyses* (1 month)
- *Report writing* (2 months).

## Limitation of the study design

During the postpartum period, it is unlikely that women would be able to take part in an interview for more than 20 minutes. Limited information will be gathered from participants during this period. Statistical methods will be used for controlling the influence of confounding variables on the association between home visits and health outcomes. The study does not intend to conduct an experimental study but aims to strengthen or broaden ongoing follow-up visit services.

## Composition and justification of budget

The major cost will be in data collection: interview time and telephone costs. Each interview is expected to take approximately 15–20 minutes to complete.

*Personnel*: research assistant (RA): The RA will review hospital records to obtain information relating to obstetrics history and home follow-up visits. She will be employed to conduct telephone interviews and data entry using the SPSS program. Initial training will be provided. She will be required to assist in communicating with relevant organisations and to conduct administrative tasks.

*Maintenance*: Telephone and fax will be used to communicate with community organisations and key persons. Data will be collected by using a telephone interview method. Postage is needed for a summary of the study results to be mailed out to the participants, if requested.

*Travel and others*: Travel is required to conduct a pilot study using a personal interview method during the initial stages of the study.

## BENEFITS OF THE STUDY

Results of the study will be presented to the Hospital ABC staff at their departmental monthly meeting. A paper will be presented at the annual Australia Public Health Association conference. Research articles will be submitted to be published in international journals such as the *Journal of Advanced Nursing and Midwifery*. Grants will be sought from external sources.

If a difference in health outcomes between private-insured and public-insured women is identified, the implications for healthcare insurance will justify the grants to be sought from private healthcare insurers such as MBF. Any materials developed as the result of this project can be licensed with a commercial value.

## BUDGET

| Budget item | Amount ($) |
| --- | --- |
| Personnel (RA step 2, $24.52 p.hr total 467 hours) | 12 162.00 |
| Maintenance (telephone and facsimile) | 819.00 |
| Travel | 282.00 |
| Postage | 90.00 |
| Printing questionnaires | 648.00 |
| GST (applied to selected non-personnel items only) | 184.00 |
| Total | 14 185.00 |

## REFERENCES

Armstrong, K. L., Fraser, J. A., Dadds, M. R. & Morris, J. (1999). A randomized, controlled trial of nurse home visiting to vulnerable families with newborns. *J Paediatr Child Health* 35(3), 237–44.

Australian Institute of Health & Welfare. (1994). *Australia's Mothers and Babies 1991*. Sydney: AIHW National Perinatal Statistics Unit.

AIHW. (1996). *Australia's Mothers and Babies 1993*. Sydney: AIHW National Perinatal Statistics Unit.

AIHW. (1999). *Australia's Mothers and Babies 1997*. Sydney: AIHW National Perinatal Statistics Unit.

Brooten, D., Roncoli, M., Finkler, S., Arnold, L., Cohen, A. & Mennuti, M. (1994). A randomized trial of early hospital discharge and home follow-up of women having cesarean birth. *Obstet Gynecol* 84(5), 832–8.

Brumfield, C. G., Nelson, K. G., Stotser, D., Yarbaugh, D., Patterson, P. & Sprayberry, N. K. (1996). 24-hour mother-infant discharge with a follow-up home health visit: Results in a selected medicaid population. *Obstet Gynecol* 88(4 Pt 1), 544–8.

Carty, E. M. & Bradley, C. F. (1990). A randomized, controlled evaluation of early postpartum hospital discharge. *Birth* 17(4), 199–204.

Cox, J., Holden, J. M. & Sagovsky, R. (1987). Detection of post-natal depression. Development of the 10-item Edinburgh Postnatal Depression scale. *British Journal of Psychiatry* 150, 782–6.

Cronenwett, L. R. (1985a). Network structure, social support, and psychological outcomes of pregnancy. *Nursing Research* 34, 93–9.

Cronenwett, L. R. (1985b). Parental network structure and perceived support after birth of first child. *Nursing Research* 34, 347–52.

Frank-Hanssen, M. A., Hanson, K. S. & Anderson, M. A. (1999). Postpartum home visits: Infant outcomes. *J Community Health Nurs* 16(1), 17–28.

Ghilarducci, E. & McCool, W. (1993). The influence of postpartum home visits on clinic attendance. *J Nurse Midwifery* 38(3), 152–8.

Grullon, K. E. & Grimes, D. A. (1997). The safety of early postpartum discharge: A review and critique. *Obstet Gynecol* 90(5), 860–5.

Jirojwong, S. (1995). Psychosocial factors relating to the use of antenatal services among pregnant women in Southern Thailand. PhD dissertation, Faculty of Medicine, Dentistry and Health Sciences, University of Melbourne.

Jirojwong, S. & Skolnik, M. (1990). Types of antenatal care and other related factors associated with low birth weight in Southern Thailand. *Asia Pacific Journal of Public Health* 4(2–3), 132–41.

Johnson, T. S., Brennan, R. A. & Flynn-Tymkow, C. D. (1999). A home visit program for breastfeeding education and support. *J Obstet Gynecol Neonatal Nurs* 28(5), 480–5.

Lieu, T. A., Braveman, P. A., Escobar, G. J., Fischer, A. F., Jensvold, N. G. & Capra, A. M. (2000). A randomized comparison of home and clinic follow-up visits after early postpartum hospital discharge. *Pediatrics* 105(5), 1058–65.

Meikle, S. F., Lyons, E., Hulac, P. & Orleans, M. (1998). Rehospitalizations and outpatient contacts of mothers and neonates after hospital discharge after vaginal delivery. *Am J Obstet Gynecol* 179(1), 166–71.

Personal communication, anonymous. (2000). Rockhampton, 6 July 2000.

Queensland Health. (1999). *1998 Annual Report*. Brisbane: Queensland Health.

Serwint, J. R., Wilson, M. H., Duggan, A. K., Mellits, E. D., Baumgardner, R. A. & DeAngelis, C. (1991). Do postpartum nursery visits by the primary care provider make a difference? *Pediatrics* 88(3), 444–9.

Weiss, R. S. (1974). The provision of social relationships. In Z. Rubin (ed.), *Doing Unto Others*. Englewood Cliffs, NJ: Prentice-Hall.

Williams, L. R. & Cooper, M. K. (1993). Nurse-managed postpartum home care. *J Obstet Gynecol Neonatal Nurs* 22(1), 25–31.

## APPENDIX 3.2
# EXAMPLE OF A QUALITATIVE RESEARCH PROPOSAL

**Title**: Health literacy and self-management of gestational diabetic: a study among Vietnamese, Cambodian, Thai and Laotian women in Sydney.

**Researchers**: Dr Sansnee Jirojwong, Associate Professor Virginia Schmied, Dr Jane Cioffi, Professor Maree Johnson, Professor Rhonda Griffiths, Associate Professor Hannah Dahlen.

## AIM

This is a qualitative in-depth study that aims to explore Southeast Asian migrant women's health literacy relating to gestational diabetes. It will describe how Vietnamese, Cambodian, Thai and Laotian women use information from health professionals to self-manage their illness during the perinatal period. The impact of information from other sources including their family and community on self-managing the illness also will be explored.

## BACKGROUND

### Gestational diabetes and Southeast Asian migrant women

Gestational diabetes (GDM) is a form of diabetes which develops during pregnancy in some women. Women with the disease will have high blood sugar for the first time during their pregnancy and this high blood sugar will disappear after birth. The symptom can recur in later pregnancies (AIHW 2006).

For pregnant women who appropriately manage the illness, complications including cesarean birth and having a large baby can be reduced (Koklanaris et al. 2007; Lee et al. 2007). They also have reduced risk of developing diabetes later in life (Gomez et al. 2008). Studies have shown that women who have gestational diabetes have a greater risk of developing type 2 diabetes. Many researchers (AIHW: Thow & Waters 2005; Hoffman et al. 1998; Lee et al. 2007) have found that approximately 10% of women with gestational diabetes will be diagnosed with type 2 diabetes within five years after the birth of their child and 50% will develop the diabetes within 25 years following the birth.

Southeast Asian-born women tend to have a higher rate of gestational diabetes than the rate in Australian-born women (AIHW: Thow & Waters 2005; Cheung et al. 2001; Doery et al. 1989). The rate of some migrant groups can be up to three times higher than the rate of GDM in Australian-born women. For example, the rate of gestational diabetes in Cambodian (6%) and Filipina (7%) migrant women in Australia was found to be twice the rate of all pregnant women (3.5%), while Vietnamese-born women have a rate of 10%, which is three times higher than the rate of all pregnant women (Beischer et al. 1991; Doery et al. 1989; Moses et al. 1994).

Early detection and lifestyle modification are important strategies to reduce the severity and complications of gestational diabetes. Insulin or its derivatives is also used to control the GDM in some groups of women. If there are options, Asian-born women tend to choose oral medication rather than injectable insulin to control their blood sugar (Jacobson et al. 2005). Little is known about how Southeast Asian women understand and experience gestational diabetes. No published information describes how women gain information to manage their illness and how women understand the influence of the illness on the pregnancy, birth and health outcomes for both mother and infant. No published information explains how these women interpret their symptoms and use this to change their lifestyles. One small study using survey design in Victoria was reported recently at the Population Health Congress. This study found that Vietnamese and Arabic women with gestational diabetes had less knowledge about the disease, its management and impact when compared to Indian migrants and a group of Australian-born women (Razee et al. 2008). The influence of the women's family members and their communities on the management of the women's health is also reported.

This study is informed by the concept of health literacy. Health literacy is defined by the US National Library of Medicine as the degree to which individuals have the capacity to obtain, process and understand basic health information and services needed to make appropriate health decisions. It includes the ability to understand instructions on prescription drug bottles, appointment slips, medical education brochures and doctor's directions. Tasks include locating health information, evaluating information for credibility and quality, and analysing relative risks and benefits of various options of managing their illness.

### Statement of the problem

Vietnamese, Cambodian, Thai and Laotian women have a high risk of having gestational diabetes (AIHW: Thow & Waters 2005; Cheung et al. 2001; Doery et al. 1989). There is a gap of knowledge about how these women interpret their symptoms and use their interpretation to monitor or reduce the severity of diabetes. The impact of information gained from healthcare professionals, their family and their community on their perception of the disease and self-management is not known.

### Significance of the problem

Diabetes is one of the national chronic disease priorities. Southeast Asian pregnant women have a higher rate of gestational diabetes. They also have a higher risk of having type 2 diabetes than Australian-born women (AIHW: Thow & Waters 2005; AIHW 2006). Early and appropriate self-management of the disease by the women will have long-term effects on reducing the severity of the disease and its complications (Gomez et al. 2008).

The results of this study will help identify barriers and facilitating factors that influence the ability of Southeast Asian-born pregnant women to understand and use information to manage their illness. These self-managements include their diet, physical activities and medication, when applicable. Their understanding of illness management on their infant's health will also be explored. This is particularly important because cultural beliefs and practices are known to strongly influence disease management and outcomes (Kleinman 1980). This study's results will be used to improve the quality of health promotion and disease prevention information so that women can use it to effectively manage their current illness. It will also have long-term effects if women can modify their lifestyles, which then reduces the risk of having diabetes later in life.

## RESEARCH QUESTIONS

The participants of this study are Vietnam, Cambodia, Thailand and Laos-born pregnant women. Specific research questions are:

- What are Vietnamese, Cambodian, Thailand and Laos-born pregnant women's knowledge, attitudes and cultural beliefs about gestational diabetes and its impact on their health and their infant's health?
- How do Vietnamese, Cambodian, Thai and Laos-born pregnant women seek, locate and understand health information about gestational diabetes from different sources (for example, health professionals, family and community)?
- How do the women interpret and evaluate information from different sources and ignore it or use it to manage their symptom during the perinatal period?
- To what extent do these women modify their lifestyles including diet and physical activities during pregnancy and following birth because of gestational diabetes and how has this been influenced by information from different sources?

## RESEARCH METHOD

### Study design

A qualitative in-depth research method will be used.

### Study participants and recruitment

Four major migrant groups (Vietnamese, Cambodian, Thai and Laotian women) will be recruited from Liverpool and Fairfield Hospitals. Women who receive care at a special antenatal clinic (endocrinology clinic) will be invited to participate in the study. We will also work with the bilingual early parental educators in this area who provide education for Vietnamese, Cambodian, Thai and Laotian women during pregnancy to identify and approach women who have gestational diabetes.

The first investigator will also use her well-established link with community organisations such as Buddhist temples to recruit additional participants by the use of a snowball method (personal contact or word of mouth). This method is effective in studies among Australian minority groups (Jirojwong & Manderson 2001). Bilingual research assistants together with the Chief Investigator (CI 1) will recruit women and conduct the interview in their own language.

### Sampling procedure and sample size

There will be 10–12 women of each migrant group included in the study. They will be the first or the second generation migrant women from Vietnam, Cambodia, Thailand and Laos. The total of 50 participants will have gestational diabetes and will be interviewed in their own language either during their pregnancy or within three months after birth.

Women will be recruited at the Liverpool and Fairfield Hospitals endocrinology antenatal clinic. Hospital staff will identify women who are eligible to be included in the study. The researcher will approach and invite women to take part in the study. Arrangements will be made to interview participants at a time and location convenient to them. An interview will be tape-recorded and will be no longer than one hour.

In addition, personal contact through community organisations such as Buddhist temples and community organisations will be used. The number of participants will be sufficient to saturate the data and identify themes.

### Collection of data

Three research assistants (RAs) who are bilingual in Vietnamese-English, Khmer-English or Laotian-English will be employed to assist with data collection. The first CI is an accredited interpreter in Thai–English and will interview Thailand and Laos-born women. Training of the RAs will be conducted prior to the data collection. Personal interviews will be audio-recorded and transcribed verbatim. Field notes and diary will be used to record observation information.

The participants will participate in a personal in-depth interview at the hospital clinic, their own home or a location nominated by them. The interview will explore how women understand gestational diabetes and its impact on their health and their infant's health, what are the sources of information that they use to manage the symptom and the impacts of their environments including home, work, social gathering and community organisations on their self-management. Their beliefs, relating to lifestyle modification and medication when applicable to their health and their baby's health during their perinatal period, will be explored. Field notes and diary will be used as other sources of information.

Data will be analysed using content analysis to identify themes and categories (Miles & Huberman 1994). The steps described by Miles and Huberman will be used. The study results will be presented to relevant organisations and individuals. The results will be further used to design structure a questionnaire which will be applied in a larger study among Asian-born pregnant women.

## BUDGET

The requested project budget is $16 360.00.

| Request | Amount $ |
| --- | --- |
| Personnel | 13 441.30 |
| Bilingual research assistants (Vietnamese, Cambodian, Thai and Laotian) (300 hr will be used to conduct interviews and also transcribe the recordings) HEW 5.1 rate/hr = $34.34, plus on cost 16.5% (total = $40.01/hr) (a) Interview 50 participants, 1 hr/person = 50 hr (b) Recruitment of participants (additional 30 min/participant, total = 25hr) (c) Communication with team members and meetings = 20 hours & attend training sessions for reliability = 5 hours (total = 25 hr) (d) Transcribe the recorded interviews – verbatim, 4 hr / 1 hr interview (200 hr) | 12 001.83 |
| Administrative assistance 40 hours (help with filing and communications) HEW 4.1 rate/hr = $30.89, plus on cost 16.5% (total = $35.99/hr) | 1 439.47 |
| Travel | 1 320.00 |
| Interview each participant 40 km round trip × 50 participants × $0.66/km | 1 320.00 |
| Maintenance | 1 600.00 |
| Computer accessories (memory sticks, disks) | 400.00 |
| Consumables | 200.00 |

*(Continued)*

*(Continued)*

| Request | Amount $ |
|---|---|
| Fax, mail and other communication, $50/mth × 4 mth | 200.00 |
| Digital recorder (Each $200.00 × 4) | 800.00 |
| TOTAL Requested | 16 360.00 (note 1) |

Note 1 Round to the nearest absolute figure.

## Timeline for funds to be expended in 2008

| Activities | Month | | | | | | | | | | | |
|---|---|---|---|---|---|---|---|---|---|---|---|---|
| | 1 July 08 | 2 | 3 | 4 | 5 | 6 | 7 Jan 09 | 8 | 9 | 10 | 11 | 12 |
| Literature review | | | | | | | | | | | | |
| Gaining ethical clearance, confirmation of the study with participating organisations and key contact persons | | | | | | | | | | | | |
| Employing and training research assistants | | | | | | | | | | | | |
| Data collection (RAs and SJ) | | | | | | | | | | | | |
| Data analysis (SJ and the team) | | | | | | | | | | | | |
| Writing grant application for external fund (SJ and the team) | | | | | | | | | ARC linkage | | | |
| Writing the final report (SJ and the team) | | | | | | | | | | | | |
| Writing manuscripts for publication (SJ and the team) | | | | | | | | | | | | |

## Projected outcomes of the project

By mid-2009, the following outcomes will be achieved:

- The results of this study will support an external grant application. Targeted grant agencies are Diabetes Australia, the Kidney Foundation and ARC linkage grant.
- At least two research manuscripts will be submitted to refereed journals.
- The results of the study will be presented at two international conferences (Public Health Association of Australia and International Council of Nurses Conference).
- The ongoing work will attract at least one new higher degree research student for 2009.
- An interdisciplinary collaborative research team will be formed with researchers from Victoria University and Monash University.
- Links will be strengthened with community organisations including Khmer Workers Forum, Lao Buddhist Society, Australia and Health Promotion Service, Sydney South West Area Health Service.

# REFERENCES

Australian Institute of Health & Welfare: Thow, A. M. & Waters, A.-M. (2005). *Diabetes in Culturally and Linguistically Diverse Australians: Identification of Communities at High Risk*. AIHW cat. no. CVD 30. Canberra: AIHW.

AIHW. (2006). *Australia's Health 2006*. Canberra: AIHW.

Beischer, N. A., Oats, J. N., Henry, O. A., Sheedy, M. T. & Walstab, J. E. (1991). Incidence and severity of gestational diabetes mellitus according to country of birth in women living in Australia. *Diabetes* 40 Suppl 2, 35–8.

Cheung, N. W., Wasmer, G. & Al-Ali, J. (2001). Risk factors for gestational diabetes among Asian women. *Diabetes Care* 24(5), 955–6.

Doery, J. C. G., Edis, K., Healy, D., Bishop, S. & Tippett, C. (1989). Very high prevalence of gestational diabetes in Vietnamese and Cambodian women (letters to the editor). *Med J Aust* 151, 111.

Gomez, M., Colagiuri, R., Buckley, A., Eigenmann, C. & Thomas, M. (2008). Evaluating type 2 diabetes prevention programs in culturally and linguistically diverse communities (CALD)—What's needed? Paper presented at the Population Health Congress 2008: A Global World, Practical Action for Health and Well-being, 6–9 July 2008, Brisbane, Queensland.

Hoffman, L., Nolan, C., Wilson, J. D., Oats, J. J. & Simmons, D. (1998). Gestational diabetes mellitus: Management guidelines. The Australasian Diabetes in Pregnancy Society. *Med J Aust* 169(2), 93–7.

Jacobson, G. F., Ramos, G. A., Ching, J. Y., Kirby, R. S., Ferrara, A. & Field, D. R. (2005). Comparison of glyburide and insulin for the management of gestational diabetes in a large managed care organization. *Am J Obstet Gynecol* 193(1), 118–24.

Jirojwong, S. & Manderson, L. (2001). The feeling of sadness: Migration and subjective assessment of mental health among Thai women in Brisbane, Australia. *Transcultural Psychiatry* 38(2), 167–86.

Jirojwong, S., Ritchie, B., Russell, E. & Walker, S. (2000). Outcomes with Home Follow Up Visit After Postpartum Hospital Discharge. Research proposal submitted to Central Queensland University, Rockhampton.

Jirojwong, S., Schmied, V., Cioffi, J., Johnson, M., Griffiths, R. & Dahlen, H. (2008). Health Literacy and Self Management of Gestational Diabetic: A Study Among Vietnamese, Cambodian, Thai and Laotian Women in Sydney. Research proposal submitted to College of Health and Science, University of Western Sydney, Sydney.

Kleinman, A. (1980). *Patients and Healers in the Context of Culture*. Berkeley: University of California Press.

Koklanaris, N., Bonnano, C., Seubert, D., Anzai, Y., Jennings, R. & Lee, M. J. (2007). Does raising the glucose challenge test threshold impact birthweight in Asian gravidas? *J Perinat Med* 35(2), 100–3.

Lee, A. J., Hiscock, R. J., Wein, P., Walker, S. P. & Permezel, M. (2007). Gestational diabetes mellitus: Clinical predictors and long-term risk of developing type 2 diabetes: A retrospective cohort study using survival analysis. *Diabetes Care* 30(4), 878–83.

Miles, B. M. & Huberman, A. M. (1994). Introduction: Three approaches to qualitative data analysis. In B. M. Miles & A. M. Huberman (eds), *An Expanded Sourcebook: Qualitative Data Analysis*. London: SAGE Publications, pp. 8–12.

Moses, R. G., Griffiths, R. D. & McPherson, S. (1994). The incidence of gestational diabetes mellitus in the Illawarra area of New South Wales. *Aust NZ J Obstet Gynaecol* 34(4), 425–7.

Razee, H., Cheung, W., Ploeg, H., Smith, B., Blignault, I. & McLean, M. (2008). Physical activity and nutritional behaviour in women with recent gestational diabetes. Paper presented at the Population Health Congress 2008: A Global World, Practical Action for Health and Well-being, 6–9 July 2008, Brisbane, Queensland.

## FURTHER READING

Allen, D. & Lyne, P. (2006). *The Reality of Nursing Research Politics, Practices, and Processes*. London and
    New York: Routledge.
Brinkmann, S. (2009). Literature as qualitative inquiry: The novelist as researcher. *Qualitative Inquiry*
    15(8), 1376–94.
Burns, N. P. D. & Grove, S. K. (2007). *Understanding Nursing Research: Building an Evidence-Based Practice*.
    St Louis, MI: Elsevier Saunders.
Chung, K. C. & Shauver, M. J. (2008). Fundamental principles of writing a successful grant proposal.
    *Journal of Hand Surgery* 33(4), 566–72.
Darbyshire, P., Downes, M., Collins, C. & Dyer, S. (2005). Moving from institutional dependence to
    entrepreneurialism: Creating and funding a collaborative research and practice development position.
    *Journal of Clinical Nursing* 14(8A), 926–34.

## USEFUL WEBSITES

EndNote
<www.endnote.com>
Reference Manager
<www.refman.com>
Zotero
<http://libguides.mit.edu/zotero>
These links will provide information on how to use and purchase bibliographic software products.
<www.youtube.com/watch?v=t2d7y_r65HU>
This YouTube presentation or video outlines: What is the role of a literature review in research? What does it
    mean to 'review' the literature? Get the big picture of what to expect as part of the process.
<www.lib.ncsu.edu/tutorials/lit-review>

## REFERENCES

Abrams, S. E. (2012). Purpose, insight and the review of literature. *Public Health Nursing* 29(3), 189–90
Ayres, L. (2007). Qualitative research proposals—Part I: Posing the problem. *Journal of Wound, Ostomy and
    Continence Nursing* 34(1), 30–2.
Bliss, D. Z. (2005). Writing a grant proposal—Part 6: The budget, budget justification, and resource
    environment. *Journal of Wound, Ostomy and Continence Nursing* 32(6), 365–7.
Clevenger, L. (1994). The effect of head covering on rewarming and shivering in cardiac surgical patients.
    *Critical Care Nursing Quarterly* 17, 73–85.
Cowin, L., Johnson, M., Craven, R. G. & Marsh, H. W. (2008). Causal modeling of self-concept, job
    satisfaction, and retention of nurses. *International Journal of Nursing Studies* 45, 1449–59.
Cox, J. L., Holden. J. M. & Sagovsky, R. (1987). Detection of postnatal depression: Development of the
    10-item Edinburgh Postnatal Depression Scale. *British Journal of Psychiatry* 150, 782–6.
Craven, R. G., Marsh, H. W. & Burnett, P. (2003). Cracking the self-concept enhancement conundrum:
    A call and blueprint for the next generation of self-concept enhancement research. In H. W. Marsh,
    R. G. Craven & D. McInerney (eds), *International Advances in Self Research*, vol. 1. Greenwich, CT:
    Information Age Publishing, pp. 91–126.
Endacott, R. (2008). Clinical research 6: Writing and research. *International Emergency Nursing* 16(3),
    211–14.
Engberg, S. & Bliss, D. Z. (2005). Writing a grant proposal—Part 1: Research methods. *Journal of Wound,
    Ostomy and Continence Nursing* 32(3), 157–62.
Falk, G. W. (2006). Turning an idea into a grant. *Gastrointestinal Endoscopy* 64(suppl.), S11–S13.

Foster, R. L. (2013). Extracting and synthesizing information from a literature review. *Journal for Specialists in Pediatric Nursing* (18) 85–8.

Francis, B. J., Bork, E. C. & Carstens, P. S. (1979). *The Proposal Cookbook. A Step by Step Guide to Dissertation and Thesis Proposal Writing*, 3rd edn. USA: Action Research Associates.

Hamilton, H. & Clare, J. (2004). Reviewing the literature: Making 'the literature' work for you. *Collegian: Journal of the Royal College of Nursing Australia* 11(1), 8–11.

Harper, P. J. (2007). Writing research proposals: Five rules. *HIV Nursing* 8(2), 15–17.

Harrison, D. (2012). Tips to help you find, apply for and get grants. *Neonatal, Paediatric and Child Health Nursing* 15(1), 26–27.

Houser, J. (2008). *Nursing Research: Reading, Using, and Creating Evidence*. Sudbury, MA: Jones & Bartlett.

Inouye, S. K. & Fiellin, D. A. (2005). An evidence-based guide to writing grant proposals for clinical research. *Annals of Internal Medicine* 142(4), 274–82.

Marsh, H. W. & Ayotte, V. (2003). Do multiple dimensions of self-concept become more differentiated with age? The differential distinctiveness hypothesis. *Journal of Educational Psychology* 95(4), 687–706.

Marsh, H. W. & Perry, C. (2005). Self-concept contributes to winning gold medals: Causal ordering of self-concept and elite swimming performance. *Journal of Sports Exercise Psychology* 27, 71–91.

Martin, C. J. & Fleming, V. (2010). A 15-step model for writing a research proposal. *British Journal of Midwifery* (18)12, 791-8

Myors, K., Johnson, M. & Langdon, R. (2001). Coping styles of pregnant adolescents. *Public Health Nursing* 18(1), 24–32.

Nieswiadomy, R. M. (2002). *Foundations of Nursing Research*. Upper Saddle River, NJ: Prentice Hall.

Nieswiadomy, R. M. (2008). *Foundations of Nursing Research*. Upper Saddle River, NJ: Pearson/ Prentice Hall.

Nieswiadomy, R. M. (2012). *Foundations of Nursing Research*. Upper Saddle River, NJ: Pearson/ Prentice Hall.

Parahoo, K. (2006). *Nursing Research: Principles, Process and Issues*. Basingstoke, UK: Palgrave Macmillan.

Pierce, L. L. (2009). Twelve steps for success in the nursing research journey. *Journal of Continuing Education in Nursing* (40)4, 154–62.

Polit, D. F. & Beck, C. T. (2010). *Essentials of Nursing Research: Appraising Evidence for Nursing Practice*. Philadelphia: Wolters Kluwer Health/Lippincott Williams & Wilkins.

Polit, D. F. & Beck, C. T. (2012). *Nursing Research: Generating and Assessing Evidence for Nursing Practice*, 9th edn. Philadelphia: Wolters Kluwer Health/Lippincott Williams & Wilkins.

Proctor, E. K., Powell, B. J., Hamilton, A. M. & Santens, R. L. (2012). Writing implementation research grant proposals: Ten key ingredients. *Implementation Science* 7(96). <www.implementationscience.com/ content/7/1/96>.

Rew, L. (2011). The systematic review of the literature: Synthesizing evidence for practice. *Journal for Specialists in Pediatric Nursing* 16(1), 64–9.

Schmelzer, M. (2006). How to start a research proposal. *Gastroenterology Nursing* 29(2), 186–8.

Singh, M. D., Cameron, C. & Duff, D. (2005). Writing proposals for research funds. *Axon* 26(3), 26–30.

Stevens, D., Johnson, M. & Langdon, R. (2000). A comparison of two warming techniques in surgical patients with mild or moderate hypothermia. *International Journal of Nursing Practice* 6(5), 268–75.

Taylor, J. & Johnson, M. (2010). How women manage fatigue after childbirth. *Midwifery* 26, 367–75.

Vivar, C. G., McQueen, A., Whyte, D. A. & Armayor, N. C. (2007). Getting started with qualitative research: Developing a research proposal. *Nurse Researcher* 14(3), 60–73.

CHAPTER 4

# ETHICAL AND LEGAL CONSIDERATIONS IN RESEARCH

Keri Chater

Keri Chater

## KEY TERMS

human research
  ethics committees
confidentiality
risk
beneficence
non-maleficence
human rights
anonymity
vulnerable people

## CHAPTER LEARNING OBJECTIVES

After reading this chapter you will be able to:

- explain the historical development of human research ethics committees

- define and delineate key terms in ethics such as beneficence, non-maleficence, confidentiality, anonymity, risks and rights of participants in the research process

- discuss the process of gaining informed consent

- recognise the needs of vulnerable groups in research

- appreciate the need to examine potential power relationships in research.

## Introduction

Health research can be conducted in a laboratory with animals, or in a virtual or real situation. Most health research projects that interest us are conducted in a real situation, in a community or a healthcare environment, where people volunteer their information. This information can be collected by researchers or research assistants. Quite often, the information or data of an individual can be private and should not be shared with anyone except the research team. Occasionally the media report on ethical issues such as that researchers do not disclose harm to their participants. For example, in 1987 there was a report in *Metro Magazine* of a Dr Green who withheld treatments to women with carcinoma in situ at New Zealand's National Women's Hospital from 1966 onwards (Skegg 1986). It should be noted that benefits of treatments for cervical cancer were known at that time. Therefore, researchers and users of research should be aware and appreciate the ethical and legal issues relating to research.

## History of ethics committees

In many countries, including Australia, all research undertaken has to adhere to a strict set of legal and ethical guidelines, and nursing research is no different. Ethical comportment in research had its genesis in the Nuremberg Trials after the Second World War (Annas & Grodin 1992). This was mainly a response to the atrocious Nazi experiments carried out on innocent people without their consent (Caplan 1992).

Although the Nuremberg Trials were held to try criminals for different types of war crimes, the 'Doctors' trial' proved to be exceptionally complex because the judges were not only concerned with the criminal element of the medical experiments but also with the much broader ethical elements of the research that was carried out. In the opening address for the Doctors' Trial on 9 December 1946 it was stated:

> The defendants in the dock are charged with murder, but this is no mere murder trial…To kill, to maim, and to torture is criminal under all modern systems of law. These defendants did not kill in hot blood, nor for personal enrichment…They are not ignorant men. Most of them are trained physicians and some of them are distinguished scientists. Yet these defendants, all of whom are fully able to comprehend the nature of their acts, and most of whom are exceptionally qualified to form a moral and professional judgment in this respect, are responsible for wholesale murder and unspeakably cruel tortures. (Taylor 1992, p. 67)

The Nuremberg Code was a document that arose from the findings of these trials, which listed 10 points for the conduct of ethical research. Point 1 was that research participants need to be able to give 'free, voluntary, and informed consent' (Grodin 1992, p. 135), and this has been the guiding ethical principle adopted today.

The Nuremberg Code was formalised in law in the International Covenant on Civil and Political Rights and adopted by the United Nations General Assembly in 1976. The Nuremberg Code also informed the Declarations of Helsinki I and II (McClimens & Allmark 2011), which emphasised informed consent and relationships of dependency between a researcher and a participant and a participant's competence to decide to take part in the research.

Subsequently, these legal and ethical guidelines for undertaking research have formed the bases of international and national **human research ethics committees** (HRECs). In Australia, the overriding committee is called the Australian Health Ethics

**Human research ethics committees:** Established to approve human research ethics applications.

Committee (AHEC), which is a sub-committee of the statutory body, the National Health and Medical Research Council. In New Zealand, the National Ethics Advisory Committee (NEAC) has a statutory function to advise the New Zealand Minister for Health on issues relating to ethical conduct of research, and the Health Research Council of New Zealand (HRC) reviews and assesses ethical applications for undertaking research.

## Roles of research councils and the conduct of health research

Both Australia and New Zealand have national ethics committees that formulate policies and oversee the implementation of ethical conduct in human research. These committees are statutory and exist by Act of Parliament. They also provide guidelines for the various levels of HRECs, which are found in many tertiary education, health and social organisations.

For the purpose of nursing research, the main committees nurse researchers will come into contact with are those based in universities or hospitals. All universities and major hospitals have an ethics committee. Many government departments, including those associated with social services, have their own ethics committees.

### The role of the human research ethics committee

Generally, a HREC is composed of a minimum of eight people with equal representation of men and women, with the majority of membership being from outside the institution. The external membership of the committee should represent the community, have an interest in health and medical research, but not undertake research. One member should represent health professions, for example a nurse or allied health person. Another member should represent and perform pastoral care in the community, for example a religious leader or an Indigenous leader. Other membership includes a lawyer and representatives of researchers who are currently undertaking research and submitting or reviewing research proposals (NHMRC 2007).

There are two major roles of a HREC at an organisational level: first, to protect the public, and second, to support and encourage research. In order to protect the public, all proposed research must be approved by an ethics committee. Research that involves humans and collects data by interviewing, reviewing health records or surveying will require approval from a HREC of the relevant institution. If patients are participants and the research is conducted by nurses, an ethical clearance application will need to be submitted to the hospital or health organisation where the nurses are working or the patients are being treated.

For a novice researcher, it is recommended to limit the research project to one organisation. For example, a qualitative research project may limit participants to being recruited from one educational institution or a location outside their place of employment. Therefore, only one ethics application will need to be submitted to the ethics committee of the researcher's employment organisation. If the study participants are patients, the ethics committee of the relevant health organisation needs to approve the study. The more organisations required to approve the project, the greater the number of ethics applications that will have to be submitted. Researchers need to be aware of the time required for the review process and take this into account in their project management.

In Australia, the National Ethics Application Form (NEAF) is completed online. HREC members often access the form electronically. For multicentre studies, a lead

HREC reviews the ethics application and approves the project at the initial site, and then the researcher seeks approval from each of the other sites by supplying evidence of the initial approval from the lead committee. Although this does reduce the number of applications to be processed, depending on the number of sites the timeframe for ethical approval from multiple HRECs could still be one year or more depending on the number of sites involved.

To submit an application to the ethics committee, some relevant protocols have to be followed. Large organisations will have these available in electronic form at their relevant websites. A small organisation will have an administrative unit to review and approve a research project conducted in the organisation. Examples of ethics authorities in Australia and New Zealand that have protocols for seeking research ethics approval and their links are listed under Useful websites. The main protocol or form required will have detailed information on the research project. The researcher needs to outline the nature of the research question and details of the research method (Richardson-Trench et al. 2011). It is important to describe how research participants' **confidentiality** will be protected, what **risks** and benefits are associated with participating in the research, and how participant consent will be obtained. Information in the participant information sheet must include the participants' right to ask questions relating to the study, the researcher's name and contact details, the right of the participant to withdraw from the research without any negative effect on care provided to them, and how data will be managed and used by the researcher (Atkins et al. 2011).

> **Confidentiality:** When the researcher promises to protect the identity of the participant by allocating either a code number or a pseudonym to the participant.

> **Risk:** The level of either emotional or physical discomfort a potential participant may experience when being involved in research.

## TIPS AND SKILLS

If you are receiving funding to support your research, this must be clearly stated in the research application. The HREC will want to know who is the funding body and the amount of funding (White 2012), in particular if this will impact on the study's findings. If you are carrying out research in other countries as well as your own, you will need to provide evidence that ethics approval has been sought and gained in those locations.

Aside from the actual ethics application there are two additional forms the researcher will need to submit to the ethics committee. The first is called a Plain Language Statement (PLS) but may also have other names. The PLS outlines, in simple language, exactly what the research is about. More importantly, it outlines what the person will be participating in, what is expected of the participant and how the researcher will protect the participant's privacy. Once the potential participant has read and understood what the study is about and their level of involvement, they may agree to participate. If the person agrees to participate, this is where the second form, the consent form, becomes important. The consent form is a standardised form that can be modified to reflect the nature of the research. Also, some institutions combine the information in the PLS and the consent form. This document may also go by various names such as the Participant Information and Consent Form (PICF).

Box 4.1 is an example of how a PLS can be set out. It also covers all the areas that need to be addressed in the process of informing a potential participant. At the bottom of the PLS, there is a statement regarding the participant's right to contact the ethics committee that approves the research project. Examples of a PLS and a consent form are shown in Appendix 4.1.

## Box 4.1

**INVITATION TO PARTICIPATE IN A RESEARCH PROJECT**
**(Fill in the project title)**
Who is conducting this research?
What is the research project about?
Why am I being asked to participate?
What do I need to do when participating in this project?
What are the possible risks and benefits for me?
Will there be a future benefit?
Will my participation be confidential?
Is my participation voluntary?
What are my rights and risks as a participant?
What will happen to the results?
Contact details of the researcher
Contact details of the ethics committee

# Ethical principles and research conduct

## Informed consent

Informed and voluntary consent to participate in research is the first principle of the Nuremberg Code (McClimens & Allmark 2011) and remains a cornerstone of research ethics. Consent to participate in research or indeed any nursing or medical intervention is based on the principle of autonomy (Berglund 2012). For a potential participant to be informed, there needs to be a set of requirements in place. First, all the information about the research, including risks and benefits, must be provided to the participant, the same as for carrying out a nursing procedure. Second, the participant needs to understand what the study involves. This is particularly important for people whose first language is not English. Third, the participant must have the capacity to consent to the research, which has implications for minors or people with cognitive impairment. Fourth, consent must be voluntary; this means that the participant freely consents to be part of the study and has the right to withdraw at any time (Leedy & Ormond 2010). Finally, the actual consent form must be signed by the participant and witnessed by the researcher.

As researchers, how do we ensure that our participants are informed and able to consent? Generally there are a number of steps to be followed. The researcher makes contact with each potential participant through the chosen methodological strategies. These can include making contact by telephone or emailing the person to give a brief overview of the research. If the person is interested, the researcher makes a time to meet them and mail or email the research information to them before the meeting. The PLS is either read out or given to the participant before gaining their consent.

Once the potential participant has been informed and is aware of all the risks and benefits of participating in the research (Berglund 2012), they will be asked to sign a consent form (see Appendix 4.1). Consent forms contain standardised information with some variation depending on each organisation's requirements. Specific information in the consent form has to be modified to fit with the research protocol, such as methods used to collect the data from participants and how the data will be used.

## TIPS AND SKILLS

Evidence-based nursing research has gained popularity within the disciplines of nursing and midwifery. There are many different types of evidence-based research including, but not limited to, systematic reviews of the literature, quantitative and qualitative research, and randomised controlled trials (Houghton et al. 2010).

With any type of research, whether it be conducted as part of an evidence-based research project or not, all are required to go through the same ethics approval protocols and address the same type of ethical issues as those mentioned in this chapter.

### Beneficence and non-maleficence

When undertaking research there needs to be a favourable risk:benefit ratio, which means that the benefit to the participant will outweigh the risk of being involved in the research. The researcher has the obligation to maximise the benefit of participation and minimise the risk. In ethical terms, this is called **beneficence** (Johnstone 2009). The word 'beneficence' comes from the Latin *beneficus* from *bene* meaning 'good' or 'well', and *facere*, to do, so beneficence means doing good, being generous, etc. During the research process the researcher needs to be aware that what they are asking the participant to do will be of benefit to them.

> **Beneficence:** A term referring to someone who is 'doing good'.

However, the benefit of research to the participant may not be immediately obvious and this needs to be made clear to the participant. For example, what the researcher is asking the participant to do is to contribute to the growing body of knowledge of nursing. In addition, by their participation they will be contributing to the improvement of nursing care and health outcomes of future clients who have a health condition similar to theirs. Their participation is thus of benefit to the discipline of nursing and to society in general.

It is important that the researcher also ensures that they do no harm. In ethics, this is termed **non-maleficence**. 'Maleficence' comes from the Latin *maleficus* and means doing harm or evil. The researcher needs to ensure that the person participating in the research will not be harmed or will be able to weigh up the benefits and risks associated with the research. Non-maleficence therefore means doing no harm.

> **Non-maleficence:** A term referring to someone who is 'doing no harm'.

Beneficence and non-maleficence are not the same, although they are often confused or used interchangeably. The confusion is mostly due to individual interpretation (Berglund 2012). Simply put, beneficence is the act of doing a good or beneficial act, whereas non-maleficence means that as nurses we consciously do not act to harm a person. The complexity of this can be very easily demonstrated below.

As nurses, we all have to give someone a potentially painful injection or carry out a painful procedure. We know that our nursing action may cause pain (maleficence) and we also know that the action will be beneficial (beneficence). But as nurses we also know that our patients need to be informed about the procedure we are about to undertake and also need to consent to it as well as be aware of the risks and benefits. This is the same with research.

## •.THINKING DEEPLY

### Beneficence and maleficence

There are times in research where the participant may experience harm or discomfort. This may include physical harm such as having an injection or giving blood, or psychological harm such as reliving an unpleasant experience. This appears to be contrary to the ethical principle of non-maleficence or do no harm.

As the nurse researcher, how can you gauge the risk or harm of your research on the participant and put in place mechanisms to minimise this?

You will need to explain the level of risk as well as how you will minimise this in your ethics application. Once a research strategy involves invasive procedures such as taking blood or taking a biopsy then the level of risk is deemed to be high. Section 2.1.8 of the Australian National Statement on Ethical Conduct in Human Research (NHMRC 2007) states that 'the greater the risks to participants in any research for which ethical approval is given, the more certain it must be both that the risks will be managed as well as possible, and that the participants clearly understand the risks they are assuming' (p. 18).

### Rights

**Human rights:** In research this applies to the participant being fully informed about the research as well as being able to withdraw from participating at any stage.

The rights of the participant are based on the broader notion of **human rights**, which include the right to respect for human dignity. There are two aspects to this (Johnstone 2009). First, the participant has the right to full disclosure. This means that the researcher must disclose all aspects of the research including what is to be involved in it: the risk and benefits; protection of the participant's identity; persons who will access the data; time commitment to the research; the right to withdraw at any time without prejudice; and who to contact if they have any further questions. One other aspect to be included is the methods used to handle and store the data. The participant will also need to know if the researcher is going to publish the findings or present them at a conference. All this information should be verbally explained and contained in the PLS.

Second, human dignity includes the right to be free from coercion. The participant must feel free to withdraw without penalty. Likewise there must not be any excessive reward for participating. Along with this, the researcher and the participant should not be in a dependent relationship because this could be misconstrued as coercion. Dependent relationships can also be seen as power relationships (NHMRC 2007). Examples are nurse researchers researching their patients or nurse academics researching their students. Both forms of research are legitimate, but researchers will have to take extra care in explaining how they will address the issues of dependency and power relationships.

### Privacy and confidentiality

Participants also have the right to privacy. They have the choice of what information to share and what not to share. As well as this, they need to know that what is shared will be treated with respect and kept in confidence.

There are two common ways to maintain participant confidentiality. One is to assign a number to each participant's data—participant 1, 2, 3 and so on. Another is to give each participant a pseudonym. The name of each person will be replaced with another name so that they will not be recognised in any research report. The issue of confidentiality is less likely to occur in quantitative research when the number of participants is large and the data are presented in an aggregated form.

In addition, the researcher needs to assure the participant of **anonymity**. Anonymity is generally assured when a survey technique is used to gather data. Survey techniques are commonly used with quantitative research. If the survey has no identifying marker and the researcher does not know who returned the survey then the participant is truly anonymous to the researcher.

**Anonymity:** Lack of personal identifiable information; the state of having no name.

A major interesting methodological and ethical issue is found when a focus group interview, collaborative research or a group observation is used to collect qualitative data (see also Chapter 7). Generally, participants in these types of research are people considered to be key stakeholders, meaning people who have recognised expertise in a specific area of nursing. Alternatively, they may be a group of people who experience a common illness or circumstance. This creates an interesting ethical issue because not only does the researcher hear and collect information from the participants but so do the other members of the group, who may or may not know each other.

In order to ensure confidentiality and anonymity here, the researcher will have to outline in the PLS the 'ground rules' for participating as well as reiterate the rules at the beginning of and possibly throughout the research. These rules are about human dignity, maintaining privacy of the information shared by participants, and not discussing the membership of the group outside that forum; they include respect for the comments of others in the group, and allow each member to have equal time when discussing the matter under research. Ho (2012) argues for reciprocity and attention to power relations based on feminist principles as one method of assuring autonomy during the research process.

## TIPS AND SKILLS

When you are undertaking a literature review on nursing research topics for your assignments, pay particular attention to the ethical aspects outlined in the research article. Note how the researchers gained ethics approval and what ethical issues were addressed. In particular, pay attention to how privacy and confidentiality were addressed.

One mistake that researchers often make is to assure both anonymity and confidentiality when submitting ethics protocols for approval. Anonymity and confidentiality are different. If your research method involves participants filling out a survey and posting it back or delivering it to an assigned spot, and if the survey has no identification markers, then the participant will be anonymous. This means that the researcher has no way of identifying the participant.

On the other hand, if your research method is face-to-face interviews, the researcher knows who the participant is. In this situation anonymity cannot be guaranteed. What the researcher has to assure the participant in the PLS is how the participant's confidentiality will be ensured.

## Implications for evidence-based practice

Wong and Chan (2007) conducted a qualitative study in Hong Kong and explored the experiences of Chinese family members of terminally ill patients. The patients were in a palliative care unit. Twenty family members were interviewed and the results showed that they had anticipatory grief with reactions including anger, unease, sadness and helplessness. This was quite acute when the patients were first admitted to the palliative care unit.

Nurses can apply the above evidence in their practice. Despite the complexity of the study and a range of ethical issues, these can be addressed.

## Data management throughout the research study and beyond

Another aspect of rights is that participants need to know how the information collected will be managed. There are two aspects to management of data. The first is how the researcher, particularly in qualitative research, will faithfully interpret the participant's views, and the second is the physical management of the data (Kerridge et al. 2009).

Participants need to be assured that their views will not be misrepresented or misquoted. These are both methodological and ethical issues. When the researcher embarks on a research project, the methodology chosen is the one most suitable to address the research question. This methodology will have clear steps guiding how data will be analysed and interpreted.

The physical management of data refers to the approach used to secure the data during the research process as well as into the future. Ethics committees generally stipulate the period that data needs to be stored and the method used to destroy the data. If the data are interview transcripts, observation notes, diary or survey questionnaires, these must be kept for five years after the research is concluded. If the research involves higher levels of risk, for example blood samples, then generally the data or sample blood needs to be kept for 15 years (NHMRC 2007).

As well as the length of time kept, it is essential to maintain the security of the data. For non-computer-based data such as transcripts, surveys, tape-recordings or photos, these data need to be kept in a locked cupboard. Signed consent forms or any other information that could identify the participant need to be kept separately from the actual data in another locked cupboard. This information needs to be conveyed to the participants, as well as a statement of exactly who will access the data and how long the data will be kept. Organisations such as universities will have policies on these issues. For example, the Central Queensland University requires data to be kept for five years. Generally, people who access the data are the research team, which may include the research assistant or the student's supervisors.

Almost all researchers use computers now and data are often stored electronically on a computer. The management of data on a computer will be stipulated by the institution in which the research will be conducted. Generally, they will be stored on a computer and need to be protected. Some ways to protect your computer-based data are by firewalls, cryptography, digital signatures and passwords (Atkins et al. 2011).

Technology is growing rapidly and there are many online survey tools available for use. As well, more and more hospitals and other institutions are using computer technology to store patient data. Each institution will have protocols in place for each type of data collection and storage of the collected data.

## Implications for evidence-based practice

Nurse and midwife researchers need to be aware of the ethical implications associated particularly with randomised controlled trials or RCTs as by the very nature of the trial one group of patients will be receiving the intervention, be it nursing, surgical or pharmacological, and the other group will be forgoing the intervention. However, NHMRC guidelines state that the control group must be treated with the appropriate standard of care and interventions.

If research has been carried out and there is clear evidence that the intervention or treatment has a positive or improved outcome, it may possibly be implemented. However, as Koschel and associates (2012) discovered, researching and implementing evidence-based practice may prove difficult unless there is managerial and infrastructure support.

## Vulnerable groups and power relationships between researcher and participant

It can be argued that any person who is in hospital is vulnerable. Being sufficiently unwell to require hospitalisation, or having test results that may influence a life-changing condition, contributes to a person's vulnerability to outside factors. As nurses, we are aware of this vulnerability and also of power relationships at play between the nurse, other healthcare professionals and the patient. Professional codes of conduct as well as codes of ethics guide the behaviour of professionals, including the potential for the imbalance of power relationships and how to ameliorate it.

Are these codes of conduct the same for research? As stated earlier, in the ethics application submitted to an institution the potential power relationships need to be explicitly identified. Each identified ethical issue needs to be addressed and strategies for managing it clearly explained.

What about conducting research with groups who are considered vulnerable because of their health status or life situation? Examples of recognised **vulnerable people** include people residing in aged care facilities with mental health problems, people with dementia, the terminally ill, people who are intellectually challenged, migrants without English (Nyamathi et al. 2007), victims of violence, war or terrorism. Displaced persons are particularly vulnerable and all researchers need to be aware of the unintentional risk for this group when asking them to participate in a research project. Efforts need to be made to minimise power relationships and any element of risk to the participants.

It should be noted that there are specific guidelines in both Australia and New Zealand (see below) about ethical conduct when undertaking research with Indigenous people. However, no specific guidelines are available for research with people who

**Vulnerable people:**
Individuals who are marginalised and discriminated against in society because of their social situation—class, ethnicity, gender, age, illness, disability or sexual preference.

have mental health issues or dementia. These vulnerable populations may be left out of research for fear that ethics approval will be difficult to obtain (Keogh & Daly 2009; Gibson et al. 2013).

Since approval to conduct research with vulnerable groups is difficult to gain, it is up to the researcher to provide very clear guidelines on how participant consent will be obtained and how the research will be ethically conducted. Heggestad and associates (2013) acknowledge that gaining consent from people living in aged care facilities may be difficult. They recognise that many older people, particularly those with dementia, may not be able to consent in the traditional format but may be able to give 'assent' or verbal consent. Keogh and Daly (2009) argue that the problem with researching mental health service users stems from ethics committees' differing interpretations of 'capacity to consent' given the mental health condition and its severity. Gibson and associates (2013) have highlighted the dilemma of gaining ethics approval when conducting research with people who have experienced suicidal ideation. The boundary between research and therapy may blur. They argue that this is not a reason to exclude this vulnerable group from research but rather to question what is meant by 'level of risk' and how to address it.

The main point here is that working with people with diminished capacity to consent should not exclude them from participating in research. As an adjunct to this, nurse researchers need to devise strategies that can include vulnerable people in research as well as ameliorate perceived power relationships.

Keogh and Daly (2009) have devised strategies for facilitating informed consent with vulnerable populations. As well as allowing the potential participant time to read or hear the information about the research, they suggest encouraging them to ask questions and stressing the voluntary nature of the research; they add that it is helpful to use 'a professional researcher/gatekeeper to make judgements in relation to each individual's capacity to consent…[as well as]…including ongoing assessment of participant understanding, continuous information giving, repeatedly seeking permission and evaluating participant willingness to continue involvement' (p. 280).

## THINKING DEEPLY

### Working with vulnerable people

If your research involves people who are considered vulnerable and who may have a limited capacity to consent, how are you the researcher going to address this in your ethics application? The ethics committee will want this information very clearly spelt out.

Both Australia and New Zealand have specific guidelines for working with Indigenous peoples (see Useful websites) and this information should guide your application. Of key importance is how you are going to acknowledge and ameliorate power relations.

## Indigenous peoples as participants in nursing and midwifery research

As stated earlier, one of the researcher's roles is to minimise power relationships in their research project. What is of particular importance is the relationship between the researcher and the vulnerable group. Nurse researchers must be especially aware of protecting the human rights of these groups.

Australia and New Zealand are multicultural societies with Indigenous populations. The need to respect the values, cultures and spiritual beliefs of clients is an integral part of nursing care (Fry & Johnstone 2008; Staunton & Chiarella 2008). Similar principles are applied in conducting research among Indigenous people. However, special considerations relating to historical context and the nature of culture and clan need to be taken into account. The Australian guidelines for conducting research with Aboriginal and Torres Strait Islander communities (NHMRC 2006) and the New Zealand guidelines for ethical conduct in research with Maori communities (Health Research Council of New Zealand, New Zealand Government 2008) have to be clearly adopted in all research protocols involving Indigenous people.

The explicit nature of the guidelines for working with both Aboriginal and Torres Strait Islanders and Maori has emanated from the knowledge that colonisation of both countries by the British had a major impact on their health and welfare. In Australia, the British considered that the country was empty—'no one's land' or terra nullius. This set the tone for less than adequate treatment of Indigenous peoples and their dispossession from the land (Australian Institute of Aboriginal and Torres Strait Islander Studies 2008). In New Zealand, the British acknowledged that the land was occupied and supported this in a document called the Treaty of Waitangi (McHugh 1991).

Regardless of the differing approaches by the British at the time of settlement, it is acknowledged that Indigenous populations in both countries have lower life expectancy, increased health risks, less access to resources (Eckermann et al. 2006; Johnstone 2009) and less control over personal life decisions than non-Indigenous populations. The poor health, social outcomes and historical context need to be acknowledged in research protocols that include Indigenous populations as participants.

In Australia, these guidelines have been extended by adding specific statements on research values. These values include acknowledging spirit and integrity, reciprocity, respect, equality, survival and protection, and lastly responsibility (NHMRC 2006). Not only do these value statements have to be present in the research application but also there has to be clear evidence of how each value will be addressed in the research process.

In New Zealand, specific guidelines are in place for research with Maori for the same reasons. The Health Research Council of New Zealand also bases their research strategy with Maori on the Treaty of Waitangi, specifically Articles Two and Three, which outline Maori control over resources as well as a fair share of benefits from society (Health Research Council of New Zealand, New Zealand Government 2004). The implications of this for research are that there needs to be an acknowledgment of the traditional power imbalances between Indigenous and non-Indigenous peoples and that researchers and Indigenous peoples need to share in the processes and the outcomes of the research.

# SUMMARY

- Ethics committees were established to inform participants and to minimise harm. Prior to data collection, researchers need to seek ethical approval from their relevant committee.
- There are several ethical principles that need to be considered throughout the research process: informed consent, beneficence and non-maleficence, rights and power relationships between the researcher and the participants. Careful planning is required when research is conducted among disadvantaged groups such as children, elderly people and minority groups.
- Ethical issues can arise throughout the research process, from choosing a topic to data storage and publication or presentation of findings.

---

### PRACTICE EXERCISE 4.1

Discuss the principles of informed consent and how they apply to nursing as well as nursing research.

ANSWER: The principle of informed consent applies equally to nursing and to nursing research and is based on the individual's autonomous ability to make an informed choice. There are five components to informed consent:

- disclosure of all relevant information
- comprehension or understanding of this information
- competency to decide or make a choice
- freedom from coercion or voluntary participation
- the actual signed consent form.

---

### PRACTICE EXERCISE 4.2

Explain the difference between confidentiality and anonymity.

ANSWER: When undertaking interviews or running focus groups the researcher actually sees the participants. Because of this the participant cannot be anonymous. Therefore the researcher has to promise confidentiality. This means that the participant's name will be changed and replaced with a coded number or a pseudonym to protect confidentiality. Alternatively, if the research involves quantitative surveys that are not coded in any way so that the researcher cannot identify the participant, then this is considered to be anonymity.

---

### PRACTICE EXERCISE 4.3

Discuss the reasons behind the need for a Plain Language Statement.

ANSWER: Often a formal ethics application contains technical or medical terms that may not be understood by the average person in the street. A Plain Language Statement is designed to make the research understandable to the average person. It should contain no jargon and should address all components of the proposed research.

PRACTICE EXERCISE 4.4

Critically discuss the need for different research protocols for working with Indigenous populations.

ANSWER: Both Australia and New Zealand have Indigenous populations who have experienced colonisation and cultural displacement. Within these groups there is a lower than average life expectancy and a higher than average incidence of illness. This is acknowledged by both countries' governments. Because of this history of colonisation both Australia and New Zealand acknowledge that the Indigenous populations require different approaches to health research. Because of this the national ethics bodies of both countries have developed specific guidelines in collaboration with Indigenous peoples that highlight respect for culture and tradition as well as collaboration in the research process.

PRACTICE EXERCISE 4.5

Explain the need for secure storage of data and why it is kept for a specific period of time.

ANSWER: Data from research are to be kept securely for specific periods depending on the nature of the research. If the research involved interviews or surveys then the data are to be kept securely for five years. If the research was invasive, for example taking blood or tissue, then the data is to be stored for 15 years. Data need to be kept for these lengths of time, and securely, to prevent theft in order to maintain confidentiality. As well as this, data is to be kept for the specified periods in case there are any challenges to the research process or methodology. Occasionally a researcher may be audited to ensure strict adherence to ethical standards.

## APPENDIX 4.1
## EXAMPLE OF PLAIN LANGUAGE STATEMENT AND CONSENT FORM IN ENGLISH

**SYDNEY SOUTH WEST**
AREA HEALTH SERVICE
**NSW⊕HEALTH**

University of
Western Sydney

Dr Sansnee Jirojwong
College of Health and Science
School of Nursing, Hawkesbury Campus
Locked Bag 1797
Penrith South DC NSW 1797
Email s.jirojwong@uws.edu.au
Phone (02) 45701918, 0427733004, Fax (02) 45701420

### INFORMATION SHEET FOR WOMEN WITH GESTATIONAL DIABETES

**Health literacy and self-management of gestational diabetes: A study among Vietnamese, Cambodian, Thai and Laotian women in Sydney**

#### Invitation

You are invited to take part in this research which is being conducted by Drs Sansnee Jirojwong and Jane Cioffi, Associate Professors Virginia Schmied and Hannah Dahlen, and Professors Maree Johnson and Rhonda Griffiths from the University of Western Sydney. You are being invited as a participant because you have high blood sugar or diabetes in pregnancy.

#### What is the purpose of this research?

The purpose of this study is to explore how the first- or second-generation Australian-Vietnamese, Cambodian, Thai and Laotian women in Sydney use information from health professionals to self-manage their blood sugar from the time they know that they have the condition until about three months after birth of their baby. We would also like to know other sources of information about this condition that you seek and use to self-manage your health.

It is hoped the information gained in this study will improve maternity and health services for women who have high blood sugar in pregnancy.

#### Who can participate in the research?

Women who can participate in this study are those who have high blood sugar in their pregnancy and were born in Vietnam, Cambodia, Thailand or Laos or whose parents were born in one of these countries. We will be asking about how women understand about gestational diabetes or high blood sugar in pregnancy and its impact on their health and their infant's health. We will also ask how women seek, locate and understand health information about this high blood sugar from different sources and use or do not use it to manage their health.

Your decision to participate is completely voluntary. If you decide to participate you can withdraw at any time without having to give a reason. If you decide not to participate, or you wish to withdraw from the project at any time, your decision will not disadvantage you. If you choose to withdraw, we will remove any information about you from our record. Your decision whether or not to participate will not prejudice your present or future care or your relationship with Sydney South West Area Health Service as it will not be known to any healthcare provider.

## What would you be asked to do?

If you agree, you will be asked to participate in an individual face-to-face interview. An interview will be conducted using your own language by a bilingual research team member. The aim of this interview is to explore how you manage your high blood sugar using information from various sources and what you understand about high blood sugar in pregnancy and its impact on your health and your baby's health. Key broad questions will be used to facilitate this interview. The following are examples of the questions that will be asked:

- When you were told that you have high blood sugar, what was your feeling?
- How do you feel now?
- In your opinion, what is the effect of having high blood sugar on your own health and the health of your baby?
- What do you think are long-term effects of having high blood sugar on your own health and your baby's health?
- Where and how did you find information that can be used to manage your blood sugar?

The interview will not last more than one hour. You can nominate the place and time convenient for this interview. With your permission, the interview will be audio-recorded.

## What are the risks and benefits of participating?

This study involves discussing having high blood sugar in your pregnancy and the sources of information you use or do not use to manage your health. It is possible that the discussion during this interview may relate incidents or stories that may cause you distress or discomfort. You may feel distressed talking about an incident. We feel that there is only a small chance that this may occur. If it does, we will encourage you to seek support from an available counselling or support service such as your church, temple or healthcare workers. We also will provide the contact numbers and details of support workers for additional support if you need this. If you are uncomfortable during the discussion, remember that participation in this study is completely voluntary and you can withdraw at any time without any consequences. You can also ask for the tape-recording to be stopped at any time or you can review the tape and ask for your words to be changed.

Women may benefit from this study by having the opportunity to talk about issues that are important to their health and their baby's health. We hope that the knowledge generated by this study will be used to improve the quality of maternity and health services for these women.

## How will your privacy be protected?

We would ask you not to identify yourself during the recording of the interview. This is to protect your privacy. No identifying information will be kept about you. The audio recordings and hand-written and transcribed notes will be de-identified, thus removing all reference to individuals and institutions. If necessary, we will use fictitious names to ensure your privacy. The audio recordings and notes will be securely stored at the University of Western Sydney and destroyed seven years after publication. Individual participants and institutions will not be identifiable in any publications arising from this project.

## How will the information collected be used?

The information will be used in a report that will be submitted to the University of Western Sydney who have funded the study. A report will be provided to all participating organisations, hospitals and area health services. We also plan to write papers for publication in professional journals outlining the research and the findings and to present the results at professional conferences. Confidentiality of individual participants and organisations will be assured.

### What do you need to do to participate?

Please read this Information Statement and be sure you understand its contents before you consent to participate. After you have read this information, and you have questions you wish to ask, or any issues you wish to discuss, please feel free to contact Dr Sansnee Jirojwong (Principal Researcher), on telephone 45701918, 0427733004.

**You are making a decision whether or not to participate. Your signature on the consent form indicates that, having read the information provided above, you have decided to participate.**

**Thank you for considering this invitation**

Signature ...............................................

Dr Sansnee Jirojwong

University of Western Sydney

Date ....... /....... /.......

### Complaints about this research

This research has been approved by the Sydney South West Area Health Service Human Research Ethics Committee (Western Zone), Reference ................. Should you have a concern about your rights as a participant, or you have a complaint about the manner in which the research is conducted, this may be given to the researcher, or, if an independent person is preferred, to the Ethics Secretariat (Western Zone), SSWAHS Area Health Service, Locked Bag 7017, LIVERPOOL, BC, NSW 1871, telephone (02) 96120614, fax (02) 96120611, email jennie.grech@sswahs.nsw.gov.au.

You will be given a copy of this form to keep.

Dr Sansnee Jirojwong

College of Health and Science

School of Nursing, Hawkesbury Campus

Locked Bag 1797

Penrith South DC NSW 1797

Email s.jirojwong@uws.edu.au

Phone (02) 45701918, 0427733004, Fax (02) 45701420

## SYDNEY SOUTH WEST
### AREA HEALTH SERVICE
## NSW⊕HEALTH

University of
Western Sydney

### CONSENT FORM

**Health literacy and self-management of gestational diabetes: a study among Vietnamese, Cambodian, Thai and Laotian women in Sydney**

1  I ............................................... of ...................................................................................., aged .............. years, agreed to participate as a subject in the study described in the subject information statement attached to this form.

2  I acknowledge that I have read the Subject Information Statement, which explains why I have been selected, the aims of the study and the nature and the possible risks of the investigation, and the statement has been explained to me to my satisfaction.

3  Before signing this Consent Form, I have been given the opportunity to ask any questions relating to any possible physical and mental harm I might suffer as a result of my participation. I have received satisfactory answers to any questions that I have asked.

4  I consent to participate in an individual face-to-face interview which will be audio-taped.
5  My decision whether or not to participate will not prejudice my present or future treatment or my relationship with Sydney South West Area Health Service or any other institution cooperating in this study or any person treating me. If I decide to participate, I am free to withdraw my consent and to discontinue my participation at any time without prejudice.
6  I agree that research data gathered from the results of the study may be published, provided that I cannot be identified.
7  I understand that if I have any questions relating to my participation in this research, I may contact the study researcher, Dr Sansnee Jirojwong, on telephone 02-45701918, 0427733004, who will be happy to answer them.
8  I acknowledge receipt of a copy of this Consent Form and the Subject Information Statement.

Complaints may be directed to the Ethics Secretariat (Western Zone), Sydney South West Area Health Service, Locked Bag 7017, LIVERPOOL BC, NSW, 1871 (phone 9612 0614, fax 9612 0611, email jennie.grech@sswahs.nsw.gov.au).

Signature of subject                              Signature of witness

......................................              ......................................

Please PRINT name                             Please PRINT name

......................................              ......................................

Date ...... / ...... / ......                       Date ...... / ...... / ......

Signature(s) of investigator(s)                Please PRINT Name

......................................              ......................................

Date ...... / ...... / ......

✂-------------------------------------------------------------------------------------

**Where relevant to the research project, please check the box below.**

I wish to have a plain English statement of results
posted to me at the address I provided below:        ☐ YES    ☐ NO

**Mailing Address**

Name (Please print) ...............................................................................................

Address ................................................................................................................

.................................................................................. Postcode ...........................

## FURTHER READING

Atkins, K., Britton, B. & de Lacy, S. (2011). *Ethics and Law for Australian Nurses*. Cambridge: Cambridge University Press.

Berglund, C. (2012). *Ethics for Healthcare*, 4th edn. Melbourne: Oxford University Press.

Courtney, M. & McCutchen, H. (2010). *Using Evidence to Guide Nursing Practice*, 2nd edn. Australia: Churchill Livingstone Elsevier.

Leedy, P. & Ormond, J. (2010). *Practical Research Planning and Design*, 9th edn. Boston: Pearson Education International.

Richardson-Trench, M., Taylor, B., Kermode, S. & Roberts, K. (2011). *Research in Nursing*, 4th edn. Australia: Cengage Learning.

## USEFUL WEBSITES

The Monash Centre for the study of Ethics in Medicine and Society:

<www.cems.monash.org>

The Monash Centre for the study of Ethics in Medicine and Society is concerned with both education and research. Its focus is on ethics and cultural values.

Australia, Australian Health Ethics Committee:

<www.nhmrc.gov.au/about/committees-nhmrc/australian-health-ethics-committee-ahec>

Code of Ethics for Nurses in Australia and Code of Ethics for Midwives in Australia:

<www.nursingmidwiferyboard.gov.au/Codes-Guidelines-Statements/Codes-Guidelines.aspx>

The code of ethics for nurses and for midwifes has been developed as a guide for ethical comportment in both nursing and midwifery: Code of Professional Conduct for Nurses in Australia and Code of Professional Conduct for Midwives in Australia. There is a Code of Conduct for Nurses and a separate Code for Midwives practising in Australia that can be obtained from the above site.

National Statement on Ethical Conduct in Research Involving Humans:

<www.nhmrc.gov.au/_files_nhmrc/publications/attachments/e35.pdf>

The National Statement is a guide for all current and future researchers and specifies the ethical issues that need addressing when undertaking research.

Values and Ethics: Guidelines for Ethical Conduct in Aboriginal and Torres Strait Islander Health Research:

<www.nhmrc.gov.au/_files_nhmrc/publications/attachments/e52.pdf>

These guidelines, to be read in conjunction with the National Guidelines, are specific to outreaching with Aboriginal and Torres Strait Islanders.

Congress of Aboriginal and Torres Strait Islander Nurses (CATSIN):

<www.catsin.org.au>

CATSIN is specifically set up to address particular issues relating to Aboriginal and Torres Strait Islander nurses.

Nursing Council of New Zealand:

<www.nursingcouncil.org.nz>

This is the peak body representing nurses and midwives in New Zealand.

Code of Conduct for Nurses:

<http://nursingcouncil.org.nz/News/A-new-Code-of-Conduct-for-nurses> (follow link to PDF file)

Reviewed by the Nursing Council of New Zealand in 2012, this document is designed to protect the health and safety of the public by setting standards of clinical competence, ethical conduct and cultural competence for nurses.

The above link will lead you to a number of guidelines for New Zealand Nurses including *Guidelines: Professional boundaries to be read in conjunction with the Code of Conduct* and *Guidelines for Cultural Safety, the Treaty of Waitangi and Maori Health in Nursing Education and Practice*. These guidelines were established by the New Zealand Nursing Council and are specifically designed to raise cultural awareness of the health of Maori.

New Zealand National Ethics Advisory Committee:

<www.neac.health.govt.nz>

The National Ethics Advisory Committee (NEAC) provides advice to the Minister of Health on ethical issues relating to health and disability. It also determines nationally consistent standards for conducting research.

Health Research Council of New Zealand:

<www.hrc.govt.nz>

The Health Research Council of New Zealand is responsible for managing the New Zealand government's investment in health research.

## REFERENCES

Annas, G. & Grodin, M. A. (eds) (1992). *Nazi Doctors and the Nuremberg Code: Human Rights and Human Experimentation.* New York: Oxford University Press.

Atkins, K., Britton, B. & de Lacy, S. (2011). *Ethics and Law for Australian Nurses.* Cambridge: Cambridge University Press.

Australian Institute of Aboriginal and Torres Strait Islander Studies. (2008). *The Little Red, Yellow, Black Book*, 2nd edn. Canberra: Aboriginal Press.

Berglund, C. (2012). *Ethics for Healthcare*, 4th edn. Melbourne: Oxford University Press.

Caplan, A. (1992). How did medicine go so wrong? In A. Caplan (ed.), *When Medicine went Mad.* Totowa, NJ: Humana Press, pp. 53–92.

Eckermann, A.-K., Dowd, T., Chong, E., Nixon, L., Gray, R. & Johnson, S. (2006). *Binan Goonj: Bridging Cultures in Aboriginal Health*, 2nd edn. Sydney: Churchill Livingstone.

Fry, S. & Johnstone, M. J. (2008). *Ethics in Nursing Practice*, 3rd edn. Malden, MA: Blackwell Publishing.

Gibson, S., Benson, O. & Brand, S. (2013). Talking about suicide: Confidentiality and anonymity in qualitative research. *Nursing Ethics* 20(1), 18–29.

Grodin, M. A. (1992). Historical origins of the Nuremberg Code. In G. Annas & M. A. Grodin (eds), *Nazi Doctors and the Nuremberg Code: Human Rights and Human Experimentation.* New York: Oxford University Press, pp. 121–44.

Health Research Council of New Zealand, New Zealand Government. (2004). Health Research Strategy to Improve Maori Health and Wellbeing. Auckland: Health Research Council of New Zealand.

Health Research Council of New Zealand, New Zealand Government. (2008). Guidelines for researchers on health research involving Maori. <www.hrc.govt.nz/sites/default/files/Guidelines%20for%20HR%20on%20Maori-%20Jul10%20revised%20for%20Te%20Ara%20Tika%20v2%20FINAL[1].pdf>

Heggestad, K., Nortveldt, P. & Slettebo, A. (2013). The importance of moral sensitivity when including persons with dementia in qualitative research. *Nursing Ethics* 20(1), 30–40.

Ho, A. (2012). CBCAR and a relational approach to research ethics. In C. Pavlish & M. Pharris (eds), *Community-based Collaborative Action Research.* Burlington, MA: Jones & Bartlett Learning, pp. 333–56.

Houghton, C. E., Casey, D., Shaw, D. & Murphy, K. (2010). Ethical challenges in qualitative research: Examples from practice. *Nurse Researcher* 1, 15–25.

Johnstone, M. (2009). *Bioethics: A Nursing Perspective*, 5th edn. Sydney: Churchill Livingstone.

Keogh, B. & Daly, L. (2009). The ethics of conducting research with mental health service users. *British Journal of Nursing* 18(5), 277–81.

Kerridge, I., Lowe, M. & Stewart, C. (2009). *Ethics and Law for the Health Professions*, 3rd edn. Sydney: Federation Press.

Koschel, A., Cross, M., Haines, H., Ervin, K., Skinner-Louis, D. & Carbone, D. (2012). Research and evidence based practice in a rural Victorian cohort. *Australian Journal of Advanced Nursing* 30(2), 13–19.

Leedy, P. & Ormond, J. (2010). *Practical Research Planning and Design*, 9th edn. Boston: Pearson Education International.

McClimens, A. & Allmark, P. (2011). A problem of inclusion in learning disability research. *Nursing Ethics* 18(5), 633–9.

McHugh, P. (1991). *The Maori Magna Carta: New Zealand Law and the Treaty of Waitangi*. Auckland: Oxford University Press.

NHMRC (National Health and Medical Research Council). (2006). *Exploring What Research Means: Resource Package for Aboriginal and Torres Strait Islander Communities and Organisations*. Canberra: Australian Government.

NHMRC. (2007). *National Statement on Ethical Conduct in Human Research*. Canberra: Australian Government.

Nyamathi, A., Koniak-Griffin, D. & Greengold, B. (2007). Development of a nursing theory and science in vulnerable populations research. In J. Fitzpatrick (ed.), *Annual Review of Nursing Research: Vulnerable Populations*, vol. 25, pp. 3–26.

Perely, S., Fluss, S., Bankowski, Z. & Simon, F. (1992). The Nuremberg Code: An international overview. In G. Annas & M. A. Grodin (eds), *Nazi Doctors and the Nuremberg Code: Human Rights and Human Experimentation*. New York: Oxford University Press, pp. 121–44.

Richardson-Trench, M., Taylor, B., Kermode, S. & Roberts, K. (2011). *Research in Nursing*, 4th edn. Australia: Cengage Learning.

Skegg, D. C. G. (1986). Cervical screening. *New Zealand Medical Journal* 99, 26–7.

Staunton, P. & Chiarella, M. (2008). *Nursing and the Law*, 6th edn. Sydney: Churchill Livingstone.

Taylor, D. (1992). Opening statement of the prosecution December 9, 1945. In G. Annas & M. A. Grodin (eds), *Nazi Doctors and the Nuremberg Code: Human Rights and Human Experimentation*. New York: Oxford University Press, pp. 121–44.

White, E. (2012). Challenges that may arise when conducting real-life nursing research. *Nurse Researcher* 19(4), 15–20.

Wong, M. S. & Chan, S. W. (2007). The experiences of Chinese family members of terminally ill patients: A qualitative study. *Journal of Clinical Nursing* 16(12), 2357–64.

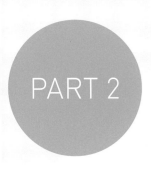

# PART 2
# QUALITATIVE RESEARCH METHODS

Ann and Bob have had discussions with an experienced researcher at the School of Nursing and Midwifery of the local university. The constructive feedback they have received on their proposal has helped them maintain focus and direction for their intended project. They continue to maintain contact with their mentor for ongoing guidance and support.

It is now crunch time—the development of a research question/s is now required. After a review of literature relating to chest pain has been completed, and patient characteristics have been taken into account, Ann and Bob conclude that the decision by patients to re-present at the emergency department is based on their personal and socio-cultural beliefs. Serious discussions have occurred between Ann and Bob. Their philosophy of caring and healthcare has influenced their decision to explore the question of the use of emergency departments.

In order to explore the beliefs of this group of patients as to why they continue to re-present to the ED, Ann considers looking to a qualitative research design as a suitable research method. In this part of the book, Chapters 5 to 8 focus on various aspects to be considered when conducting qualitative research. In particular, Chapter 5 describes sampling used in qualitative research while Chapter 6 discusses a range of research designs used to carry out different forms of qualitative research. In deciding on which specific research design will be most appropriate, Ann will be required to review each design in relation to their research question. Frequently used research designs, rather than advanced or developing research designs, are Ann and Bob's primary concern. Choosing an appropriate research design is one aspect of the research process; knowing how to go about the correct process of data collection is another important consideration for Ann. Chapter 7 introduces you to several data collection methods from which the researcher needs to choose in order to collect the correct type of data to answer the research question. Chapter 8 provides extensive information about qualitative data analysis while a short section on the use of a computer program is also given.

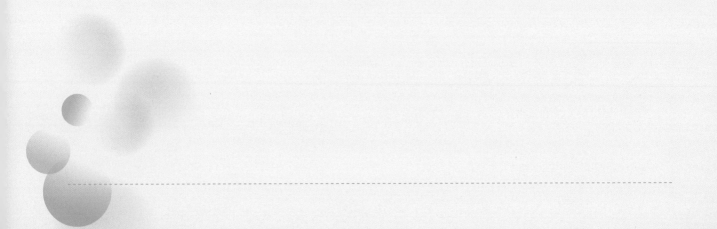

CHAPTER 5

# SAMPLING IN QUALITATIVE RESEARCH

Anthony Welch

## CHAPTER LEARNING OBJECTIVES

By the end of this chapter you will be able to:

- describe different types of sampling methods used in qualitative research
- identify reasons for choosing different sampling methods in qualitative research
- outline characteristics of specific sampling methods and how they would be applied to qualitative designs.

## KEY TERMS

case study sampling
convenience
   sampling
intensity sampling
networking
opportunistic
   sampling
purposive sampling
snowballing or
   chain sampling
theoretical sampling

## Introduction

Making the correct choice about what types of data will be required to answer the research question and the sampling methods by which such data are obtained is critical to all research. This chapter introduces you to various methods of sampling in qualitative research and different combinations of sampling methods used in qualitative studies. Examples of the different sampling methods are provided. When possible, underlying reasons for choosing such methods to answer research questions are demonstrated. This chapter is devoted to humans as research participants, not to other sources such as historical documents, objects or works of art.

## What is sampling?

Sampling is the process by which the researcher identifies and selects individuals, groups, communities or texts or other data sources to be included in a study in order to answer the research question. Sampling methods vary depending on the purpose of the study, the research question, the study, the type of data and the process of data analysis. Figure 5.1 shows how sampling methods are related to other activities of the research process (see also Chapter 3).

Figure 5.1    Sampling methods and their relationship with other research activities

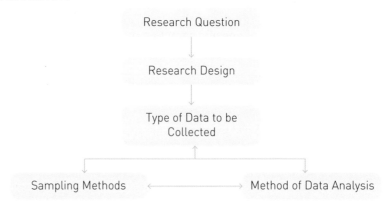

Sampling is a key activity in the research process requiring considerable thought in choosing the methods best suited to gathering the correct type of data. Although on the surface it appears to be an easy task, choosing which sampling method or combination of methods for a particular research study can be a complex process. For qualitative research, the sampling stage may not be as clearly determined at the commencement of the study as quantitative research because of the different designs in qualitative research. However, the process of sampling in qualitative research needs to be consistent with the particular research design and the type of data required to answer the research question. Therefore, the researcher needs to have a sound understanding of what type of data can be obtained by each sampling method.

Before introducing you to various sampling methods in qualitative research, it is important to be aware of fundamental values that underpin sampling methods. These values are outlined in Box 5.1. As you read through each value statement, it will become apparent that the focus is primarily about the importance of, and commitment to, bringing the everyday world to people's awareness. These four fundamental values provide a guide for the researcher when making choices about the most appropriate method/s of sampling for a given qualitative research study.

## Sampling methods in qualitative research

Under the broad umbrella of qualitative research, there are a number of sampling methods used by researchers. Before exploring how different methods of sampling apply to particular qualitative research designs, let us first consider the range of sampling methods. Each is outlined in Figure 5.2 and has been designed over time so that different types of information can be obtained. The list of sampling methods is not exhaustive.

Figure 5.2   Sampling methods in qualitative research

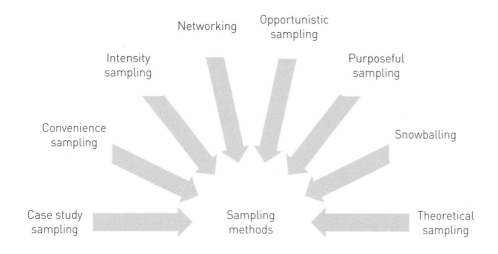

## Case study sampling

**Case study sampling** is the selection of cases (individuals, groups or organisations) 'that best [represent] the phenomenon being studied' (Taylor et al. 2007, p. 206). What constitutes a case for a particular study is identified at the time of designing the study. Cases become a part of the sampling process. They are selected on the basis that they

**Case study sampling:** The selection of cases that are most appropriate to the subject under investigation.

will be the best source of data to answer the research question. The selection of cases can change during the course of a study.

For example, you are conducting a study of a phenomenon in hospitals. You select two hospitals as your sample. After gathering information about the hospitals and how they work, you may decide to focus more specifically on particular areas within them such as clinical units. You may later decide to sample clinical staff as additional cases because of their importance in how the clinical units run and their relationship with the studied phenomenon. This can also work the other way, by beginning with nurses or midwives, then moving to clinical units and the hospital depending on the type of data you need.

⊗▐▊▊▊▊▊▊▊▊▊▊▊▊▊▊▊▊▊▊▊▊▊▊▊▊▊▊▊▊▊▊▊▊▊▊▊▊▊▊▊▊▊▊▊▊▊

## TIPS AND SKILLS

The use of case studies as the sampling approach for a particular study requires the researcher to be strategic in what cases they choose. The researcher has to see a clear direction in which the study needs to go.

- - - - - - - - - - - - - - - - - - - - - - - - - - - - - - - - - - - - - - - - - - - - - - - - - - - -

## Convenience sampling

**Convenience sampling:** The selection of participants easily accessible to the researcher.

**Convenience sampling** is the use of easily accessible participants for a study. For example, you have decided to study the phenomenon of caring. You can choose any group of health professionals, but you decide on nurses because they are the largest group of professionals and easy to access. The choice is more about convenience than the type of data you want. The use of such a method is not without its problems, the main one being the potential to compromise obtaining in-depth information of participants' experiences. Careful consideration should be given to the use of this method in undertaking quality research.

## Intensity sampling

**Intensity sampling:** Selection of cases that have been identified as having an intense experience of a studied phenomenon.

**Intensity sampling** is concerned with cases (individuals, groups, organisations) that have had an intense experience of a particular study phenomenon. The experiences can include loneliness, grieving the loss of another, feeling ostracised by a group, living through the process of forced closure of a facility and living through redundancy. To use intensity sampling, researchers need to know what a typical experience of the particular phenomenon is and then be able to identify people who have had intense experiences of that phenomenon.

This method requires sound judgment in the decision-making process. Intensity sampling is used in heuristic research where the researcher has had an intense experience of a phenomenon stimulating their desire to undertake an in-depth self-exploration of the experience with the aim of illuminating in-depth understandings of such a phenomenon.

## Networking

**Networking:** Involves the researcher either knowing or recruiting participants by asking colleagues or associates.

**Networking** requires researchers either knowing or recruiting participants by asking colleagues or associates. This method is usually used when the researcher has limited knowledge about suitable potential participants or has exhausted all avenues in participant recruitment.

An example of networking could be a nurse, working in the area of wound care and undertaking a study of the experience of living with a chronic wound, who would have knowledge of potential participants through her professional network. Another example could be a nurse who is not working in the area of wound care with limited knowledge of potential participants asking colleagues working in the area for assistance in locating potential participants for the study.

## Opportunistic sampling

**Opportunistic sampling** or what has been referred to by Patton (2002) and DiCenso and colleagues (2005) as 'the on-the-spot decisions' takes advantage of accessing new sources of data. This method is commonly used in ethnographic studies where the researcher is often confronted with making decisions about what to observe, who to interview, what type of data to collect and what direction they should take as the study progresses. The challenge for the researcher is to take advantage of each opportunity as it emerges and be prepared to follow where the data lead. The sampling process is dynamic and fluid. The researcher is generally not in a position to set in place a structured, systematic, time-sequenced approach to data sampling.

> **Opportunistic sampling:** On-the-spot decisions about sampling to take advantage of opportunities during actual data collection.

Opportunistic sampling requires the researcher to be open to new opportunities for sampling. The researcher needs to be focused, yet flexible in gathering appropriate data in order to answer the research question.

For example, a researcher undertakes a study about first-time mothers. There is an opportunity to interview the new mother (in her home) about what such an experience means to her. She talks about the importance of having a husband who has been with her during her pregnancy through to the arrival of their first-born child. While having a quiet informal conversation with the mother after the formal interview, her husband arrives home. He is interested in what the study is about and interested to talk about his experience of being there for his wife during this exciting and challenging period of their lives. The researcher asks the husband if he would be willing to be part of the study. His information is used as a part of the data.

## TIPS AND SKILLS

Opportunistic sampling requires the researcher to be open and flexible in accessing new sources of data. Careful consideration needs to be given to the type of information collected through this sampling process as it can influence the direction of the study.

## Purposive sampling

This sampling method is the process of identifying and deliberately selecting the cases that the researcher believes will provide 'information-rich' data (Collingridge & Gantt 2008; Schneider et al. 2003). These could be, for example, participants with particular experiences, organisations and communities with particular characteristics, particular events that you wish to study or particular documents you wish to review as part of your study.

> **Purposive sampling:** Used where the researcher recruits participants to the study based on some attribute that the researcher feels is appropriate.

The aim of this method is to gain in-depth understanding of the phenomenon being studied. The use of this sampling method requires the researcher to have knowledge of the group or setting they wish to study and its potential to contribute to the research. For example, if you are undertaking a study about becoming first-time mothers, you may wish to attend antenatal classes conducted at a local healthcare clinic (with the permission

92

of the clinic) to speak informally to the mothers-to-be about their experiences and ask them whether they would be interested in participating in your study. The choice of who will be invited to be part of the study is that of the researcher.

## TIPS AND SKILLS

Purposive sampling is the most common sampling process used in qualitative research. The aim of using this method is to include participants who can provide the best source of data for the study. It requires the researcher to have knowledge of the suitability of potential participants who can provide in-depth descriptions of the studied phenomenon.

## Snowballing

**Snowballing or chain sampling:** Involves starting with one or two participants and then relying on them to identify and refer to the researcher other potential participants who meet the inclusion criteria for the study.

**Snowballing** or what has also been termed **chain sampling** or nominated sampling begins with the researcher identifying one or two participants who have had the inclusion criteria of the study. The researcher then asks those participants if they know other individuals who would be suitable participants. This form of sampling is also commonly used in qualitative research. In a study that explored 10 men's experiences of living day by day with depression, Welch (2007) was able to recruit six of the 10 by using snowballing. The researcher initially identified four participants through a newspaper advertisement. After the four participants were interviewed, they were asked if they knew other men who had experienced depression and might be willing to be participants. Of these, three knew of others. The researchers then asked these participants to contact the others to ascertain their interest in being part of the study. If they were, would they be prepared to contact the researcher? This process was found to be most effective in obtaining an appropriate sample for this study.

## Theoretical sampling

**Theoretical sampling:** A process where findings from a small number of cases determine theoretically important aspects that direct subsequent sample or case selection.

Theoretical sampling is one of the sampling methods frequently used in grounded theory to 'focus and feed the process of constant comparison' (Birks & Mills 2011, p. 10). To sample theoretically involves the researcher carefully accessing participants and then analysing their data. The preliminary results will help identify other sources of information-rich data. Theoretical sampling begins at the point of initial analysis of data that uncovers important theoretical insights which provides direction to future sampling methods for data collection (Draucker et al. 2007; Higginbottom 2006). The process of theoretical sampling continues throughout the course of the study.

For example, a researcher wants to formulate a theory of being a first-time mother. After analysing the first three women's data, 'the presence of a spouse' emerges as a possible theme. The identification of this theme suggests to the researcher that in order to generate further data, future potential participants need to be selected who have a spouse. In the course of interviewing further participants a second theme of 'absence of a spouse' emerges. The researcher then decides to gather further information from this group of women. The combined data is then analysed to develop concepts and categories that become part of the development of a theory.

Table 5.1 shows the sampling methods described earlier, relevant research design and researchers' skills required to complete the study project efficiently and successfully.

**Table 5.1**  Sampling methods, qualitative research designs and researcher skills

| Sampling method | Used in which research design | Researcher skills required |
| --- | --- | --- |
| Case study sampling | Case-based studies can be used in historical, critical social theory and narrative research | Ability to identify typical cases according to the aim of the study |
| Convenience sampling | A range of qualitative research designs (e.g. phenomenology and feminism) | Needs to be discerning in the choice of participants and the type of data to be included in the study |
| Intensity sampling | Case study research (see above) and heuristics | Knowledge of what is normal or typical of the phenomenon in order to identify participants who have had an intense experience of that phenomenon. In heuristics, the researcher-participant need to be able to engage in self-reflection, critical analysis and immersion in the study phenomenon |
| Networking | A range of qualitative research designs including phenomenology and critical social theory | Ability to identify reliable persons with knowledge of potential participants |
| Opportunistic sampling | Commonly used in ethnography | Sound judgment to ensure that the opportunities for new data are in line with the focus of the study and the appropriate type of data |
| Purposive sampling | Most of qualitative research designs including phenomenology, grounded theory, hermeneutics, critical social theory, action research and heuristics | Knowledge of the target population and potential participants who can provide 'information-rich' data |
| Snowball sampling | A range of qualitative research designs including phenomenology and critical social theory | Ability to make informed judgments about potential participants recommended by previous participants |
| Theoretical sampling | Used in grounded theory | Ability to make decisions about the type of information needed for ongoing analysis in order to build a theory |

## Bias in sampling

Bias has the capacity to distort and compromise the data and the study findings. It exists in all research (see also Chapter 9), and qualitative research is no exception. Arguments put forward in qualitative research about bias include the need to control all elements

**●.THINKING DEEPLY**

Researchers need to know the best sampling method for their study. You are about to undertake a study concerning the lived experience of caring for a person with heart failure. What type/s of sampling methods would you consider to be appropriate for this study?

After reflecting on the focus of the study, you decide to include the person's cultural context as you believe that a person's lived experience has to be considered in their cultural and social context. Due to this change in focus for your study, what sampling methods would be most appropriate for this study (see also Chapter 6)?

of bias. They include preconceptions at any stage of the research project, beliefs and assumptions by the researcher about the study phenomenon, and viewing bias as a natural and legitimate part of life, and therefore of research.

In any study which the author, as a mental health researcher, has undertaken, the potential for bias has always been present. Controlling my bias about what I am researching is of paramount importance. For example, a number of years ago I was conducting a study about how people with a mental illness cope with daily living. At the beginning of the study when I was selecting potential participants, I found myself wanting to interview only those people who had rich, positive experiences about coping rather than those who were simply coping and barely existing each day, even though they met the study inclusion criteria. It was only during the sampling process that I realised I was excluding participants who met the inclusion criteria on the ground that they had not had a positive experience of coping. The study was stopped as my level of bias was compromising the integrity of the study.

The particular position one takes about bias will significantly influence how one goes about choosing the research design and the sampling methods in order to gather data to answer the research question. Dealing with bias is a necessary consideration in any study, irrespective of the chosen research design. It is important that the researcher acknowledge the presence of bias in their study and demonstrate how they address this (Denzin & Lincoln 2011).

Figure 5.3 shows the key elements to be considered when selecting a sampling method in qualitative research.

**●.THINKING DEEPLY**

The notion of bias is frequently raised in qualitative research. If you were asked the question 'How do you deal with bias in qualitative research?' what would be your answer? Think about whether or not there is a place for bias in a qualitative research study. If yes, what strategies could you use to reduce the effect of bias?

Figure 5.3    Key elements to be considered when selecting a sampling method in qualitative research

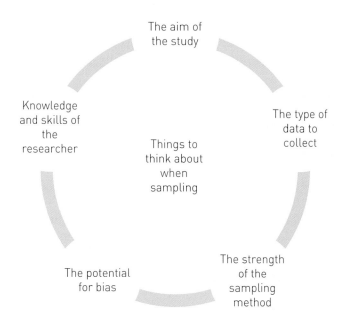

## Implications for evidence-based practice

Knowledge generated through qualitative enquiry, with its focus on human experience, has been increasingly recognised because of the importance of experiences of patients and their families in the provision of quality holistic care. The strength of study findings is closely linked to the quality of the research design. This includes the use of appropriate sampling to answer the research question. Qualitative studies that are well conducted provide sound evidence and can lead to practice change.

# SUMMARY

- Sampling is one of the key elements in undertaking good research.
- Sampling can involve one method or more depending on the study aim and the design.
- The choice of sampling method requires knowledge about potential participants and sound judgment by the researcher.
- Sampling that leads to rich data is critical for the development of insights and understandings of the study phenomenon.

## PRACTICE EXERCISE 5.1

When undertaking research about the lived experiences of any phenomena, what type of sampling method/s would be appropriate? Why would you choose such method/s?

ANSWER: Research that is concerned with lived experience is about exploring the everyday life of human beings. Phenomena include caring for another, living with hope, taking life day by day and living with a chronic illness.

The most appropriate sampling method when exploring the lived experience of individuals is purposive sampling, in which the most appropriate participant to obtain in-depth descriptions and understanding of the particular phenomenon being studied will be selected. Other sampling methods such as networking and snowballing can be used. However, the latter methods depend on other people being able to identify appropriate participants that the researcher can later contact.

## PRACTICE EXERCISE 5.2

What do you consider to be the benefits and limitations of using convenience sampling?

ANSWER: Convenience sampling allows the researcher to take advantage of available data that are easily accessible. However, the data may not be adequate to answer the research question in any depth.

## FURTHER READING

Creswell, J. W. (2007). *Qualitative Inquiry and Research Design: Choosing Among Five Approaches.* London: SAGE Publications.

Douglass, B. & Moustakas, C. (1985). Heuristic inquiry: The internal search to know. *Journal of Humanistic Psychology* 25, 39–55.

Pelto, P. J. & Pelto, G. H. (1978). *Anthropological Research: The Structure of Inquiry.* Cambridge: Cambridge University Press.

## USEFUL WEBSITES

<www.qualitative-research.net/index.php/fqs>

The Forum Qualitative Sozialforschung (Forum Qualitative Social Research) is a peer-reviewed multilingual online journal for qualitative research. You can gain access to the journal free of charge.

<http://qhr.sagepub.com>

SAGE publishes the *Qualitative Research Journal*, which can be useful for reviewing various published articles and discussion papers on various qualitative research issues.

<www.groundedtheoryreview.com>

The site of the *Grounded Theory Review*. This can be useful for readers who want to review the application of grounded theory in qualitative research.

## REFERENCES

Birks, M. & Mills, J. (2011). *Grounded Theory: A Practice Guide.* London: SAGE.

Collingridge, D. S. & Gantt, E. E. (2008). The quality of qualitative research. *American Journal of Medical Quality* 23, 389.

Denzin, N. K. & Lincoln, Y. S. (2011). *The SAGE Handbook of Qualitative Research*, 4th edn. London: SAGE.

DiCenso, A., Guyatt, G. & Ciliska, D. (2005). *Evidence-based Nursing: A Guide to Clinical Practice.* St Louis, MO: Elsevier Mosby.

Draucker, C. G., Marsolf, D. S., Ross, R. & Rusk, T. B. (2007). Theoretical sampling and category development in grounded theory. *Qualitative Health Research* 17(8), 1137–48.

Higginbottom, G. (2006). Sampling issues in qualitative research. *Nurse Researcher* 12(1), 7–19.

Patton, M. Q. (2002). *Qualitative Research and Evaluation Methods*, 3rd edn. London: SAGE Publications.

Schneider, Z., Elliot, D., LoBiondo-Wood, G. & Haber, J. (2003). *Nursing Research: Methods, Critical Appraisal and Utilisation*, 2nd edn. Australia: Mosby.

Taylor, B., Kermode, S. & Roberts, K. (2007). *Research in Nursing and Health Care: Evidence for Practice*, 3rd edn. Australia: Thomson.

Welch, A. (2007). The phenomenon of taking life day-by-day: Using Parse's research method. *Nursing Science Quarterly* 20(3), 265–72.

CHAPTER 6

# QUALITATIVE RESEARCH DESIGN

Anthony Welch

## CHAPTER LEARNING OBJECTIVES

By the end of this chapter you will be able to:

- understand the philosophical foundations of qualitative research
- describe a range of qualitative research designs
- explain different methods of conducting research within particular qualitative designs
- list the type of questions to ask when choosing a qualitative research design.

## Introduction

In the previous chapter you were introduced to different approaches to sampling in qualitative research. This chapter will introduce you to various ways by which you can undertake qualitative research. Examples of different frequently used qualitative research designs are provided and how they can be applied to health research for the professions of nursing and midwifery. Before describing the different pathways to qualitative research, we need to have an understanding of what constitutes qualitative research.

## What is qualitative research?

In order to gain an understanding of what qualitative research is all about, we first need to have some knowledge of its origins and how it has emerged as a legitimate and important method of enquiry. The development of qualitative research can be traced back to the work of Wilhelm Dilthey (1833–1911), who was motivated by a need to develop a research pathway that could explore the everyday world of human beings, such as their experiences, perceptions, attitudes and beliefs. Since then, many scholars, theorists and researchers have contributed to establishing qualitative research as a major research approach in health sciences. As we move through the chapter, you will be introduced to a number of these people and the unique contributions they have made to the development of different research designs that fall under the umbrella of qualitative research.

As a starting point, it is important to understand that qualitative research has one central aim: that of developing an understanding of how human beings—you and me—construct and make sense of the everyday world in which we live—'a social, personal and relational world' (McLeod 2001, p. 2).

Qualitative research is different from quantitative research because of a different set of fundamental values that underpin the philosophical perspectives of qualitative research. These six fundamental values (Streubert Speziale & Rinaldi Carpenter 2007) are outlined in Box 6.1.

### Box 6.1

**FUNDAMENTAL VALUES OF THE PHILOSOPHICAL PERSPECTIVE OF QUALITATIVE RESEARCH**

- A belief in multiple realities, or perspectives, to a given situation. Each person has their own unique perspective on life and each situation they encounter. Their perspectives or personal reality can change depending on their life experiences and the meaning they give to each experience.
- A commitment to selecting an approach to research that is appropriate to answer the research question.
- A commitment to the participant's viewpoint—truthfully describing what is important to the participant about their experience.
- Minimising disturbance to the natural setting or context in which the study is conducted.
- Acknowledging researcher participation in the research process: the researcher is an integral part of the research because they are the person who collects and analyses the data.
- Presenting the findings of the study in a literary style rich with expressions and descriptions of participants' experiences.

These core characteristics or fundamental values encompass a range of research designs that fall under the qualitative research paradigm (Patton 2002). There are a number of qualitative research designs. We will devote the discussion to frequently used approaches or research designs in this chapter. They include phenomenology, heuristics, grounded theory, ethnography, critical social theory, feminism, action research and bricolage.

# The types of qualitative research

Figure 6.1    Different qualitative research designs

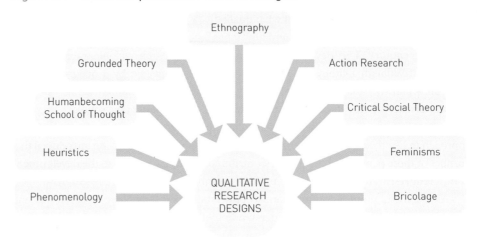

## Phenomenology

**Phenomenology:** A philosophical movement and a mode of enquiry that aims to understand the essential structures or essence of phenomena of individuals' everyday experiences.

**Phenomenology** as a scientific research method was developed as an alternative approach to the traditional natural sciences commonly referred to as positivist scientific methods or quantitative research (Denzin & Lincoln 2011). Since the initial works of such notable people as Franz Brentano (1838–1917), Carl Stumpf (1848–1936) and Edmund Husserl (1859–1938) in the 19th century, phenomenology has continued to develop as a movement, because of the ongoing expansion of philosophical views and a research method. Two major pathways or streams of phenomenological research have developed over time: descriptive phenomenology and interpretive phenomenology. Heuristics, which is another method of phenomenological enquiry, will be presented as a comparison with descriptive and interpretive phenomenological pathways.

### Descriptive phenomenology

Descriptive phenomenology is primarily concerned with obtaining in-depth, rich, concrete descriptions of people's experiences. Through these descriptions, understanding of the everyday world of human beings is obtained. Description, therefore, is considered to be fundamental to gaining insight into human experience. What the person shares with you about their experience forms the basis of your investigation, analysis and final report. The participant's raw descriptions as spoken by them are of paramount importance in conducting this form of enquiry. In this research approach, the participants are asked to describe their experience of a particular phenomenon, situation or concept of interest to the study. Such situations may include what it is like being ill, living with diabetes, coping with study at university and caring for a loved one. Concepts include such notions as resilience, hope, having faith and being compassionate.

## Interpretive (hermeneutic) phenomenology

The development of an interpretive (**hermeneutic**) phenomenology is attributed to Paul Ricoeur (1976), Martin Heidegger (1962) and Hans Gadamer (1976). The rationale for such an approach to research is that to understand the ways human beings act, experience and find meaning in their lives requires starting with description then moving beyond description to interpretation. The interpretation of information or data is referred to as hermeneutics. Hermeneutics has its origin in biblical exegesis—the interpretation of biblical and historical texts (Bleicher 1980). Heidegger argued that hermeneutics is a fundamental element of human existence: human beings are continually engaged in interpretation in order to make meaningful sense of the world in which they live.

**Hermeneutics:** The interpretation of information or data.

The foundation of interpretive phenomenology is the belief that people are sensate, meaning that we experience our world from a subjective point of view. It is our interpretation of our experiences that creates meaning for us as human beings. Think about the last time you had a conversation with friends or colleagues about a particular issue or situation. Did all agree or disagree in exactly the same way? Or was there a subtle difference in how each of you perceived and understood the issue which you discussed? The subtle differences in the way you perceived the issue or situation, although you might generally have agreed with the discussion, can be attributed to your own unique interpretation of the issue. Researchers who engage in this form of research are required to follow strict guidelines to ensure that the way the researcher has interpreted the information shared by participants clearly reflects what the participants wish to communicate about their experience. In this form of research, a more in-depth understanding or insight into the person's experience can be obtained. By way of example, Glenn and colleagues (2014) used hermeneutic phenomenology research to explore nursing care in the intrapartum setting. Interview transcripts of 13 nurses were analysed. They found that nurses' perspectives about the provision of caring practices were influenced by the complexity of the healthcare system, interactions with their team members, challenges related to documentation and respect for natural birth.

Within the overarching design of interpretive phenomenology there are a number of different approaches one can take depending on the focus of the research question and the type of study you wish to undertake from an interpretive perspective. The works of such people as Ricoeur, Gadamer and Heidegger are useful in helping you gain further understanding of these different approaches.

## THINKING DEEPLY

Phenomenological research is concerned with exploring anything (phenomena) that presents itself to human consciousness and is experienced by human beings as part of their everyday life. Unless a person has a conscious awareness of the phenomenon, it cannot be explored through lived experience.

The term 'lived experience' has been coined to highlight that the person or group of people have actually lived through the experience being investigated rather than it being a second-hand account of someone else's experience.

Although there are differences between the two approaches of descriptive phenomenology and interpretive phenomenology, some core **concepts** are shared. These are description, intentionality, essences, life-world and intuiting phenomena.

*Description* is a way of uncovering the essential nature or structure of phenomena. Within phenomenology, description is considered the primary mode of communicating experiences of phenomena—'things'—as they occur in everyday life, for instance the experience of hoping, grieving, feeling loved, living with chronic pain, caring for another and so forth. The act of describing phenomena as experienced is fundamental to phenomenological enquiry irrespective of whether you are using a descriptive or interpretive approach to enquiry.

Think about how you share your experience. More often than not, it is by describing what has happened and what the experience was like for you. The same process is applied when you are undertaking phenomenological research.

*Intentionality* is at the core of phenomenology. The term is used to refer to human consciousness or awareness. Phenomenology holds that every act is an act of consciousness or an awareness of something, whether that is perceiving an object, recalling a memory, imagining an experience or anticipating a future event (Sokolowski 2000). For instance, one does not hear without hearing something, or hope without hoping for something or care without caring for something. 'Intentionality' should not be confused with 'intention', which is about purpose and action, such as intending to buy a friend a present. Intentionality is at the centre of human experience as it is concerned with creating meaning about what is experienced.

*Essences* are the essential structures of phenomena—what makes up a phenomenon or thing. An essence is a basic unit of common understanding. For example, what is the essence or common understanding of caring? The nursing and midwifery literature often talk about the uniqueness of caring in these two disciplines. If you want to know what this uniqueness is all about you would be exploring the essence of caring as practised by nurses and midwives. One of the central aims of phenomenology, therefore, is to describe the essences or common understandings of phenomena as experienced by individuals and groups in everyday life.

*Life-world* denotes a world in which human beings live and through which they give expression and meaning to their personal existence—the world of lived experience. The inclusion of the word 'lived' denotes an experience that an individual has actually lived through. When we talk about lived-through experiences we are referring to experiences that have been reflected on in order to gain understanding of what occurred, for example taking time to reflect on your clinical practice in order to learn from the experience.

*Intuiting* refers to the process of imaginative variation of the data—to look at the data in different ways—until a common understanding of the phenomenon emerges (Sokolowski 2000).

## Heuristics

**Heuristics** is another form of phenomenological research. Heuristics has its origins in humanistic psychology with its emphasis on the primacy of human experience as a mode of discovery. The root meaning of 'heuristic' comes from the Greek *heuriskein*, meaning to discover or to find. It refers to a process of internal (personal) search through which one discovers the nature or meaning of an experience and develops methods and procedures for further investigation and analysis (Moustakas 1990, p. 9).

**Concept:** A mental idea based on observations of behaviours or characteristics, for example pain and stress.

**Heuristics:** A process of internal search with the aim of exploring and discovering personal insights and understanding of a phenomenon of intense interest to the researcher.

The aim of heuristic research is to explore a phenomenon through the personal experiences of the researcher. A fundamental requirement for undertaking heuristic enquiry is that the researcher has a personal and intense experience of the phenomenon and is willing to engage in such processes as introspective self-search, systematic enquiry and tacit knowing. The introspective self-search involves the researcher engaging in self-reflection about the phenomenon of interest. Systematic enquiry involves a rigorous approach of personal observation, of dialoguing with oneself and others in search of deeper meanings of the phenomenon under investigation. Tacit knowing is a process of allowing hunches to come to the fore, providing new insights about the phenomenon that surface in the course of the enquiry. In simple terms it can be said that the researcher is also the participant. The processes involved in heuristic enquiry are:

- *initial engagement*: the beginning point where the researcher identifies the focus of enquiry
- *immersion*: the process of intense concentration involving self-dialogue, self-searching, pursuing intuitive clues and drawing from tacit knowledge
- *incubation*: a process of stepping back, taking a detached stance and being receptive to the emergence of new insights and understandings
- *illumination*: a point of new awareness and understanding
- *explication*: the process of describing or depicting core themes
- *creative synthesis*: the process of drawing together the core themes into a comprehensive description of the phenomenon being studied (Moustakas 1990).

Although the processes are listed in a sequential manner, they are far more fluid and dynamic depending on the individual and the manner in which the researcher-participant engages with the process. The types of human experiences that you would focus on using this approach to research could include being a student nurse, feeling happy, feeling lonely, caring for another or living on death row.

**Figure 6.2**    Simple presentations of phenomenology and heuristic research designs

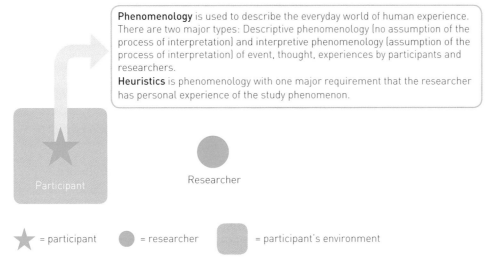

**Phenomenology** is used to describe the everyday world of human experience. There are two major types: Descriptive phenomenology (no assumption of the process of interpretation) and interpretive phenomenology (assumption of the process of interpretation) of event, thought, experiences by participants and researchers.
**Heuristics** is phenomenology with one major requirement that the researcher has personal experience of the study phenomenon.

Participant          Researcher

★ = participant     ● = researcher     ▉ = participant's environment

An arrow symbolises the data derived from participants and other sources.

## TIPS AND SKILLS

The aim of heuristic research is to explore a phenomenon through the personal experiences of the researcher and/or co-researchers. The researcher is both researcher and participant.

What do you consider to be the differences between phenomenological research and heuristic research?

What is important in both phenomenology and heuristic research is the value one places on the importance of lived personal experience as a legitimate and powerful means of knowledge development.

## Grounded theory

**Grounded theory:**

A systematic process of enquiry in which the researcher engages in a process of constant comparative analysis of data at each stage of the research process in order to generate theories about the phenomenon of concern.

**Grounded theory** is a qualitative research method the aim of which is to generate theory about a particular phenomenon of interest through the study of basic social processes and social systems present in human interactions (Birks & Mills 2011) (see Figure 6.3).

Although the development of grounded theory has been attributed to Barney Glaser and Anselm Strauss, two sociologists from the University of California, the foundations on which grounded theory is based can be traced back to the works of John Dewey, an American pragmatist, George Herbert Mead, an American philosopher, sociologist and psychologist, and the behaviourist movement of the time (Hall, Griffiths & McKenna 2013). 'Mead focused on behaviour, reflecting the pragmatists' view that knowledge is created through action and interaction of self-reflecting beings' (Hall et al. 2013, p. 19). Through self-reflection on action human beings learn about themselves and their behaviours with others. Herbert Blumer, a student of Mead, expanded Mead's ideas about human behaviour focusing on the significance of meaning in understanding behaviour. For Blumer, meaning is at the centre of behaviour as individuals interpret their experiences and construct meaning in order to make sense of their interactions with others and the environment in which they live. The name given to this process by Blumer was symbolic interactionism.

The three assumptions underpinning symbolic interactionism stipulated by Blumer (1969, p. 2) are:

- human beings act toward things on the basis of the meanings that these things have for them
- the meaning of such things is derived from, and arises out of, the social interaction that one has with one's fellows
- these meanings are handled in, and modified through an interpretive process used by the person in dealing with the things he encounters.

Symbolic interactionism is considered the cornerstone of grounded theory.

Since the original works of Glaser and Strauss (1967) in which the grounded theory method was developed, a number of modifications or iterations to the method have been proposed. The main contributors to the modifications have been Glaser (1992), Strauss and Corbin (1990), Charmaz (2006) and Birks and Mills (2011). The modifications to the original grounded theory method are shown in Table 6.3.

Figure 6.3   Simple presentations of grounded theory research design

**Grounded theory** requires an essential process for collecting and analysing data to construct a theory which is grounded in the data. **Symbolic interactionism** is widely used as a school of thought as an underpinning or framework to interpret the data.

Data generated mainly from the participants who interact with and are influenced by various aspects in the study environment.

Researcher

Participant

 = participant    = researcher    = Participant's environment

 = other persons or aspects as the participant's environment

An arrow symbolises the data derived from participants and other sources.

**Table 6.1**   Modifications to grounded theory

| Theorist | Modification/refinements |
|---|---|
| Glaser and Strauss | The generation of theory without any particular commitment to specific kinds of data, lines of research or theoretical interests (Glaser & Strauss 1967). |
| Glaser | Continued to remain true to the original method developed by Glaser and Strauss (1967) but placed more emphasis on discovery, emergence of categories and strict adherence to each step of the method. |
| Strauss and Corbin | Moved towards verification with an emphasis on technical procedures and less emphasis on the constant comparative method. |
| Charmaz | Constructivist approach brings together traditional positivist/objectivist methods and post-positivist interpretive approaches to grounded theory research (Charmaz 2006). |
| Birks and Mills | Reconceptualised coding as initial, intermediate and advanced and positioning the researcher within the context of grounded theory. Introducing storytelling and using theoretical coding in a different way. |

Despite various modifications to Glaser and Strauss's (1967) classic grounded theory method, processes that are generally considered essential are the following:

• theoretical sampling, which involves making decisions about whom to interview or what to observe next. These decisions are determined by theory generation, and that implies starting data analysis with the first interview, and writing down memos early

- constant comparative data analysis, the ongoing comparison of data: 'incident to incident, incident to codes, codes to codes, codes to categories, and categories to categories' (Birks & Mills 2011, p. 11)
- theoretical sensitivity, which has two elements: the level of the researcher's sensitivity, which reflects the person's level of insight into both self and the area of study; and the researcher's use of theory that guides their everyday thought (Birks & Mills 2011)
- memo writing
- identification of a core category
- the formulation of an explanatory theory (see also Chapters 7 and 8).

## TIPS AND SKILLS

When choosing grounded theory as your research method it is important to remember that there have been a number of modifications to the original method which have resulted in different versions. Once you make a choice of a particular version for your study, it is important to remain true to that approach.

## Ethnography

**Ethnography:**
A qualitative research method designed to explore cultural patterns of behaviour—social interactions and associated meanings—for individuals, groups and communities.

**Ethnography** has its origins in anthropology with its focus on the study of humans from evolutionary and social perspectives (*New Webster's Encyclopaedia of Dictionaries* 1990). Ethnography is defined by Fetterman (1989, p. 11) as 'the art and science of describing a group or culture' with particular attention on understanding the patterns and meanings of human behaviour such as belief systems, myths, rituals, symbols, customs, roles, events, social interactions and group interrelationships that form the basis of everyday life of a cultural group. At the core of an ethnographic study is 'to get at the implicit (back-stage) culture in addition to the explicit, public (front-stage) aspects of culture' (Germain 2001, p. 284) and to learn from the members that make up the cultural group.

Initially ethnographic studies were concerned with exploring traditional cultures about which little was known, such as tribal rituals, parenting behaviours in ancient civilisations and patterns of communicating in different cultural groups. In contemporary society the focus of ethnography is on contemporary social issues such as poverty, marginalised groups, homeless persons and organisational systems such as the healthcare system. An example of a recent ethnographic study is that of Denison and colleagues' (2013) study of Aboriginal women and healthcare workers in Canada. The aim of the study was to explore the influence of the threat of child removal on Aboriginal women's experience in accessing healthcare services. They found that Aboriginal women whose children are involved with the child protection system often experience complex sociopolitical and economic challenges, which interact with the threat of the child being removed. Such threats did not affect women's decisions to seek healthcare services for their children, but the experience of racism, prejudice and discrimination in mainstream healthcare agencies and the fear of the child being removed from the mother influenced the women's decisions to access healthcare for themselves.

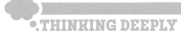

**THINKING DEEPLY**

Ethnographic research is concerned with the art and science of describing patterns of living and human interaction of a group or culture. An example of an ethnographic study in healthcare could be looking at the patterns of caring provided by different healthcare professionals.

Figure 6.4    Simple presentations of ethnography and ethnonursing

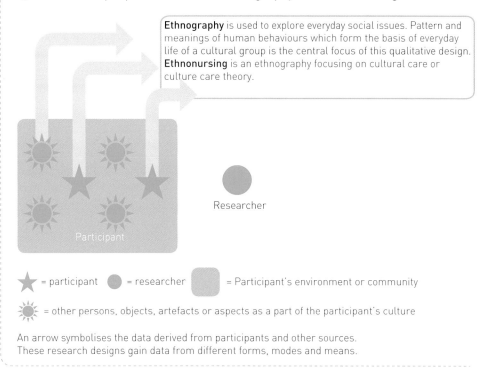

**Ethnography** is used to explore everyday social issues. Pattern and meanings of human behaviours which form the basis of everyday life of a cultural group is the central focus of this qualitative design. **Ethnonursing** is an ethnography focusing on cultural care or culture care theory.

Researcher

Participant

★ = participant     ● = researcher     ▢ = Participant's environment or community

☀ = other persons, objects, artefacts or aspects as a part of the participant's culture

An arrow symbolises the data derived from participants and other sources.
These research designs gain data from different forms, modes and means.

Like other qualitative designs, a number of different approaches to ethnographic enquiry have evolved. These include classical ethnography, systematic ethnography, interpretive ethnography and critical ethnography.

*Classical ethnography* focuses on obtaining a complete description of all aspects of a cultural group: patterns of living of the people that make up a cultural group.

*Systematic ethnography* is concerned with describing the structure of a culture rather than patterns of social interactions of the cultural group.

*Interpretive ethnography* aims to explore the meanings of social and cultural interactions. The construction of meaning is the bedrock for human understanding. In order to understand human behaviour, therefore, it is necessary to explore the meaning behind what the person is doing.

*Critical ethnography* is the study of society that gives particular attention to uncovering social inequalities, oppression and injustices, with the aim of raising social awareness and instituting change (Patton 2002).

Other ethnographic research approaches warrant mention: autoethnography and ethnonursing.

**Autoethnography:** The study of oneself within the context of the culture in which one lives.

**Ethnonursing:** A research method used to explore and describe care patterns in cultures.

**Autoethnography** is concerned with the study of one's own culture through personal experience. The person's experience provides the conduit or means of exploring and gaining insights into the culture in which the person lives.

**Ethnonursing** as a research method was developed by Madeleine Leininger (1985, 1988). Its focus is on cultural care patterns—care expressions and practices within a culture. The premises underpinning cultural care theory are that care is fundamental to health and well-being, and the act of caring involves multiple universal and diverse elements. Therefore, in order to provide holistic, humanistic cultural care, elements that need to be considered include 'worldview, ethno-history, religious [philosophical and spiritual] orientation, kinship patterns, material cultural phenomena, the political, economic, legal, educational, technological, and physical environment, language, and folk and professional care practices' (Leininger 1991, p. 23). Leininger's Sunrise model was developed as a conceptual framework to depict the various dimensions of her cultural care theory.

**Figure 6.5   The Sunrise model**

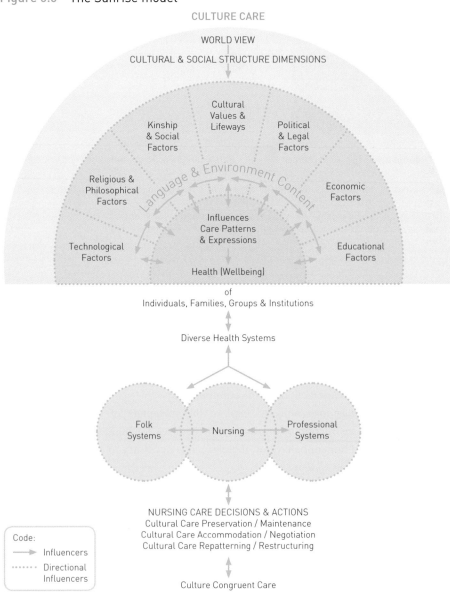

## Critical social theory

**Critical social theory** focuses on uncovering social inequality and the reasons for social change. Critical theorists attempt to confront social injustices by critiquing the socio-political ideologies, conventional social structures and uncontested social beliefs that form the fabric of a society, shaping people's experiences, interactions with others and the way we view the world (Patton 2002).

The development of critical social theory can be traced to the seminal works of Karl Marx (1818–83). The fundamental issue for Marx was that those who hold economic hegemony (control) are able to shape the lives of those who do not. The issues of control, power, oppression, manipulation and social injustice implicit in Marxism have formed the foundation for much of contemporary critical social research. As a movement, critical social theory has its origins in the Institute for Social Research established in 1924 in Frankfurt, Prussia under the patronage of Felix Weil aided by Kurt Gerlach.

Over time, critical social theory has become eclectic in orientation as a result of different ideological positions put forward by its theorists. Examples of different ideological approaches to critical social theory research are *Communicative Reason* by Jurgen Habermas, Paulo Freire's *Pedagogy of the Oppressed*, and *Negative Dialectic* by Theodor Adorno.

## Feminism

**Feminism** is a term concerned with women's issues first coined by Charles Fourier, a French philosopher, in 1837. The word 'feminism' was first used in France and the Netherlands in the latter part of the 19th century. The feminist movement gradually spread to the UK and the USA in the early part of the 20th century where the suffragettes began the fight for the right to vote. Thus began a global move for equality for women which has touched the four corners of the globe and in which Australia and New Zealand have been leaders.

At the centre of feminist thought is the recognition of women's experiences, beliefs, views, ways of being and ways of knowing as legitimate and authoritative sources of knowledge. Feminism is about raising awareness of gender inequality, oppression and injustice in the social world and exploring ways by which this can be rectified. It is also concerned with defending women's rights politically, economically, socially and culturally.

A range of feminisms within the feminist social movement have emerged, each with their own ideologies or beliefs about what is important to women. Feminist research has emerged as an important area of investigation in contemporary society and has been instrumental in uncovering and bringing to social awareness issues concerning social inequality for women and in mounting well-argued cases for social change and innovation.

So how do you know that a feminist approach to research is the most appropriate for your area of study? There are two key elements to consider in making the correct decision. First, is your area of investigation concerned primarily with women? Second, is the focus of your study concerned with making visible or bringing to social awareness issues relating to women's social concerns such as inequality, giving voice to women who are marginalised and oppressed, or exploring ways by which women can challenge patriarchal dominance? Keep in mind that the major difference between critical social theory and feminism is the central place of women in the research.

**Critical social theory:** A theory or an intellectual form that has criticism at the centre of its knowledge production. A broad range of ideas and frameworks are used to help people question, deconstruct and then reconstruct knowledge to uncover issues of power and social inequality.

**Feminism** refers to a range of feminist thought and approaches to enquiry concerned with the social structures and processes that lead to gender inequality and oppression with the aim of achieving emancipation and equality.

## TIPS AND SKILLS

In reading both the sections on critical social theory and feminism and viewing Figure 6.6, you can see the similarities and differences in the two approaches. Key to making the right choice of research design is to be able to identify the primary focus of the study. For example, if the focus is on issues of control, power, oppression, manipulation and social injustice but is not targeting any specific group or population such as women, then a critical social theory approach is appropriate. But if the specific group that you wish to explore is women then a feminist approach is appropriate.

Take time to examine your question. One suggestion is to write the question down and then in the next sentence provide a rationale for the question. The rationale or reason for undertaking the research will provide you with the answer about which approach is appropriate.

**Figure 6.6**    Simple presentations of critical social theory and feminism

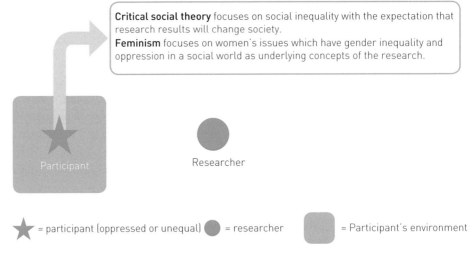

**Critical social theory** focuses on social inequality with the expectation that research results will change society.
**Feminism** focuses on women's issues which have gender inequality and oppression in a social world as underlying concepts of the research.

Participant

Researcher

★ = participant (oppressed or unequal)  ● = researcher      = Participant's environment

An arrow symbolises the data derived from participants and other sources.

## Action research

**Action research:**
A method of enquiry in which an individual or group actively engage as researchers in a process of change to address actual or emergent problems in their specific area of practice.

**Action research** has its origins in the work of J. L. Moreno, a physician who undertook community research with groups of prostitutes in Vienna during the early 1900s. The prostitutes were considered by Moreno as participants and co-researchers. The term 'action research' as a mode of enquiry was coined by Kurt Lewin, who described a program of community research projects involving community groups in the USA to address post-Second World War social problems (Lewin 1946). Action research, as the name suggests, investigates an identified area or issue of concern to and by a group of interested people with the aim of generating solutions or interventions to bring about change. Action researchers go to the site of the problem and work with the people concerned as co-researchers. The processes for action research include a repeated cycle of enquiry, intervention and evaluation. Street and Robinson (1995) have developed a schematic representation for the conduct of action research based on Lewin's original model and their own experiences in working on nursing projects.

Figure 6.7   Simple presentation of action research

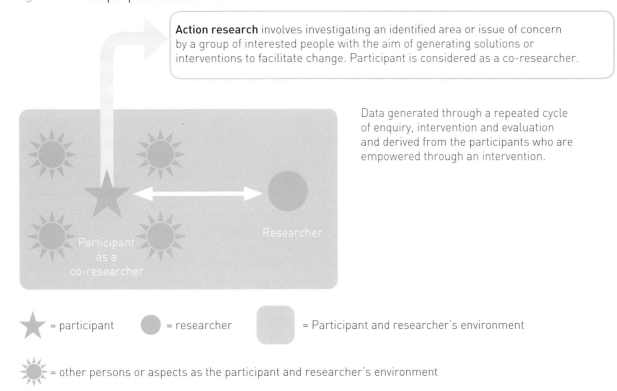

**Action research** involves investigating an identified area or issue of concern by a group of interested people with the aim of generating solutions or interventions to facilitate change. Participant is considered as a co-researcher.

Data generated through a repeated cycle of enquiry, intervention and evaluation and derived from the participants who are empowered through an intervention.

Participant as a co-researcher

Researcher

= participant       = researcher       = Participant and researcher's environment

= other persons or aspects as the participant and researcher's environment

An arrow symbolises the data derived from participants and other sources.

From its original work by Lewin (1946), action research has witnessed a number of modifications in response to different aims. Examples of the forms of action research and specific aims are given in Table 6.2.

**Table 6.2**   Action research

| Forms of action research | Focuses/aims |
| --- | --- |
| Technical action research | Improve techniques and procedures through practitioner collaboration. |
| Practical action research | Improve existing practices and develop new ones. |
| Emancipatory action research | Take responsibility for actions that free the group from practice constraints through initiating change by transforming political, social and economic conditions (Taylor et al. 2007). |

An example of this research design is that of Ullrich and colleagues' (2014) action research study which explored the similarities and differences in the nursing practice in nutritional care between a residential aged care facility and a hospital. They collected data from various sources including interviews, note-taking and observations. Results showed that how nurses chose to participate in the provision of nutritional care and assert their autonomy when changing practice to nutritional care affected the quality of the resident/patient mealtime experience. Operational efficiency in an organisation influenced the choices that nurses made about the type of intervention used to improve nursing practice in nutritional care. Nurses required management approval for practice change in providing nutritional care.

## Bricolage

**Bricolage:** A research method that creatively amalgamates or synthesises a range of methodologies and strategies deemed appropriate by the researcher in pursuit of the most robust and accurate explication of findings.

**Bricolage** has emerged over the past few decades in response to a perceived need by researchers to move beyond adopting a singular philosophical position and its stipulated method and instead embracing a broad sweep of philosophical perspectives and methodological strategies from which to utilise the most appropriate methods for the collection and analysis of data (McLeod 2001). The person using such an approach is described as the bricoleur, a French word meaning 'someone who works with his hands, and uses [different] means compared to those of the craftsman' (Weinstein & Weinstein 1991, p. 161). The idea of researcher-as-bricoleur was introduced by Levi-Strauss (1966) to describe 'a person who makes something new out of a range of materials that previously made up something different' (Crotty 1998, p. 50). The bricoleur is one who 'produces a bricolage, that is a set of pieced-together representations that are fitted to the specifics of a complex situation' (Denzin & Lincoln 2011, p. 4). The researcher-as-bricoleur uses strategies or methods (whether or not they go against conventional approaches to enquiry) deemed by the researcher as appropriate to ensure that the study is conducted in the best possible manner. In other words, procedures for information-gathering and analysis are not predetermined but are selected depending on which particular strategies will lead to the most truthful, rich and informative findings.

A number of nurse scholars have written about the application of bricolage to nursing practice. Mary Gobbi (2005), in her paper titled 'Nursing practice as bricoleur activity: A concept explored', suggests that the professional nurse as part of daily practice acts as a bricoleur in sifting through the most appropriate knowledge, skills, resources and strategies required to perform an intervention that is outside traditional practices because of the uniqueness of the situation and often conflicting influences. It is essentially like thinking on your feet in situations that have not been planned or anticipated. Such situations are part of everyday nursing practice. In summing up the place of bricolage within the context of nursing, Gobbi states:

> As practitioners... clinical care demands that they effectively manage the tensions and paradoxes of the different information sources and realities that emanate from each specific care situation. Furthermore, they have exhibited several characteristic features of the bricoleur. Namely, they manage complex, large and diverse tasks with the tools at hand; they get the job done, even it becomes a different one en-route; they put something of themselves into their care which is particularised to the person concerned; they are multiskilled and reflexive; and they have the capacity for ingenuity and inventiveness. (2005, p. 124)

The notion of researcher-as-bricoleur has not been without conjecture and criticism by adherents of traditional qualitative research methods. The main criticism is the apparent lack of a rigorous, systematic research method. However, argument in defence of a bricolage approach cites the numerous modifications made over time to such qualitative research methods as phenomenology, grounded theory and ethnography, as previously discussed. It may well be that future developments in qualitative research see the researcher-as-bricoleur as a generally accepted approach to research.

## Box 6.2

**REMOTE CARE**

Mrs Morgan is a 55-year-old Aboriginal woman who has been admitted to hospital for management of chronic pain as a result of a long history of decubitus leg ulcers. Mrs Morgan lives in a remote community in north-west Queensland. Prior to hospitalisation she has been treated by the flying doctor service, which has a scheduled monthly service to her community. On admission Mrs Morgan speaks of the difficulties in living daily with chronic pain. In talking with the nurse, she speaks of many members of her community who have similar problems, especially chronic pain as a consequence of long-term illness. She also reveals that there is little assistance provided by her local community or the government in attempting to stem the increase in the number of individuals who are developing long-term illness. When questioned about her ability to self-manage her illness and chronic pain, Mrs Morgan informs the nurse that women have no authority in their community to make changes or even to suggest to the elders what changes would be appropriate in order to improve the health of the community. She states further that she would like to be involved in making a change in the way things are done to enhance both individuals' and the community's quality of life. The nurse reflects on what Mrs Morgan has shared with her and comes to realise that she has no understanding of how this community is organised, including how members relate to each other, what are the important values of the group, and what processes are involved in making the community work together on a daily basis. At the end of the admission interview the nurse decides that there is a lot she does not know or understand about Mrs Morgan's and others' experience of pain and life in a remote Aboriginal community, the place of women in this society, how the social fabric of the community works, and what it means to be a nurse caring for this group of people.

From this case scenario think about what possible research studies could be conducted. Examples of possible studies could include:

1  The experiences of living daily with chronic pain.
2  Women's experiences of having no authority to be involved in bringing about changes to enhance quality of life in remote Aboriginal communities.
3  An exploration of the barriers to bringing about a change in community attitudes to long-term illness.

Questions that will assist you in undertaking research in this area could include:

1  What is the lived experience of coping with chronic pain as a result of long-term illness?
2  How can women in remote Aboriginal communities bring about community change for community health improvement?
3  What are the important values and social processes that hold Mrs Morgan's community together on a daily basis?

In relation to the specific questions presented above, identify the most appropriate research pathway or design to answer each of the research questions.

## Implications for evidence-based practice

In recent times there has been considerable debate about how best to evaluate qualitative research in terms of its applicability to clinical practice. Because of the nature of qualitative research, which is concerned with exploring the lived world of people in their everyday situations, identifying outcomes that can be measured for their effectiveness has proved to be problematic. However, there have been developments in establishing guidelines to evaluate the usefulness of qualitative research to clinical practice. The Joanna Briggs Institute has adopted the FAME scale developed by Alan Pearson, which consists of four dimensions: Feasibility, Appropriateness, Meaningfulness and Effectiveness (JBI 2003). Janice Morse (2003) has developed a comprehensive evaluation framework in which she stipulates a number of evaluation criteria and their dimensions. The Cochrane Collaboration also has the qualitative and implementation methods group. The group focuses on methods and process required in the synthesis of qualitative evidence. They have also developed the Cochrane Protocols for Qualitative and Implementation Research (Cochrane Collaboration 2014).

Qualitative research has much to offer the world of clinical practice, but in order to be accepted as a legitimate mode of enquiry by the scientific community, evidence of applicability to practice needs to be demonstrated. Qualitative researchers have taken on this challenge.

# SUMMARY

- Qualitative research has emerged in the past six decades as a substantive and credible scientific mode of enquiry.
- Since its inception in the early 19th century a number of qualitative research designs have been developed.
- Each design has its unique philosophical framework, particular focus, and methods of data collection and analysis.
- There is a range of research pathways from which to choose that fall under the umbrella of qualitative research.
- The researcher—neophyte or experienced—needs to have a sound knowledge about the various research pathways before selecting a particular approach to answer the research question.
- Qualitative research is a useful means of conducting research, especially for healthcare professionals, who work with individuals, families and communities across the health–illness spectrum, and across the human life cycle.

## PRACTICE EXERCISE 6.1

Discuss how grounded theory could be a useful research method for investigating the following areas of clinical practice:

a   Pain management (How do we provide appropriate pain management for our patients?)
b   Clinical decision-making (How do we go about making clinical decisions?)
c   Providing culturally safe care (How do we provide culturally safe care?)

ANSWER: The aim of grounded theory is to generate a framework or theory with explanatory power about an area of interest of which there is limited knowledge and understanding. The questions posed above may seem to be well researched, but when you search the literature on each topic you will notice that there is still considerable debate about best practice. Grounded theory can help fill such knowledge gaps by developing a theoretical understanding of such areas of professional practice.

## PRACTICE EXERCISE 6.2

In what ways can ethnography be used in nursing and healthcare research?

ANSWER: Ethnography is concerned with the study of a particular social or culture setting including the behaviours, meanings, attitudes and beliefs of a particular group of people within a cultural context. Ethnography can be used in nursing and healthcare research to explore patterns of caring, nurse–patient interactions, team collaboration and the decision-making practices of health professionals. What is important is that the notion of culture is central to the study.

PRACTICE EXERCISE 6.3

What aspects of nursing could benefit by using a critical social theory or feminist research perspective?

ANSWER: The aim of critical social theory and feminist research is to uncover or bring to the attention of others oppressive activities in society such as the oppression of women, masculine domination, marginalisation of minority groups, disempowerment of the poor and issues of social injustice, with the intent of emancipating or empowering such groups to be in charge of their own destiny. Nursing could benefit by conducting research about the status of women in nursing, exploring power relationships between medicine and nursing, or researching the issue of control between nurses and patients.

PRACTICE EXERCISE 6.4

What do you consider are areas of nursing and midwifery practice that could benefit by undertaking an action research project?

Action research is concerned with finding solutions to problems and bringing about practice change. Some of the areas in which you as a nurse could use action research include improving the nursing management of patients with diabetes, working with hospital management to improve hospital policies and developing strategies for improved discharge planning.

What do you consider some of the useful ways in which qualitative research can contribute to advancing nursing and midwifery knowledge?

HINT: Review the first few sections of this chapter.

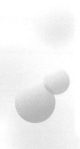

## FURTHER READING

Denzin, N. K. & Lincoln, Y. S. (eds) (1994). *Handbook of Qualitative Research.* Thousand Oaks, CA: SAGE Publications.

Leininger, M. (1985). *Qualitative Research Methods in Nursing.* New York: Grune & Stratton.

Liamputtong, P. (2009). *Qualitative Research Methods*, 3rd edn. Melbourne: Oxford University Press.

Ricoeur, P. (1976). *Interpretation Theory: Discourse and the Surplus of Meaning.* Fort Worth, TX: Texas Christian University Press.

## USEFUL WEBSITES

<www.qualitative-research.net/index.php/fqs>

The Forum Qualitative Sozialforschung (Forum Qualitative Social Research) is a peer-reviewed multilingual online journal for qualitative research. You can gain access to the journal free of charge.

<www.humanbecoming.org>

The International Consortium of Parse Scholars focuses on a humanbecoming school of thought. This is an important qualitative approach which has been used in nursing research. It aims to contribute to human health and quality of life through research and practice.

<http://qhr.sagepub.com>

SAGE publishes the *Qualitative Research Journal*, which can be useful for reviewing various published articles and discussion papers on various qualitative research issues.

<www.groundedtheoryreview.com>

The site of the *Grounded Theory Review.* This can be useful for readers who want to review the application of grounded theory in qualitative research.

## REFERENCES

Birks, M. & Mills, J. (2011). *Grounded Theory: A Practice Guide.* London: SAGE.

Bleicher, J. (1980). *Contemporary Hermeneutics.* London: Routledge & Kegan Paul.

Blumer, H. (1969). *Symbolic Intervention, Perspective and Method.* Englewood Cliffs, NJ: Prentice Hall.

Charmaz, K. (1990). Discovering chronic illness: Using grounded theory. *Social Science & Medicine* 30, 1161–72.

Charmaz, K. (2006). *Constructing Grounded Theory: A Practical Guide Through Qualitative Analysis.* London: SAGE Publications.

Cochrane Collaboration. (2014). *Cochrane Qualitative and Implementation Methods Group.* <http://cqim .cochrane.org>.

Crotty, M. (1998). *The Foundations of Social Research: Meaning and Perspective in the Research Process.* Sydney: Allen & Unwin.

Denison, J., Varcoe, C. & Browne, A. J. (2013). Aboriginal women's experiences of accessing health care when state apprehension of children is being threatened. *Journal of Advanced Nursing* 70(5).

Denzin, N. K. & Lincoln, Y. S. (2011). *The SAGE Handbook of Qualitative Research.* London: SAGE.

Dilthey, W. (1977). *Descriptive Psychology and Historical Understanding.* The Hague: Martinus Nijhoff.

Fetterman, D. M. (1989). *Ethnography: Step by Step.* Newbury Park, CA: SAGE Publications.

Gadamer, H. G. (1976). The universality of the hermeneutical problem. In L. E. Hahn (ed.), *The Philosophy of Hans-Georg Gadamer.* Chicago: Library of Living Philosophers vol. XXIV.

Germain, C. P. (2001). Ethnography. In P. Munhall (ed.), *Nursing Research. A Qualitative Perspective*, 3rd edn. Sudbury, MA: National League for Nursing.

Glaser, B. G. (1978). *Theoretical Sensitivity.* Mill Valley, CA: Sociology Press.

Glaser, B. G. (1992). *Emergence vs Forcing: Basics of Grounded Theory Analysis.* Mill Valley, CA: Sociology Press.

Glaser, B. G. & Strauss, A. L. (1967). *The Discovery of Grounded Theory: Strategies for Qualitative Research*. Mill Valley, CA: Sociology Press.

Glenn, L. A., Stocker-Schnieder, J., McCune, R., McClelland, M. & King, D. (2014). Caring nurse practice in the intrapartum setting: Nurses' perspectives on complexity, relationships and safety. *Journal of Advanced Nursing*.

Gobbi, M. (2005). Nursing practice as bricoleur activity: A concept explored. *Nursing Inquiry* 12(2), 117–23.

Hall, H., Griffiths, D. & McKenna, L. (2013). From Darwin to constructivism: The evolution of grounded theory. *Nurse Researcher* 20(3), 17–21.

Heidegger, M. (1962). *Being and Time*. New York: Harper & Row.

Husserl, E. (1962). *Ideas: General Introduction to Pure Phenomenology*. New York: Macmillan.

JBI (Joanna Briggs Institute). (2003). *About us*. <http://joannabriggs.edu.au/about/history.php>.

Leininger, M. (1978). *Transcultural Nursing: Concepts, Theories, and Practices*. New York: John Wiley & Sons.

Leininger, M. (1985). *Qualitative Research Methods in Nursing*. New York: Grune & Stratton.

Leininger, M. (1988). Leininger's theory of nursing: Cultural care diversity and universality. *Nursing Science Quarterly* 1(4), 152–60.

Leininger, M. (1991). The theory of culture care diversity and universality. In M. Leininger (ed.), *Culture Care Diversity and Universality: A Theory of Nursing*. New York: National League for Nursing Press, pp. 5–68.

Levi-Strauss, C. (1966). *The Savage Mind*. Chicago: University of Chicago Press.

Lewin, K. (1946). Action research and minority issues. *Journal of Social Issues* 2, 34–46.

Marx, K. (1961). *Selected Writings in Sociology and Social Philosophy*, 2nd edn, ed. T. B. Bottomore & M. Rubel. Harmondsworth: Penguin.

McLeod, J. (2001). *Qualitative Research in Counselling and Psychotherapy*. London: SAGE Publications.

Merleau-Ponty, M. (1962). *Phenomenology of Perception*, transl. C. Smith. New York: Humanities Press.

Merleau-Ponty, M. (1989). *Phenomenology of Perception*, ed. C. Smith, transl. J. O'Neill. Evanston, IL: Northwestern University Press.

Morse, J. M. (2003). A review committee's guide for evaluating qualitative proposals. *Qualitative Health Research* 13, 833–51.

Moustakas, C. E. (1990). *Heuristic Research: Design, Methodology, and Application*. Newbury Park, CA: SAGE.

Natanson, M. (1973). *Edmund Husserl: Philosopher of Infinite Tasks*. Evanston, IL: Northwestern University Press.

*New Webster's Encyclopedia of Dictionaries* (1990). Melbourne: Budget Books.

Patton, M. Q. (2002). *Qualitative Research and Evaluation Methods*, 3rd edn. London: SAGE Publications.

Polit, D. F. & Beck, C. T. (2004). *Nursing Research: Methods, Appraisal, and Utilization*, 7th edn. Philadelphia: Lippincott Williams & Wilkins.

Ricoeur, P. (1976). *Interpretation Theory: Discourse and the Surplus of Meaning*. Fort Worth, TX: Texas Christian University Press.

Ricoeur, P. (1981). *Hermeneutics and the Social Sciences*, ed. and transl. J. Thompson. Cambridge: Cambridge University Press.

Smith-Young, J., Solberg, S. & Gaudine, A. (2014). Constant negotiating: Managing work-related musculoskeletal disorders while remaining at the workplace. *Qualitative Health Research* 24(2), 217–31.

Sokolowski, R. (2000). *Introduction to Phenomenology*. Cambridge: Cambridge University Press.

Spradley, J. P. (1980). *Participant Observation*. New York: Holt, Rinehart & Winston.

Strauss, A. & Corbin, J. (1990). *Basics of Qualitative Research: Grounded Theory Procedures and Techniques*. Newbury Park, CA: SAGE.

Strauss, A. & Corbin, J. (1998). *Basics of Qualitative Research: Techniques and Procedures for Developing Grounded Theory*, 2nd edn. Thousand Oaks, CA: SAGE Publications.

Street, A. F. & Robinson, A. (1995). Advanced clinical roles: Investigating dilemmas and changing practice through action research. *Journal of Clinical Nursing* 10(3), 372–9.

Streubert, H. J. & Carpenter, D. R. (1995). *Qualitative Research in Nursing: Advancing the Humanistic Imperative*. Pennsylvania: J. B. Lippincott Company.

Streubert Speziale, H. J. & Rinaldi Carpenter, D. R. (2007). *Qualitative Research in Nursing: Advancing the Humanistic Imperative*, 4th edn. Philadelphia: Lippincott, Williams & Wilkins.

Taylor, B., Kermode, S. & Roberts, K. (2007). *Research in Nursing and Health Care: Evidence for Practice*, 3rd edn. Australia: Thomson.

Ullrich, S., McCutcheon, H. & Parker, B. (2014). Nursing practice in nutritional care: A comparison between a residential aged care setting and a hospital setting. *Journal of Advanced Nursing* 21 January.

Weinstein, D. & Weinstein, M. A. (1991). Georg Simmel: Sociological flaneur bricoleur. *Theory, Culture and Society* 8, 151–68.

CHAPTER 7

# DATA COLLECTION: QUALITATIVE RESEARCH

Anthony Welch and Sansnee Jirojwong

## KEY TERMS

participant
  observation
focus group
unstructured
  interview
semistructured
  interview
structured interview
open-ended
  question
bracketing
probing question
closed-ended
  question
triangulation

## CHAPTER LEARNING OBJECTIVES

By the end of this chapter you will be able to:

- identify data collection methods used in qualitative research
- align data collection methods with different approaches to qualitative research
- discuss the different approaches to interviewing
- discuss the use of triangulation as a means of data collection
- discuss the concepts of rigour and trustworthiness in relation to data collection methods in qualitative research.

## Introduction

Fundamental to credible research—research that produces appropriate, accurate and reliable data—is the method/s by which data are collected. Research studies can be meticulously designed and rigorously carried out, but unless the method/s of data collection are consistent with the chosen research question and research design, and gathered in a competent and transparent manner, the findings of a study may be challenged for accuracy, completeness and therefore credibility. Qualitative research is no exception. This chapter introduces you to the various methods and processes of data collection used in qualitative research.

Within the qualitative research paradigm there are various research designs that a researcher can use in search of new knowledge and understanding (see Chapter 6). Depending on the question being asked, the theoretical framework underpinning the study, the research design, the type of data and the method/s by which such data are collected vary. What is important is the relationship of these three elements of research.

Figure 7.1   The relationship of research design, type of data and data collection method

| The Research Design | ⟹ | The Types of Data | ⟹ | The Methods by which Data are Collected |
|---|---|---|---|---|

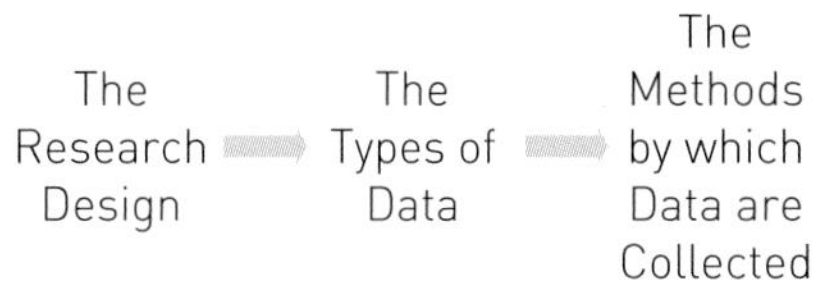

## Preparing for the process of data collection

An essential aspect of any study is to ensure that the data collection method is consistent with the research question, the philosophical underpinnings of the research design, and the best approach by which 'rich' data can be accessed to answer the research question. This requires careful planning by the researcher. In planning the process of data collection for a particular qualitative study, three elements are of primary importance: a review of literature on the topic or phenomenon, participant selection and the methods by which data will be collected.

Figure 7.2   Key elements of the data collection process

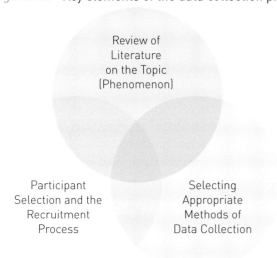

## Review of the literature

An important component of the data collection process is to review what is already known about the topic to be investigated and therefore to provide a context for the study. A review of literature is 'a systematic and rigorous exploration of the extant (existing) literature related to the concept(s) of interest' (Schneider et al. 2003, p. 28) to the researcher. In some instances the review of literature may lead to refining the research question, clarifying the research design, altering the process(es) of participant selection and choosing methods for data collection.

In qualitative research there is debate about the timing of a literature review. For instance, in phenomenological research, carrying out a literature review at the beginning of the study may lead to researcher bias. In grounded theory, however, a review of literature is made simultaneously with other methods of information-gathering such as interviews and **participant observation**.

## Selecting participants

In qualitative research the process by which participants are selected is based on obtaining rich in-depth information on the research topic, the setting in which the study is to take place and who the participants are. Depending on the target group, different sampling methods to accessing participants can be used (see Chapter 5).

# Choosing a mode(s) for data collection

The choice of which mode(s) of data collection is to be used is important for the type of data to be collected. Each mode provides a particular form of data. Modes of data collection in qualitative research include individual and **focus group** interviews, observation, narrative descriptions, case studies, histories, field notes, audio and audiovisual recordings, expressions of life or artistic representations such as art, poetry and music, and bricolage. Each of these modes provides unique avenues to accessing knowledge about an identified phenomenon or an issue of concern in the everyday world of human beings.

What is critical is ensuring that the right mode(s) is chosen for the type of study being undertaken and for the type or form of information required to answer the research question. A brief description of each of the types or forms of data collection used in qualitative research follows.

## Interviewing

Interviews are the most commonly used method of collecting data in qualitative research. Over time different interview methods have evolved to elicit particular forms of information. The interview methods can be perceived as 'on a continuum of structure ranging from highly structured to an unstructured' format (Taylor et al. 2006, p. 232). The use of a particular interview method is determined by the purpose of the study—the type of knowledge to be generated and the preferred means by which such information can be accessed. A number of terms have been assigned to particular methods of interview that have included '**unstructured**' or 'informal conversational'; '**semi-structured**', 'focused' or 'the general interview guide approach'; and '**structured**' or 'the standardised open-ended interview' (Patton 2002). However, the use of different terms to describe a particular method can be problematic for the novice researcher.

---

**Participant observation:** A method of qualitative research in which the researcher understands the contextual meanings of an event or events through participating and observing as a subject in the research. The degree of sharing in activities between the researcher and the participant ranges from full participation to onlooker.

---

**Focus group:** A form of qualitative research in which a group of people are asked about their perceptions, opinions, beliefs and attitudes towards a study topic. Questions are asked in an interactive group setting where participants are free to talk with other group members.

Clarification of the different terms assigned to a particular interview method requires discussion.

**Unstructured interview:** A method of interview where questions can be changed or adapted to meet the participant's understanding or belief. Questions can be influenced by each individual person's responses.

## TIPS AND SKILLS

The use of a particular method of interview or interview format is determined by the purpose of the study.

Figure 7.3    Frequently used methods of interview

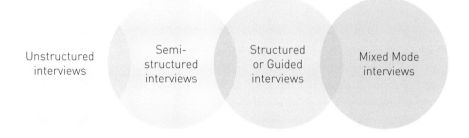

### The unstructured interview

Unstructured interviews can be used in a variety of contexts to elicit in-depth knowledge of a particular topic or experience. The essential format of an unstructured interview involves either presenting a statement or posing a question and asking the participant to comment from their perspective. The initial statement or question is the central focus of the enquiry. Any additional questions asked by the researcher are generated from the participant's comments or descriptions for the purpose of clarification and/or elaboration to ensure that the information is accurate and a good understanding or comprehension of what the participant is saying is achieved. 'What might be rude to ask or be glossed over in friendly agreement in ordinary conversation—even with intimates—becomes grist for exploration' (Charmaz 2006, p. 26). The interview is not controlled by the researcher but moves with the flow of what the participant wishes to share about the topic under investigation. The term 'unstructured' is generic in nature—an interview approach that can be used in a range of qualitative research designs. Examples of research designs in which unstructured interviews usually form an important part of the information-gathering process include phenomenology, ethnography and grounded theory (see Chapter 6).

**Semistructured interview:** A flexible set of questions which allow new questions to be brought up during the interview as a result of what the participant says. The interviewer in a semi-structured interview generally has a framework of the topic to be explored.

**Structured interview:** A formalised set of questions used to collect quantitative research data when the order in which questions are asked of survey respondents is standardised. It is also known as a standardised interview or a researcher-administered survey.

### The phenomenological interview

The phenomenological interview is a relatively new term that owes its origins to the North American phenomenological movement of the mid- to late 20th century. The phenomenological interview has become the 'tool' for accessing the experiences lived by human beings in the context of their everyday lives.

The goal of the phenomenological interview is to obtain a first-person description of a specified experience. Such an experience might focus on being ill, grieving the loss of a loved one or caring for a disabled child. The interview begins by asking the participant a question. The question is broadly stated to maximise the opportunity for the participant to respond in their own way by providing as full and rich a description of the phenomenon as possible. Such a question might be: What is your experience of being ill? Further questioning or comment by the researcher is concerned with seeking clarification about what the participant has described, or asking the participant to elaborate. An example of each type of question follows:

*Clarifying question:* You mentioned that being ill is a frustrating experience. Can you tell me what you mean by a frustrating experience?

*Elaborating question:* You mentioned you have been ill on a number of occasions. Can you tell me about those experiences?

What is essential to a phenomenological interview is to remain truthful to the subjective experiences of the participants. The researcher does not deviate by asking questions of particular interest to themselves which are not directly related to the focus of the study, but moves with the flow of the participant's description of the phenomenon of enquiry. In other words, 'all questions flow from the dialogue as it unfolds rather than having been predetermined in advance' (Pollio et al. 1997, p. 30). 'Why' questions are avoided because phenomenological enquiry is not concerned with causation. The introduction of a 'why' question has the potential to shift the focus of the discussion away from the actual experience of the phenomenon into unrelated areas that may ultimately compromise the findings.

Participants are viewed as co-researchers rather than research subjects (Giorgi 1989). The researcher is, in effect, a facilitator, assisting the participant to reflect on and provide the most comprehensive description of their experiences possible. Questions that facilitate an expanded discussion that contributes to achieving an information-rich, detailed description of participants' experiences could be:

'What was that experience like?'

'What was going through your mind at the time?'

'How did you feel when that occurred?'

In keeping with the principles of a rigorous and transparent approach to phenomenological research, two strategies or procedures have been identified to 'prevent, or at least minimise, the imposition of the researcher's presuppositions, and constructions on the data' (Crotty 1998, p. 83): the use of **open-ended questions** and the application of '**bracketing**'. The only form of questioning throughout the interview process should be open-ended. To bracket is to attempt to acknowledge and set aside any pre-understandings of the phenomenon to be studied before data-gathering starts and to remain vigilant throughout the study to ensure that the data are not contaminated by the intrusion of the researcher's own agenda and bias.

### Informal conversational interview

The informal conversational interview provides the researcher with 'maximum flexibility, spontaneity, and responsiveness to individual differences and situational changes' (Patton 2002, p. 343). Here the field of enquiry is regarded by the researcher as an open terrain for exploration. This form of information-gathering is sometimes referred to as unstructured or ethnographic interviewing. The term 'unstructured' is not to suggest that there is no intent or focus; on the contrary, although the interview is essentially a casual conversation, there is always 'a specific but implicit research agenda' (Fetterman 1989, p. 48). The researcher uses an informal approach as a means of accessing information.

Using an informal conversational interview approach, at the start of the study the researcher poses what Spradley and McCurdy (1972) term 'a grand tour question... designed to elicit a broad picture of the participant's...world, to map the cultural [or

---

**Open-ended question:** A form of question that requires the participant to answer in their own words. It allows a spontaneous, unstructured response and is sometimes called a subjective question.

---

**Bracketing:** The process of bringing to awareness, acknowledging and setting aside the researcher's assumptions and biases about the phenomenon being studied.

social] terrain' (p. 51). Such questions could be: Could you tell me about your family? Can you show me around your nursing unit? Such an interview approach is most useful in ethnographic research.

As part of data collection the researcher engages in a sifting-searching process of enquiry because the open nature of the interview means that the information given by each participant will be particular to that person in content and delivery. Over a number of interviews with various participants a large amount of information is generated that requires synthesising and clarifying. One means by which this can be achieved is through repeat interviews. If repeat interviews are required with participants, the format and direction of the questions may change from the original interview as more specific information is sought. The use of predetermined questions in this later stage of clarifying information may be necessary in order to build on existing knowledge of what is being studied and to situate that knowledge within a context.

Conducting an unstructured or informal conversational interview appears on the surface not difficult. However, it requires great skill from the interviewer in several areas: interpersonal communication; the ability to ask sensitive and **probing questions** without intruding into the personal space of another; the ability to rapidly synthesise information on the spot and generate questions in a reflexive and timely manner; the ability to remain focused on the purpose of the study while moving with the flow of the conversation; and holding in abeyance personal biases and preconceived ideas.

### Semi-structured interview

Semi-structured interviews are on a continuum between unstructured and structured interviews. They involve asking a certain number of predetermined open-ended questions about what is being researched without becoming prescriptive. Predetermined questions act as a guide to the interview, provide a systematic framework for exploring the topic, and enhance consistency in the process of data collection when more than one participant is involved (Patton 2002; Taylor et al. 2006). Additional questions may be asked by the researcher, but these are more of a probe to encourage participants to expand on what is being discussed. Using a semi-structured interview format assists the researcher to maintain a focus on the research topic and avoid deviating into areas not covered by the predetermined question guide.

At times during the interview the participant may wish to discuss a particular point or aspect of their experience that does not appear to the researcher to relate explicitly or directly to the focus of the study. In such situations the researcher respects the need of the participant to share such aspects of their experiences by providing a space within the interview for such a discussion. Such a discussion should not be dismissed by the researcher as irrelevant or simply a moment of 'wondering' on the part of the participant. What becomes important is for the researcher to ascertain whether there is a link or relationship between what is being discussed and the actual focus of the study. This can only be achieved by asking a question, such as: 'You have just described your feelings towards your wife. How do these feelings relate to the focus of this study, which is your experience of being ill?' If the researcher does not ask how the discussion relates to the focus of the study, important information may be dismissed by the researcher and so not be included as study data.

### Structured interview

Structured interviews are generally associated with quantitative research where specific, factual and objective data are required, the questions are **closed-ended**, and

**Probing question:** A question aimed to help the participant think more deeply about the study issue. It is used to search in-depth information or to make a thorough examination of the study topic.

**Closed-ended question:** A question that limits responses to predetermined categories. A closed-ended question will normally be answered using a simple 'yes/no', or 'strongly agreed/agreed/strongly not agreed/not agreed'.

the researcher has maximum control over the interview process. However, structured interviews can also be part of the data collection process in qualitative research.

Patton referred to the structured interview in qualitative research as 'the standardised open-ended interview' (2002, p. 344). The interview format involves asking a predetermined set of questions in a particular sequence (similar to an oral survey or questionnaire). The questions are designed and sequenced in the way they will be asked during the interview. The main difference from a questionnaire is that the questions are open-ended, giving the participant the opportunity to respond in their own terms rather than being confined to restricted responses as with closed-ended questions. If any clarification is required by the researcher the actual clarifying question/s must be included in the interview transcript (Patton 2002). If more than one interview is conducted, the same fixed sequence of questions must be used. In conducting structured qualitative or standardised open-ended interviews 'the fundamental principle of qualitative interviewing [must apply, which] is to provide a framework within which respondents can express their own understanding in their own terms' (Patton 2002, p. 348).

A weakness of this approach is that the enquiry is limited to a predetermined line of questioning. Unexpected information that might surface in the course of the interview cannot be pursued by the researcher.

### Mixed mode interview: Combining different methods of data collection

Depending on the design to be used in qualitative research, this form of interviewing is generally clearly prescribed, as discussed above. However, the use of different modes for data collection within a specific interview process does not have to be limited to one form. Depending on the purpose of the interview, different modes of data collection can be used. For instance, you may decide to conduct the first part of an interview in an unstructured manner, and later use a more structured approach to ask the participant to comment on some specific questions that you had drafted before the interview, or you could reverse the process by asking those questions initially, and then provide an opportunity for the participant to share what is important to them about the topic (Patton 2002). Another approach could be to combine targeted or closed-ended questions with open-ended questions to elicit in-depth data on a specific area of interest to the researcher.

A further combination of interview strategies could include the initial interview being unstructured with a second follow-up interview being more structured, focusing on specific questions that have arisen from the analysis of the initial interview. These questions may be about seeking clarification, elaboration or making further enquiry about the context of the data provided by the participant. What is important is to ensure that the strategies used by the researcher are consistent with the intent of the study and the interview.

Figure 7.4   Interview other than one to one

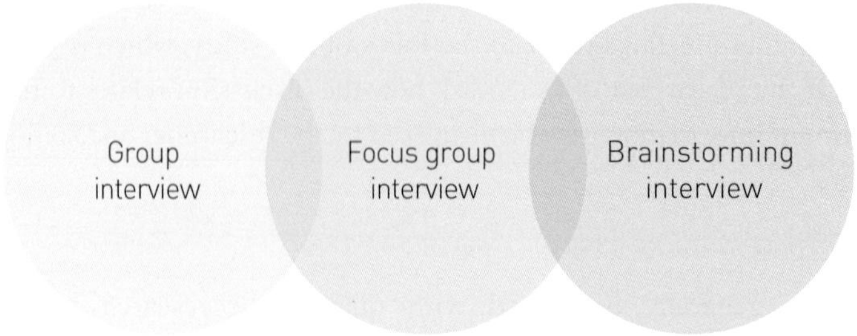

Group interview

Focus group interview

Brainstorming interview

## Group interview

Group interviews are another source of data collection in qualitative research. They can be used alone or in combination with other forms such as face-to-face interviews, participant observation or the administration of a questionnaire. The usual size of such groups is between six and eight members. Group interviews generally take two forms, focus groups or brainstorming groups, although there are various permutations to the way group interviews can be conducted.

## Focus group interview

'A focus group is a collection of people working together on a particular research issue' (Taylor et al. 2006, p. 410). Focus groups are used in both quantitative and qualitative research for collection of data. Their main purpose is to provide a forum for group members, deliberately chosen, to 'concentrate their collective intelligence' (p. 410) in responding to a particular research question or area of investigation. Focus group interviews are about 'people sharing their life experiences, preferences, intentions, and behaviours' (Fern 2001, p. 7). They provide 'the opportunity for multiple interactions not only between the interviewer and respondents but among all participants in the group' (Krueger 1994, p. 100). The format for conducting focus groups generally involves group members engaging in open discussion through the processes of attentive listening to other members' contributions, sharing their own insights and responding to what is being discussed within the group.

Because of the number of people involved in focus group interviews, and the need to maximise exploration of a particular research topic, procedural rules and processes need to be clearly defined and stated before the interview begins. This can be done by seeking the opinions of the participants about what is important for them in sharing their experiences within a group setting and working with the group to achieve a consensus. Concerns that may be raised by participating group members could be confidentiality among group members, being comfortable about speaking honestly without feeling judged, respecting each member's contributions to the discussion and feeling safe in the 'expert hands' of the interviewer.

Competence in conducting focus group interviews is therefore an important consideration for credibility in data collection. Richard Krueger (1994), an expert in focus group interviewing, suggests that the person conducting the interviews should be more of a facilitator/moderator than an interviewer. For Krueger the term moderator 'highlights a specific function of the interviewer—that of moderating or guiding the discussion…where the conversation flows because of the nurturing of the [group by the] moderator' (p. 100).

Because of the complex nature of focus group interviews, it is recommended that two members of the research team are involved, allowing one person to focus on facilitating/moderating/managing the group while the other deals with the mechanics such as recording, videoing and note-taking, or attending to the needs of group members such as debriefing people who have decided to discontinue their involvement or supporting members who have left the group in a distraught manner (Patton 2002).

## Brainstorming interview

If the intent is to canvass a broad sweep of ideas or attitudes about a particular topic in a free-flowing, creative and imaginative manner, brainstorming is an appropriate method of data collection. Such an approach to enquiry requires participants to be spontaneous and unrestricted in their responses to questions posed by the researcher-facilitator or to comments and questions from members of the group. The use of materials such as a whiteboard, computer, digital recorder or butcher's paper may be used to track the discussion and collate and synthesise the shared information.

### Narrative method

Narrative research has its origins in the human sciences. Its purpose is to gain insight into human stories or life events, with an emphasis on capturing the whole event or experience of the person or group of people (Parse 2001). During an interview narratives are captured in the participant's own language. The interview is conducted in such a way as to encourage the participant to describe the sequence of events that make up the whole story. The central assumption of narrative enquiry is that 'stories about life events shed light on the meanings of human experience' (Parse 2001, p. 43).

## Other modes of conducting interviews

In addition to forms of face-to-face interviews there are other means by which interviews can be conducted. These include telephone and internet (Skype) interviews.

### Telephone interview

A telephone interview is one alternative to a face-to-face interview; it is a less time-consuming means of data collection. The telephone interview can range from structured to unstructured depending on the type of data required for the study. What is important is to ensure that the researcher is able to obtain an accurate account of the participant's responses. This means listening attentively to what the person is saying, and being attuned to the tonal changes in voice and expression such as nuances, inflections, emphases and pauses in conversation, each of which provides a context for what the person is communicating. Because of the absence of visual contact with the person, audiotaping of the interview is recommended. If this is not possible, note-taking during and immediately after the interview by the researcher is required in order to minimise data loss. Audio-recording the researcher's account and insights of the interview would enhance the quality of data collected.

### Internet interview (Skype)

The use of Skype to conduct interviews is another alternative to face-to-face interviewing. The advantage of this approach over telephone interviewing is visual contact between participant and researcher—an important element in conducting in-depth conversational interviews. However, allowances need to be made for time delay and image distortion, which can be very disruptive to the flow of conversation and subsequent quality of data. The choice of Skype as a method of data collection should be based on the quality of data.

### Audiotaping and audiovisual recording of interviews

The preferred means of recording interviews for the purpose of research is by audiotaping and audiovisual recording. The tape-recorded interview gives the researcher the opportunity to listen to the recordings. What can be picked up through this process are the person's pauses, nuances such as emphasis on important points, and the general sense of what is being described. These are important considerations in capturing the participant's story of their experience. Audiovisual recording of interviews provides an additional source of information to that of the audiotaped interview. It is most useful in situations where the researcher is attempting to gain as full as possible a 'picture' of the interview discussion or when non-verbal cues are required for the analysis process (Taylor et al. 2006). Audiovisual recording also provides the researcher with an opportunity to revisit the interview as a learning tool for refining of interviewing skills, especially for researchers who are new to qualitative research.

## Observation

Observational methods of data collection are used in both quantitative and qualitative research. When the intent of the data collection process is to gain as complete a picture as possible of what is being studied, observation is often used. Observation as a method of data collection in qualitative research has its origins in anthropology. The practice of observation within anthropology has in more recent times been used in ethnography, ethnonursing and grounded theory. The purpose of observation is 'to seek detailed knowledge of the multiple dimensions of life within the studied milieu [natural setting] and to understand members' taken-for-granted assumptions [meanings] and rules' (Charmaz 2006, p. 21) from the perspective of those being observed.

### Choosing a form of observation for a study

Observation can take a number of forms, as presented in Figure 7.5. Depending on the type of data the researcher requires for the study, the form(s) of observation will differ. The form(s) selected by the researcher are crucial to the aims of the study and the quality of data required.

Figure 7.5   Different forms of observation

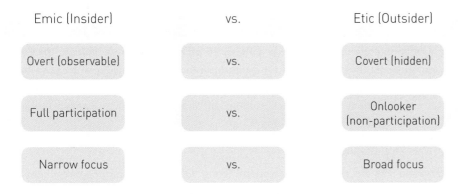

### Emic versus etic view

The word 'emic' refers to an insider's perspective or point of view. 'An emic perspective compels the recognition and acceptance of multiple realities…which is crucial to an

---

**●.THINKING DEEPLY**

The purpose of observation is to obtain information about the environment and the context of the participants' activities and interactions.

understanding of why people think and act in the different ways they do' (Fetterman 1989, p. 31). An emic perspective focuses on a particular social or cultural situation.

The companion term 'etic' refers to an outsider's perspective or point of view. A point of professional distance from the actual setting provides an objective perspective. An etic perspective allows a comparison between similar situations or cultures.

There has been considerable debate about the value of each approach, but the general consensus is that both perspectives are integral to an understanding of the setting as each perspective contributes different forms of knowledge.

### Overt versus covert observation

Overt and covert forms of observation have been used in qualitative research as methods of data collection. Overt observation requires full disclosure to the participants that they are being observed for the purpose of research. Covert observation is the non-disclosure to participants that they are to be observed as part of the study. Considerable debate has taken place over the years about the value of both forms of observation. Informing participants that their behaviour will be observed may lead to the participants not behaving in their normal everyday manner, resulting in distortion of what is observed. On the other hand, covert observation captures the natural everyday behaviour of participants. However, not disclosing the researcher's intent to observe participant behaviour has been considered to be ethically wrong (Patton 2002). There is a global move to outlaw research that engages in such apparently deceptive practices.

### Full participation versus the onlooker

Full participation requires immersion in the research setting. Ideally the researcher lives and works in the community being studied for a period of time during which they become part of the community, internalising social norms, beliefs, attitudes and ritualistic behaviours. Where possible the researcher feels, thinks and acts as one of the group (Patton 2002). Through this process of immersion the researcher is able to gain insights into and understanding of the cultural/social setting and way of life of the group or community. At the other end of the continuum the researcher adopts the position of an onlooker—someone who assumes a position of detached observer in order to gain an objective view of what is going on. The choice of what position the researcher wishes to take depends on the type of data being sought.

### Narrow versus broad focus

Observation can be narrow or broad in focus. Depending on the purpose of the study, the researcher may choose to come from either angle. In general, however, the researcher first takes a broad look at what is occurring in the research setting, noting down observations in order to gain an overview of what is taking place, such as the way members interact with each other. Once the researcher has developed a broad sense of what is going on they may decide to home in on a particular aspect in order to have an in-depth understanding. Both forms of observation complement each other and therefore are usually used in combination.

### Field notes

Field notes are an essential means of data collection, especially in situations of observation such as an ethnographic study. The purpose of field notes is to document all that the researcher observes during the enquiry. Field notes are descriptions of what has taken place and what is considered by the researcher to be important information for future reference during the process of analysis. It is primarily descriptive in nature, without interpretation. What is described may include the context of the event or situation, the interactions that take place, what is actually said, the researcher's own feelings, thoughts and reactions to what has taken place, and insights gleaned through researcher reflections (Patton 2002).

## Other methods of data collection

### Case study method

A case study approach occurs in both qualitative and quantitative studies. The focus of a case study is on a particular phenomenon or issue of concern in a particular person, a number of persons, groups or institutions over time. Methods for undertaking a case study along with data collection vary depending on the focus and parameters of the research. Case study research draws on a range of information sources that may include interviews, observation, records, historical documents and statements by others in order to assemble a comprehensive bank of data and to contextualise the information (Patton 2002). The data can be both quantitative and qualitative in nature.

### Historical method

Historical research is concerned with exploring a particular event or events and trends over time. The validity of historical research relies on the truthfulness or legitimacy of the information sources. Information sources have been categorised as primary—the original source(s) of data, and secondary—sources once removed from the primary source (Schafer 1980). Data collection therefore may involve oral history, archival documents, government reports, artworks and photography, to name a few.

### The arts as a source of data

Within the domain of qualitative research, in particular phenomenology, the arts are recognised as an avenue for data collection in advancing knowledge of the human condition—the affairs of the everyday world of human beings. The arts (referred to as 'expressions of life' by Dilthey [1977]) include but are not limited to literary works, the visual arts, music and drama. These art forms have been part of human experience throughout recorded history. Each of them has been a vehicle through which human experience has been expressed in personally significant ways (Dilthey 1977).

Figure 7.6    Different art forms as sources of data

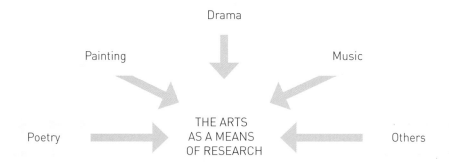

Poetry is concerned with how humans seek meaning in experience (Knights 1995). It is a mode of expression through which personal hopes and dreams, amid the uncertainties and confusions of life, are rendered intelligible. Knights (1995) suggests that poetry is a form of praxis: finding a way to speak the things a person needs to say through reflective action. Freire (1972) describes such action as critical self-insertion into the reality of one's own situation, opening up the potential for insight and personal transformation. Human experience expressed in verse is a potent means of sharing one's personal world with others.

Painting as an 'expression of life' can be traced back to the cave dwellings of our Palaeolithic ancestors living between 30 000 and 8000 BCE. Down the millennia painting has remained a major vehicle of expression through which the everyday world of human beings is portrayed. Panzine (1955, p. 9) suggests that '[a]rt follows life as the shadow follows the body'. Painting has the power to overcome distance and time and to engage the viewer in a dialogue with the 'author-painting' as if they were contemporary partners with the viewer (Gadamer 1997, pp. 545–6).

Music reaches beyond word in evoking and expressing the tones, rhythms and patterns of human existence as lived in the everyday world of humans. Music has the ability to evoke and reveal human experience that otherwise would remain silent. Music is human beings' oldest form of expression, older than word or art (Menuhin & Davis 1979). Throughout history human beings have woven the tonal world of music into the fabric of everyday life marked by experiences of birth, joy, hope, sadness, suffering and loss.

'For most of history, music has been elevated to the highest place in society…It was [and continues to be] the essential ingredient of public ceremony and celebration. It served occasions of grief. It was [and is] there for public and private fun. It marked the days. People's lives revolved [and continue to revolve] around it' (Blackwood 1991, p. 12). Langer (1953) posits that 'the tonal world of music bears a close resemblance to the ebb and flow of human feelings—a tonal analogue of emotive life' (p. 27). In other words, 'music is a mode of thought—a way of thinking in tones' (Ferguson 1982, p. 1).

Drama in the form of theatrical performance can also be included as an expression of life. Drama is both representation and illumination of life themes—love, hope, despair, tragedy. It provides a space in which the presumed and familiar can be challenged, creating a renewal of perception and awareness (Cox & Theilgaard 1994). Drama invites one to engage with the perspectival world—a world of multiple perspectives. Poole (1972) crystallises such a conception in stating: 'We are all conscious that there is only one world, but we are also quite sure that we all see it differently, we all interpret it differently, and we all attribute differing meanings to it at various times' (p. 89).

Expressions of life—poetry, painting, music and drama—are potent media for explicating human experiences that cannot be illuminated through everyday language. Dewey (1958) supports such a belief: 'In the end works of art are the only media of communication between man and man that can occur in a world of gulfs and walls that limit community of experience' (p. 105).

As expressions of life, the arts have a significant part to play in expanding understanding of the world of human beings. In research the arts have the potential to contribute to the development of new knowledge. The use of the arts is now recognised as an important source of data collection within qualitative research. Data collection using the arts can take many forms. These may be used as an adjunct to an interview where the participant is asked to share an art form that best conveys their experience of the phenomenon under study. This approach can be very useful when a participant has difficulty expressing what they wish to communicate or in situations where language is a barrier. Participants may wish to engage in an artistic expression to convey their experience such as dance, singing, drawing or making a montage (Taylor et al. 2006). Researchers may decide to use art forms such as painting or music as a vehicle for asking participants to share their thoughts and feelings about the subject matter. The arts as symbolic representations of a person's experience can be a potent source of research data.

## Implications for evidence-based practice

Qualitative research makes a significant contribution to evidence-based practice by providing in-depth information about the perceptions, expectations and experiences of healthcare consumers concerning the quality of healthcare they have received. Qualitative research complements quantitative research in providing a different source of knowledge about quality care and how the outcomes of healthcare can be evaluated.

## THINKING DEEPLY

### Self-management of gestational diabetes

Jirojwong and others (2008) explored Southeast Asian migrant women's responses and experiences of having gestational diabetes. A qualitative study was used and aimed to describe how Cambodian, Laotian, Thai and Vietnamese women use information from health professionals to self-manage their illness during pregnancy. Nineteen women participated in the study, recruited at two major hospitals in Sydney. An individual face-to-face interview was conducted at a place nominated by participants. The following broad questions were used:

- When you were told that you had high blood sugar, what was your feeling? Why did you feel that way?
- How do you feel now?
- What have you done to make you change or not change your feelings?
- In your opinion, what is the effect of having high blood sugar on your own health and the health of your baby? Give examples. (REASSURE CONFIDENTIALITY)
- In your opinion, what are the causes of your high blood sugar? There is no right or wrong answer.
- What do you think are the effects of having high blood sugar on your own health in 10 or 15 years? Give examples. (REASSURE CONFIDENTIALITY)
- What do you think are the effects of having high blood sugar on your baby's health in 10 or 15 years? Give examples. (REASSURE CONFIDENTIALITY)

An interview was about one hour and audio-recorded. Later it was transcribed verbatim. Field notes and diary were used to record observation information. Data were analysed using content analysis to identify themes and categories (Miles & Huberman 1994). The steps described by Miles and Huberman were used.

Source: Adapted from Jirojwong et al. 2008

Bricolage

Bricolage is an approach to enquiry (see Chapter 6) that uses a broad sweep of data collection methods. The researcher or bricoleur is not restricted to one stipulated approach but selects the most appropriate methods for obtaining data (McLeod 2001). Such an approach begins with the researcher engaging in a process of open receptiveness without predetermining what avenues will be required. In other words, procedures other than the initial method of data collection are not established before the enquiry but are selected depending on what particular strategies will lead to the most truthful, rich and informative data. Openness and creativity are at the core of data collection. The researcher interacts with each new piece of information, after which a decision is made about what further data are needed and what is the best way to obtain them. The methods of data-gathering are not ad hoc but a discerning, carefully thought out process.

## Triangulation in data collection

**Triangulation:** The process of integrating the results from multiple sources of data or research methods in the same study.

**Triangulation** is a process of using two or more methods for either data collection or data analysis in order to strengthen a study. The rationale for the use of triangulation has been put forward by Denzin (1978, p. 28): 'Because each method reveals different aspects of empirical reality, multiple methods…must be employed. This is termed triangulation. I…offer as a final methodological rule the principle that multiple methods should be used in every investigation.' The word is a metaphor from engineering surveying, where readings are taken from several viewpoints.

Types of triangulation that come under the umbrella of methodological triangulation include data triangulation, investigator triangulation and theoretical triangulation. For the purpose of this chapter the focus is on data triangulation.

Figure 7.7    Three major types of triangulation

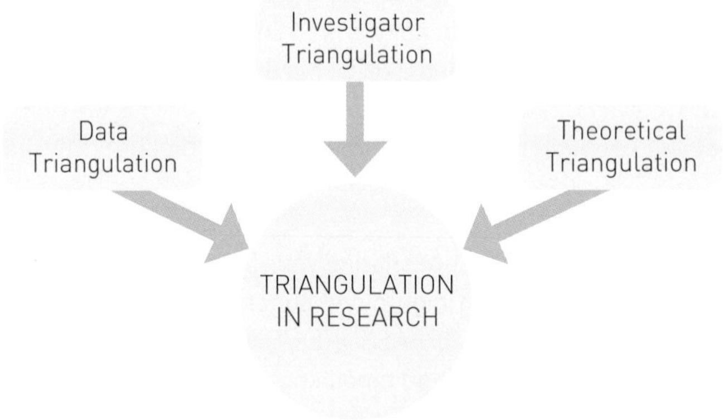

Data triangulation is concerned with the use of more than one method of data collection in one research study (Begley 1996). Within the domain of qualitative research there are a number of different approaches to this.

As outlined above, data triangulation can take a range of forms depending on the type of data sources required to answer the research question. Different combinations are often used; for example, in grounded theory data are collected from interviews (face-to-face and focus groups), observation and the researcher's field notes. In ethnographic research data are collected from interviews, observation, field notes, artefacts and the researcher's diary about their personal experiences of being immersed within a setting or culture. In phenomenological research face-to-face focus group interviews and the arts can be used in combination. Case studies often draw on a range of information sources. Contemporary documents (Bergen & While 2000) are also used.

## TIPS AND SKILLS

In using triangulation as a process for data collection it is important to ensure that the selected data collection methods are appropriate for answering the research question.

Data triangulation also includes obtaining data from individuals, groups, communities, documents, artistic expressions, photographs and diaristic accounts of participants' experiences to name a few. An example could be that if you as the researcher wanted to explore the experience of caring for a dying person at home, you might consider not only interviewing the primary carer, but also the person being cared for. You might even expand the study to include the community nurse who is also involved in the care of the person, as well as family members who live in the house.

Data collection in a mixed method research study is collected from both the quantitative and qualitative domains, for example the use of questionnaires followed by in-depth interviews or vice versa.

In using triangulation as a process for data collection it is important to ensure that selected data collection methods are appropriate for answering the research question.

## THINKING DEEPLY

Oliffe and Bottorff (2007) used photographs to assist men with prostate cancer describing their health and illness experiences. An individual interview focusing on the photographs helped the researchers collect unique data on this sensitive health issue.

### Implications for evidence-based practice

Foster and colleagues (2013) conducted a metasynthesis to explore the attitudes, experiences and implementation of family-centred care from many studies. They aimed to facilitate a better understanding of this practice from a sample of parents, hospitalised children and their healthcare providers within a paediatric critical care setting. Based on their review, a range of data collection methods including personal in-depth interview and focus group were used. Data obtained from participants about their experiences leading up to hospitalisation and admission highlighted the importance of pre-hospital and entry into hospital in providing quality person-centred care.

# Rigour and trustworthiness

The term 'rigour' refers to 'the strictness in judgement and conduct that must be used to ensure that the successive steps in a project have been set out clearly and undertaken with scrupulous attention to detail, so that the results/findings/insights can be "trusted"' (Taylor et al. 2006). The concept of rigour in qualitative research can be traced back to the works of Guba and Lincoln (1981), who believed that the terms 'validity' and 'reliability' denoting rigour in quantitative research were not the appropriate language to reflect the philosophical 'fit' in determining rigour in qualitative research. The term 'trustworthiness' was introduced by Lincoln and Guba (1985) to express the central nature of rigour in qualitative enquiry. 'Trustworthiness of the data is tied directly to the trustworthiness of the person who collects and analyses the data—and his or her demonstrated competence...[in] building a "track record" for quality work' (Patton 2002, p. 570).

In order to achieve trustworthiness in data collection in qualitative research, a number of key elements need to be demonstrated: researcher competence; transparency of the research process—the decision trail; and congruence between the selected philosophical and methodological approaches for a particular study.

Quality of research data is dependent on researcher competence. Three aspects are of particular importance here: having an informed understanding of the philosophical underpinnings of the theoretical framework to be used for the study; being able to discern the appropriate data collection strategies; and being appropriately skilled in the use of the selected data collection methods.

Beginning the process of data collection without having a solid grasp of the theoretical framework or ontology (underlying values and beliefs) informing the study has the potential to compromise the study's integrity. Each theoretical framework within qualitative research has its own underlying values and beliefs about how a study should be conducted. Failure to have such an understanding before beginning a study inevitably leads to errors in the focus of the data collection process. An example would be choosing a phenomenological approach to enquiry to explore the phenomenon of everyday lived experience of women when the intent of the researcher is to explore the broader experience of social inequality for women.

In addition to theoretical competence, the researcher also needs to be competent in selecting the appropriate data-gathering methods for the study. The methods of data collection need to be consistent with the theoretical framework underpinning the study.

Transparency in the decision-making processes of the researcher is fundamental to credibility. This can be achieved by the researcher maintaining ongoing documentation of the decision trail (audit trail) concerning data collection and analysis throughout the course of the study. In terms of data collection, any issues in the process need to be carefully documented.

A final and critical point is researcher competence in the use of data collection methods. The range of data collection methods in qualitative research can provide significant challenges to the new researcher or even to the advanced researcher who is not familiar with the processes involved in the selected data collection methods. It is therefore incumbent on the researcher to acquire the necessary competence to ensure the collection of quality data. Failure to do so has the potential to compromise the integrity of the study.

# SUMMARY

- There are various methods for collecting qualitative data.
- An important component of the data collection process is to review what is already known about the topic to be investigated and therefore to provide a context for the study.
- The choice of which mode(s) of data collection to be used for a particular study is determined by the type of information required to answer the research question.
- The choice of the most appropriate data collection method/s for a particular study needs to take into consideration the philosophy underpinning the research, the research question/s and the research design.
- Methods of data collection in qualitative research include interview, observation, case study, historical method, the arts and bricolage.
- One or more data collection methods can be used in a single study.
- Triangulation, rigour and trustworthiness are important aspects when assessing the evidence generated from qualitative research.

## PRACTICE EXERCISE 7.1

Ann and her team are preparing to conduct a research project that aims to explore the meaning of chest pain and the decision process patients used before presenting at the hospital emergency department. Major issues that they intend to explore include social support and help-seeking behaviours of the patients. The team will interview participants at their own homes. In addition to an interview schedule with open-ended questions, what else do you think could be methods of data collection?

ANSWER: Diary, hospital records, drawing to express the participants' illness experiences.

## PRACTICE EXERCISE 7.2

You have been invited to join a research team to conduct a study about pain management practices in your facility. The purpose or aim of the proposed study is to identify the ways in which nurses provide pain relief for patients with chronic pain. You are asked by the head of the research team to explore the most effective means of data collection and to give a reason for your choice(s).

ANSWER: It is assumed that this study is conducted in a healthcare setting such as a hospital or a long-term care facility. Hospital records and an individual in-depth interview with participants can be the data collection methods. Hospital records can be used as an initial point of data collection about the participants' documentation of the ways in which they have provided pain relief for their patients as well as giving important information to guide the interview process. The interview offers an opportunity to gain in-depth information about the participants' experiences of providing pain relief to patients with chronic pain. The method of an interview (unstructured interview, informal conversational interview or mixed mode interview) is influenced by the aim of the research.

## PRACTICE EXERCISE 7.3

John is a survivor of prostate cancer. He is part of a research team investigating illness experiences and help-seeking behaviours by men with positive screening for prostate cancer. List at least one issue that can influence the rigour and trustworthiness of data collected by John.

ANSWER: Personal experiences of the illness, his current health condition, method of data collection (e.g. personal in-depth interview compared to using participants' diary).

## FURTHER READING

Berg, B. L. (2007). *Qualitative Research Methods for the Social Sciences*. Boston: Pearson.

Burgess, R. G. (1987). *In the Field: An Introduction to Field Research*. London: Allen & Unwin.

Pelto, P. & Pelto, G. (1978). *Anthropological Research: The Structure of Inquiry*. Cambridge: Cambridge University Press.

## USEFUL WEBSITES

<http://qhr.sagepub.com>

SAGE publishes *Qualitative Research Journal*, which can be useful for reviewing various published articles and discussion papers on various qualitative research issues.

<www.srcd.org>

The Society for Research in Child Development which has a number of useful issues relating to research among children.

## REFERENCES

Begley, C. (1996). Using triangulation in nursing research. *Journal of Advanced Nursing* 24(1), 122–8.

Bergen, A. & While, A. (2000). A case for case studies: Exploring the use of case study design in community nursing research. *Journal of Advanced Nursing* 31, 926–34.

Blackwood, A. (1991). *Music of the World*. Oxford: Facts on File.

Charmaz, K. (2006). *Constructing Grounded Theory: A Practical Guide through Qualitative Analysis*. London: SAGE Publications.

Cox, M. & Theilgaard, A. (1994). *Shakespeare as Prompter: The Amending Imagination and the Therapeutic Process*. London: Jessica Kingsley.

Crotty, M. (1998). *The Foundations of Social Research: Meaning and Perspective in the Research Process*. Sydney: Allen & Unwin.

Denzin, N. K. (1978). *The Research Act: A Theoretical Introduction to Sociological Methods*, 2nd edn. New York: McGraw-Hill.

Dewey, J. (1958). *Art as Experience*. New York: Capricorn Books.

Dilthey, W. (1977). *Descriptive Psychology and Historical Understanding*, transl. R. M. Zaner & K. L. Heiges. The Hague: Martinus Nijhoff.

Ferguson, D. (1982). *A History of Musical Thought*. Westport, CN: Greenwood.

Fern, E. F. (2001). *Advanced Focus Group Research*. London: SAGE.

Fetterman, D. M. (1989). *Ethnography: Step by Step*. Newbury Park, CA: SAGE.

Foster, M. J., Whitehead, L., Maybee, P. & Cullens, V. (2013). The parents', hospitalized child's, and health care providers' perceptions and experiences of family centered care within a pediatric critical care setting: A metasynthesis of qualitative research. *Journal of Family Nursing* 19(4), 431–68.

Freire, P. (1972). *Cultural Action for Freedom*. Harmondsworth: Penguin.

Gadamer, H. G. (1997). The philosophy of Hans-Georg Gadamer. In L. E. Hahn (ed.), *The Library of Living Philosophers*, vol. XXIV. Illinois: Open Court.

Giorgi, A. (1989). Some theoretical and practical issues regarding the psychological phenomenological method. *Saybrook Review* 7, 71–85.

Guba, E. & Lincoln, Y. (1981). *Effective Evaluation*. San Francisco: Jossey-Bass.

Jirojwong, S., Schmied, V., Hannah, D. & Johnson, M. (2008). Health literacy and self management of gestational diabetic: A study among Vietnamese, Cambodian, Thai and Laotian women in Sydney. Research proposal submitted to College of Health and Science, Sydney: University of Western Sydney.

Knights, B. (1995). *The Listening Reader: Fiction and Poetry for Counsellors and Psychotherapists*. Pennsylvania: Jessica Kingsley.

Krueger, R. A. (1994). *Focus Group Interviews: A Practical Guide for Applied Research*, 2nd edn. Southern Oaks, CA: SAGE.

Langer, S. K. (1953). *Feeling and Form: A Theory of Art Development from Philosophy in a New Key*. London: Routledge & Kegan Paul.

Lincoln, Y. S. & Guba, E. G. (1985). *Naturalistic Inquiry*. Beverly Hills, CA: SAGE Publications.

McLeod, J. (2001). *Qualitative Research in Counselling and Psychotherapy*. London: SAGE.

Menuhin, Y. & Davis, C. (1979). *The Music of Man*. Toronto: Methuen.

Miles, B. M. & Huberman, A. M. (1994). Introduction: Three approaches to qualitative data analysis. In B. M. Miles & A. M. Huberman (eds), *An Expanded Sourcebook: Qualitative Data Analysis*. London: SAGE Publications, pp. 8–12.

Oliffe, J. L. & Bottorff, J. L. (2007). Further than the eye can see? Photo elicitation and research with men. *Qualitative Health Research* 17, 850–8.

Panzine, A. (1955). In W. Boeck & J. Sabartes (eds), *Picasso*. New York: Harry N. Abrahams.

Parse, R. (2001). *Qualitative Inquiry: The Path of Sciencing*. Boston: National League for Nursing.

Patton, M. (2002). *Qualitative Research and Evaluation Methods*, 3rd edn. Thousand Oaks, CA: SAGE Publications.

Pollio, H., Tracy, H. & Thompson, C. (1997). *The Phenomenology of Everyday Life*. Cambridge: Cambridge University Press.

Poole, R. (1972). *Towards Deep Subjectivity*. London: Allen Lane.

Schafer, R. J. (1980). *A Guide to Historical Method*. Homewood, IL: Dorsey Press.

Schneider, Z., Elliot, D., LoBiondo-Wood, G. & Haber, J. (2003). *Nursing Research: Methods, Critical Appraisal, and Utilization*, 2nd edn. Sydney: Mosby.

Spradley, J. P. & McCurdy, D. W. (1972). *The Cultural Experience: Ethnography in Complex Society*. Chicago: Science Research Associates.

Taylor, B., Kermode, S. & Roberts, K. (2006). *Research in Nursing and Health Care: Evidence for Practice*, 3rd edn. Australia: Thomson.

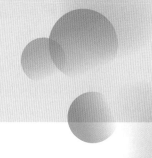

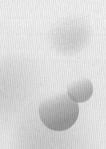

CHAPTER 8

# QUALITATIVE DATA ANALYSIS

Lisa Whitehead

Lisa Whitehead

## KEY TERMS

methodology
familiarisation
theme
code
constant
 comparison
theoretical
 saturation
audit trail

## CHAPTER LEARNING OBJECTIVES

By the end of this chapter you will be able to:

- understand the differences between various approaches to qualitative data analysis, including grounded theory, ethnography and phenomenology
- apply information on data analysis by working through the early stages of analysis
- generate awareness of processes that can be used to improve and demonstrate trustworthiness in qualitative analysis
- understand the practicalities and resource demands involved in qualitative data analysis
- become familiar with the functions of qualitative data analysis software.

# Introduction

All data that are collected in the course of a research study require some form of analysis in order to draw out collective meaning. In qualitative research, data collection can take many forms: face-to-face interviews, focus groups, photographs and explanation (photovoice), the arts objects (painting, poetry and music), video, diaries, field notes and internet-based interviews. There are a number of approaches to qualitative data analysis and the approach taken for any given study will be determined by the **methodology** guiding the study (see Chapter 6). The researcher is likely to take one of three broad approaches to qualitative analysis:

1   The number of times a particular word or concept, for example 'fatigue', occurs in narrative would be counted. The qualitative data can then be categorised and if required statistical analysis undertaken. This kind of analysis is referred to as content analysis.

2   A thematic analysis would explore data further than the first example. All data referring to a concept, for example 'stigma', would be given a code, extracted and examined in more detail.

3   In a theoretical analysis such as grounded theory, the researcher would analyse the data further to generate an emerging **theory**. The theory may be tested against existing theories or against further analysis of the data, a process referred to as analytic induction (Strauss & Corbin 1990).

Regardless of the approach to qualitative data analysis, there are a number of general considerations.

**Methodology:** The theoretical or philosophical framework that underpins and guides the research process throughout the study; the principles that embody a research approach and guide the researcher in the application of methods.

# The stages of qualitative analysis

Analysis of qualitative data usually goes through some or all of the following stages:

*   **familiarisation** with the data through reading, watching and/or listening
*   transcription of recorded material
*   organising and indexing of data for easy retrieval and identification
*   anonymisation of sensitive data
*   coding
*   identification of **themes**
*   re-coding
*   development of provisional categories
*   exploration of relationships between categories
*   refinement of themes and categories
*   development of theory and incorporation of pre-existing knowledge.

**Familiarisation:** The process of becoming familiar with the data. The process often begins by transcribing the data, reading and rereading the transcript and continuing on through the process of analysis.

# Theories and methods

Where a researcher has adopted a design, such as grounded theory, to inform a study, the process of data analysis will be driven by the framework of that design. The researcher may choose to follow general inductive principles of qualitative research and in this case may choose to draw on a generic approach such as thematic analysis. The particular approach chosen will be guided by a number of considerations including the research

**Theme:** A theme is generated when similar ideas from participants expressed in the data are brought together. The theme may be labelled using a word or expression taken directly from the data or else named by the researcher to best characterise the collection of data.

question and the data collection method. This section explores the process of data analysis as it relates to a general approach through thematic analysis and then on to three key designs in qualitative research: grounded theory, phenomenology and ethnography.

## Thematic analysis

Many qualitative researchers draw on thematic analysis to analyse qualitative data. This may be as part of a wider methodological design such as ethnography, or as a stand-alone design. There are several approaches to thematic analysis in circulation and this section will outline the general features of inductive thematic analysis.

An interview is generally prepared for analysis by a verbatim transcription. A numbering system such as line numbers is often applied to help locate text throughout the analysis and reporting processes. The transcript may be printed out for analysis or imported into a software package such as NVivo and viewed electronically. Once the text has been read a number of times and the researcher is familiar with the content, the next step is to identify specific sections of the text. This is termed 'coding' and refers to highlighting sections of the text that relate to the research question/s and/or appear to be meaningful. These sections may be a word, a phrase or a whole passage; it depends on the researcher's approach and the data as to how many data are highlighted in order to maintain the context of the situation or experience described. Once the transcript has been read a number of times, and the words, phrases or passages that describe the experience or context have been studied, the process of coding is undertaken, often on a number of transcripts, **codes** are then reviewed and, if appropriate, themes generated.

Themes may be developed in one of three ways. First, theory-driven, where the researcher seeks to explore the application of a theory to the data collected. Second, from previous research, where the researcher seeks to explore and compare themes generated through previous research. Third, inductively from the raw data, to explore the data without any consciously expressed predetermined interest. These three approaches can be considered on a continuum from theory-driven at one end to data-driven at the other. The latter approach is the most common and is discussed further below.

Inductive themes may be derived from the research aims of the study and more specific themes derived from multiple readings of the raw data. One section of text may be coded into more than one theme and sections of text may not be coded at all if they do not relate to the aims of the study (see Practice exercise 8.4). Generally, the creation and assignment of themes to the text continues through a number of readings and undergoes revision as the analysis evolves. A number of sub-themes may emerge as the meaning of an initial theme becomes more complex through the analysis of further texts. Quotations are usually selected to illustrate the essence of the theme. While there are no rules about the number of themes that may be developed in a given study, when a large number of themes are generated the researcher should carefully evaluate whether these themes are able to stand alone without overlap. Where overlap appears to exist, the researcher may be able to combine themes to enhance clarity. Depending on the aims of the study, the researcher may choose to present the themes descriptively or interpret them in the context of a theory or conceptual framework as befits the method employed in the study.

While presented as a linear, step-by-step process (Table 8.1), thematic analysis is an iterative and reflexive process.

**Code:** A name given to data that have been separated into component parts.

**Table 8.1**   Stages of thematic analysis

| Stage 1 | Stage 2 | Stage 3 | Stage 4 | Stage 5 |
|---|---|---|---|---|
| Multiple readings of the data to generate familiarisation | Recognising and noting important, interesting and relevant data | Generating themes to capture the qualitative richness of the phenomenon noted in stage 2 | Refining of themes and development of relationships between themes through reading and comparison with further data | Interpretation of themes in the context of theory or conceptual framework |

### Example of inductive coding

In a study analysing qualitative data on the role that families play in supporting a member living with heart failure (Whitehead 2009), one response to the question 'What impact has living with heart failure in your family had on your life?' was: 'I ring mum and dad every morning to check that they are OK…If I ring and no one answers the phone, I worry because I think something has happened.' This response could be considered to contain two different meaning units and could be assigned two different codes relating to two different themes. The first text segment of meaning, 'I ring mum and dad every morning to check that they are OK', could relate to a theme labelled 'Feelings of responsibility'. The second, 'If I ring and no one answers the phone, I worry because I think something has happened', could be labelled 'anxiety related to deterioration in health'. A large number of themes can be assigned to a single transcript, but often these 'open' themes are combined as analysis continues. Practice exercise 8.4 works through the process of coding using excerpts of transcripts from the heart failure study.

## Grounded theory

Grounded theory is a research design where data analysis is viewed as part of a wider approach beginning with the research question, sample selection and data collection (see Chapter 6 for a review of grounded theory). Grounded theory analysis is inductive in that the resulting theory emerges from the data through a process of structured analysis. The aim of generating theory as the final output distinguishes grounded theory from other designs that may aim to generate a description of the data or a level of interpretation. The aim of grounded theory is theoretical development (Strauss & Corbin 1998).

A 'grounded theory' consists of 'plausible relationships' (Strauss & Corbin 1998) between sets of concepts directly developed from the data analysis. Theory provides a set of testable propositions to advance understanding of the social world more clearly, rather than 'absolute truths'.

Grounded theory analysis follows a structured process and normally starts with a broad research question. It then proceeds in stages, with analysis carried out after each stage of data collection to inform understanding of the concept of interest and possibly to reframe the question and so the sampling process. A paper by Coyne and Cowley (2006) illustrates this process (see Box 8.1).

At the core of grounded theory data analysis is the concept of **constant comparison**. This involves comparing the concepts or categories emerging from one stage of data collection with those emerging from the next. The researcher looks for

**Constant comparison:**
The process whereby the data and the concepts created from analysis are compared to ensure that they are a good fit and re-evaluated if they are not.

relationships between the concepts and categories by constantly comparing them to form the basis of the emerging theory (Figure 8.1). The researcher continues with the

Figure 8.1   Description, interpretation and theoretical development

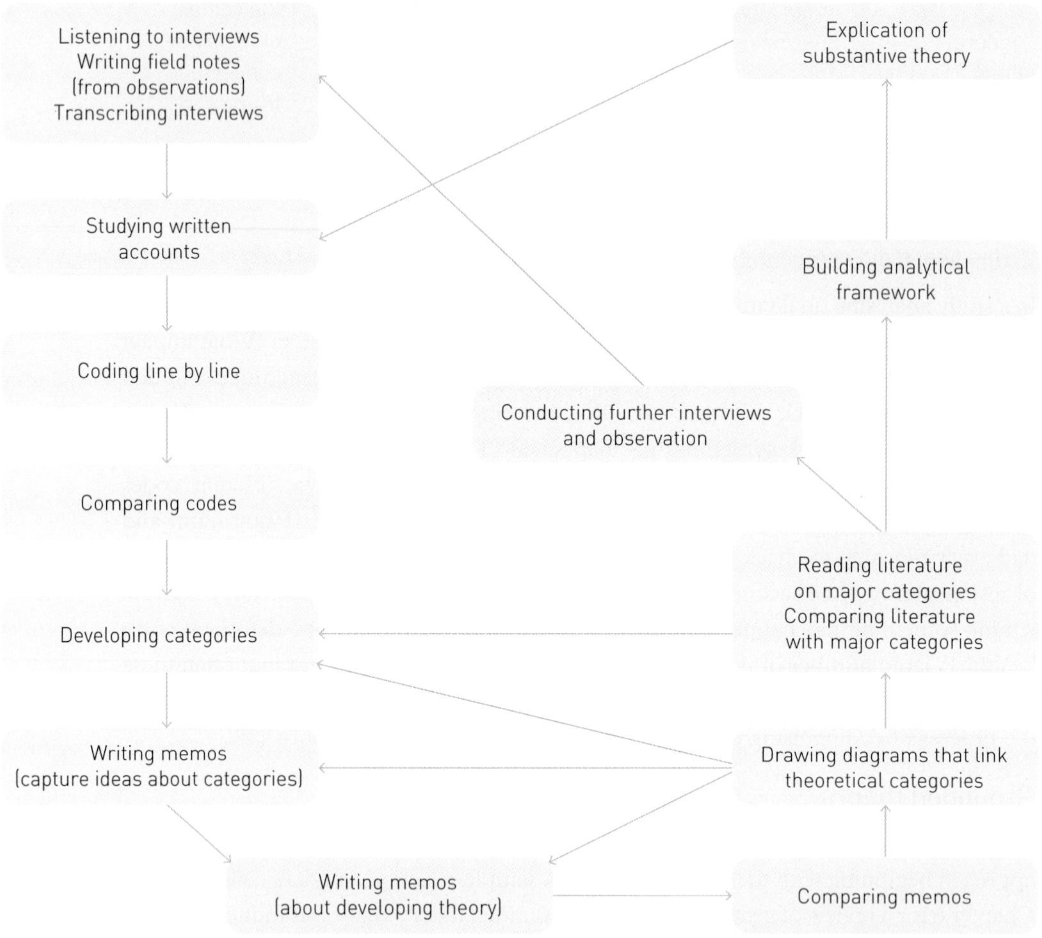

Source: Adapted from Coyne & Cowley 2006

## Box 8.1

### STAGES OF DATA COLLECTION

#### Stage 1
The study started with a broad subject area, 'parent participation in hospitalised child's care'.

#### Stage 2
The data indicated that 'time' could be a significant condition linked to categories labelled 'relationships' and 'knowing'. The links were tentative, which indicated the need for further sampling. Therefore it was decided to collect data from another research site where the children would experience lengthy admissions (longer than four days) in order to develop and extend the category of time.

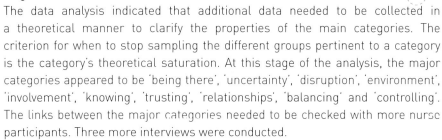

### Stage 3

The data analysis indicated that additional data needed to be collected in a theoretical manner to clarify the properties of the main categories. The criterion for when to stop sampling the different groups pertinent to a category is the category's theoretical saturation. At this stage of the analysis, the major categories appeared to be 'being there', 'uncertainty', 'disruption', 'environment', 'involvement', 'knowing', 'trusting', 'relationships', 'balancing' and 'controlling'. The links between the major categories needed to be checked with more nurse participants. Three more interviews were conducted.

### Stage 4

This phase did not involve more data collection from participants. The researcher reread all the interview transcripts and theoretically sampled for the properties of time (a major category). This helped to identify the links between time and the major categories because time emerged as a sub-category of the categories 'being there', 'disruption' and 'balancing'. This stage helped to clarify that knowing and trusting were both properties and sub-categories of balancing. Concurrent with the theoretical sampling of the data, the sampling of the literature helped to clarify the core processes in the study.

process of constant comparison until they reach **theoretical saturation**, that is, no further concepts or categories emerge from the data. The process of grounded theory analysis is cumulative and can mean revisiting the data as new ideas emerge and as data collection and analysis progress. 'Theoretical sensitivity', the ability 'to see the research situation and its associated data in new ways, and to explore the data's potential for developing theory' (Strauss & Corbin 1990, p. 44), is important and although creative, remains grounded in the process.

**Theoretical saturation:**
The point at which no further data collection or coding is required because no new instances are to be found in the data.

The analysis process in grounded theory has the following stages:

1 Open coding (initial familiarisation with the data)
2 Delineation of emergent concepts
3 Conceptual coding (using emergent concepts)
4 Refinement of conceptual coding schemes
5 Clustering of concepts to form analytical categories
6 Searching for core categories
7 Core categories lead to identification of core theory.

Testing of emerging theory by reference to wider literature and factors (such as cultural or social factors) is related to the area of study. For an example of grounded theory analysis see Wilson and Crowe (2008).

## Phenomenology

Researchers undertaking a phenomenological study draw on a variety of philosophical sources (Gadamer 1989; Heidegger 1996; Husserl 1970; Merleau-Ponty 1964). They can use an open approach to data analysis or choose one of the methods developed to guide phenomenological data analysis such as Colaizzi's (1978) seven-stage method or Giorgi's (1985) four-step method.

Researchers such as Gadamer (1989) and van Manen (1994) take an unstructured approach to data analysis with emphasis on the generation of insight that is rooted in life-world experiences and a belief that a structured process of analysis may constrain insight. Others have set out a process for data analysis, and one of the most commonly used approaches is that of Giorgi (1985), which includes:

- reading to get a narrative sense of the text as a whole, then dividing the text into 'meaning units' that differentiate changes in meaning
- expressing the meanings in more general and transferable ways
- formulating a narrative structure that highlights the common themes across experiences and cases
- illustrating the common themes with quotations and drawing out the variety of experiences within a theme.

Box 8.2 illustrates the process of analysis following Giorgi's approach (Giorgi 1986) in a study on concepts of learning (Morgan 1993). The first part contains data from the interview. Following this a basic description of the interview that aims to remain faithful to the specifics of each individual's experience was written. Three key learning concepts were identified in this description.

## Box 8.2

- Interviewer (I). Can I ask you what do you mean by learning? When you think of learning something, what does it mean to you?
- Participant (S). To gain some knowledge, I think, is learning. We're learning all the time, not necessarily by sitting down and studying. I think there are all kinds of ways. But to me learning is gaining knowledge.
- I. Can you explain what you mean by gaining knowledge?
- S. I suppose just picking up bits of information really. I think if you do it quite basically that's what it is. We do that every day in our way of life, perhaps do it to a greater degree by doing a course. We obviously want to learn more. I obviously want more knowledge about things and I've got an interest in things and I want to know as much as possible about them.
- I. So it is gaining bits and pieces of knowledge.
- S. Yes, yes.

For S, learning means to gain knowledge (1), and S affirms that we are learning all the time and that learning (2) can mean more than 'schoolwork'; indeed, S states that there are many ways to learn, but picks 'gaining knowledge' as the meaning. When pressed by the researcher concerning the meaning of 'gaining knowledge', S gives a synonymous answer: 'picking up bits of information', and he repeats it: S again expresses that learning is pervasive in life (3), but allows that it may be more apparent in a course. While S believes everyone wants to learn more, he refers to himself to answer and says that he wants to know as much as possible about things that interest him.

When choosing phenomenology (or grounded theory or ethnography) as your research method it is important to remember that there have been a number of modifications to the original method that have resulted in different versions. Once you make a choice of a particular version of your study, it is important to remain true to that approach, and this includes data analysis.

## Ethnography

Ethnography focuses on the study of cultures and subcultures. Large-scale ethnographic studies explore large-scale institutions, communities and value-systems. Small-scale ethnographic studies explore single social settings such as a community health centre or staff working in a single ward (Seneviratne et al. 2009). Data collection involves immersion in the setting through observation, interviews with key informants, and often field notes. The aim is to generate the 'emic' or insider view of the members of the culture under study. The presentation of results involves 'thick' or 'rich' description to deliver a detailed account of the patterns of cultural and social relationships.

There are two main approaches to ethnography: descriptive and critical ethnography (Thomas 1993). The approach chosen has implications for the process of analysis where the outcome of a descriptive ethnographic study is to describe cultures and groups and the outcome of critical ethnographic studies is to explore macro-social issues such as power, control and hidden agenda, drawing in a political element (Thomas 1993). Further detail on ethnography is set out in Chapter 6.

The outcome of an ethnographic analysis has been described as presenting a piece of writing that is artistic, complex and like a story so that the reader can access the complexity of data and see the social action in context (Geertz 1973). Data analysis is described as being time- and energy-intensive (Robertson & Boyle 1984) and requires that the researcher is first familiar with the data collected through field notes, interviews and/or observation. Analysis begins early, as soon as some data have been collected. Researchers then work through the stages of thematic analysis described in detail in the next section. Through the process of thematic analysis, themes are developed and related to one another, a process requiring critical thinking and skills as themes are synthesised (Fetterman 1989). Analysis of ethnographic data involves re-analysing data, moving backwards and forwards through the data, and writing and rewriting the findings. Researchers are active participants in the process of data collection and analysis, and it is necessary to acknowledge the role and influence of the researcher (see the section on trustworthiness for further details).

In presenting the analysis, quotations and examples contained in the researcher's field notes are presented for the reader as a window on the findings and to demonstrate the process of analysis through which the researcher has arrived at the finding. Ethnographic studies sometimes result in the development of theory but more commonly generate typologies or a classification system. For example, a study on communication in the operating room (Gardezi et al. 2009) identified three forms of recurring 'silences': absence of communication; not responding to queries or requests; and speaking quietly. The silences were classified as defensive or strategic and may have been influenced by larger institutional and structural power dynamics as well as by the immediate situational context. The ethnographic report, the result of the analysis, should present the main features of the group and the setting and uncover the relationships discovered through analysis. Fetterman (1998) describes this process as one 'of compression as the ethnographer moves from field notes to written text' (p. 123). It is important that the participants recognise their own social reality generated by the analysis; this would involve revisiting participants to discuss this or sending out the report for review and discussion.

Implications for evidence-based practice

In order to share good practice and to build on approaches to data analysis, it is essential that researchers provide adequate information on the approaches and processes they have used in the dissemination of the research. This will enhance the rigour and trustworthiness of the research and allow discussion on developments in the field to take place.

## Analysing visual data

Visual data may take the form of photographs, objects, hand-drawn pictures, video and works of art (painting, poetry and drama). Visual data may be collected to support other forms of data collection methods or to stand alone. Ethnographic research has a tradition of using visual data, usually photographs or symbolic presentations, often to illustrate major differences in the culture under study, for example dress (Ball & Smith 1992). Photographs, video and works of art allow the researcher to collect data that goes beyond words alone, but there are limitations to be aware of. Both represent a snapshot in time, only what the lens can capture and often staged, particularly in the case of historical photographs and works of art. If one chooses to use such forms of data permission must be sought (see also Chapter 4).

Analysis of photographs and video must consider these issues in the generalisation of any analysis to a wider field. Photographs and video can be used for a number of applications in research including documentation, for instance in wound management (Swann 2000), to evaluate teaching and learning for patients and healthcare professionals (e.g. Krouse 2001), to promote empowerment (e.g. Baker & Wang 2006) and to promote understanding, mainly of patient experience (e.g. Gaskins & Forte 1995). The process of analysis itself can take a structured or unstructured approach depending on the researcher's stance, the research question and the research methodology adopted for the study. Photographs and videos can be analysed using a structured list of questions or a coding list (e.g. Anderson & Adamsen 2001). Alternatively, the researcher may choose to take an unstructured approach and note down everything that relates to the research question (e.g. Olsson et al. 1998). In a study with older adults on the experience of pain, Baker and Wang (2006) asked people to take the photographs themselves and then write narratives to describe how the photograph depicted their experience of pain.

The use of drawings in the study of health and illness is limited and to date largely undertaken with children (Guillemin 2004). Guillemin has conducted studies with women to explore their understanding of heart disease and of menopause using drawing as a method of data collection (Guillemin 2004). Participants were first interviewed, and then asked to create a drawing. They were then asked to describe their drawing, which led to reflection on links between the drawing and statements made in the interview concerning their experience. In all such studies there has been a strong focus on the use of drawings for diagnostic or therapeutic purposes (Diem-Wille 2001).

## THINKING DEEPLY

The collection of visual data in research can generate ethical issues. This goes beyond simply the risks of taking photographs in public places. Reflect on the ethical issues that all forms of visual data can create and the implications of these during analysis. Are there ways to counteract some of the issues raised during analysis?

## Building trustworthiness in qualitative data analysis

In building trustworthiness in data analysis, a number of approaches can be taken (see also Chapter 7). The first is setting out a decision trail that documents each step of the data analysis process, effectively creating an **audit trail** (Whitehead 2004). This transparency allows others to follow and evaluate your process. The transcription of data is held by many, though not all, qualitative researchers to be important. Transcription of recorded data reduces reliance on the selective memory and recording of notes by the researcher during data collection. It also allows the sharing of raw data with others to enhance consistency in data analysis. The researcher may instigate independent coding where an independent coder is given the research objectives and some of the raw text from which the themes were developed and asked to create themes from this raw text. Another approach would be to make coding consistency checks where an independent coder is given the research objectives, the themes and descriptions of each theme without the raw text attached. The independent coder is then given a sample of the raw text, previously coded by the initial coder, and asked to assign sections of the text to the themes that have emerged. The raw text selected has sections of text from which the initial themes were derived.

> **Audit trail:** A decision trail that documents each step of the data analysis process. An audit is a process of observing and recording events or scrutinising pre-existing records for subsequent comparison to standards.

Using a qualitative data analysis program such as NVivo, the researcher may open up the data analysis process to others outside the research team to develop external credibility of the analysis process. This could include stakeholder checks, which provide the opportunity for people with a specific interest in the research, such as participants and service providers, to comment on themes or the interpretations made (Erlandson et al. 1993, p. 142). Stakeholder checks may be carried out throughout the research process, for example providing a summary of the data at the completion of interviews and allowing participants to immediately correct errors of fact or challenge interpretations. Checks may occur during subsequent interviews by asking participants to verify interpretations and data gathered in earlier interviews. Before submission of the final report, researchers may provide copies of the preliminary analysis, or specific sections of the research report, to stakeholder groups, asking for a written or oral commentary. A stakeholder check may also be conducted by providing a complete draft copy for review by participants or other persons in the setting being studied.

In qualitative data analysis most approaches recognise the role of the researcher in shaping data collection and in data analysis. In order to 'make visible' the role of the researcher in shaping data collection and analysis, the researcher's reflections on the processes used in data generation, subsequent analysis and their influences on these processes are essential for researcher credibility. For example, Whitehead states in her study of the experience of living with chronic fatigue syndrome:

> [M]y experience as a nurse taught me to recognise patients' symptoms as 'real' to them. One quote that stayed with me after my training seemed particularly relevant: 'pain is what a patient says it is and exists when he says it does' (McCaffery 1983, p. 95). Inherent in this is the acceptance, without prejudice, of what the patient says. I found the treatment that some of the participants had experienced unacceptable and detrimental to their welfare. A review of the notes at a later stage helped to show how my horizon was operating during and shortly after the interview, and prompted reflection on the horizon of the text and the prejudices that I brought, and continued to bring, to the analysis. (2004, p. 517)

## THINKING DEEPLY

How is your own background likely to shape your research interests, the way you would conduct yourself during a study and the process of analysis? If you find it hard to reflect on these alone, ask a friend or mentor to interview you about these areas. That way you will begin to explore how your current position, your past and your future expectations are likely to influence your research.

## Computer software packages for qualitative analysis

The use of computer software packages to aid qualitative data analysis has been growing since the mid-1990s. Current packages include NVivo and AtlasTi, and while they have different interfaces, all facilitate the same processes, namely data storage and management, coding, data searching and retrieval, and developing and testing theory.

Software packages allow the researcher to import raw data and file these. Data can comprise text files such as transcriptions but also visual material, such as photographs, videos and scanned documents. Files can be labelled and indexed accordingly and text files can be annotated once imported into the software.

## Coding

During analysis of the data, themes can be created easily and assigned to small or large sections of the data as the researcher chooses. Figure 8.2 shows a section of a transcribed interview with themes assigned to parts of the text within NVivo.

As analysis evolves, themes can be renamed, deleted or moved into a hierarchical framework without losing any of the data or any analysis. An example of a coding scheme for a study on the experience of fatigue in chronic illness is set out in Figure 8.3.

Following inductive analysis, the tree nodes (higher-order nodes) were developed. The theme of the impact of fatigue has been 'exploded' to show the sub-themes within the main theme of the impact of fatigue.

## Data searching and retrieval

Computer programs allow the researcher to search the text for particular words or phrases. Data coded under each theme can be displayed easily and if attributes have been assigned to each participant such as gender, occupation and age, the researcher can display data coded under a theme by a given attribute, for example all data coded under the theme 'stigma' for men under the age of 35 years.

Figure 8.2    NVivo screenshot of a transcribed interview

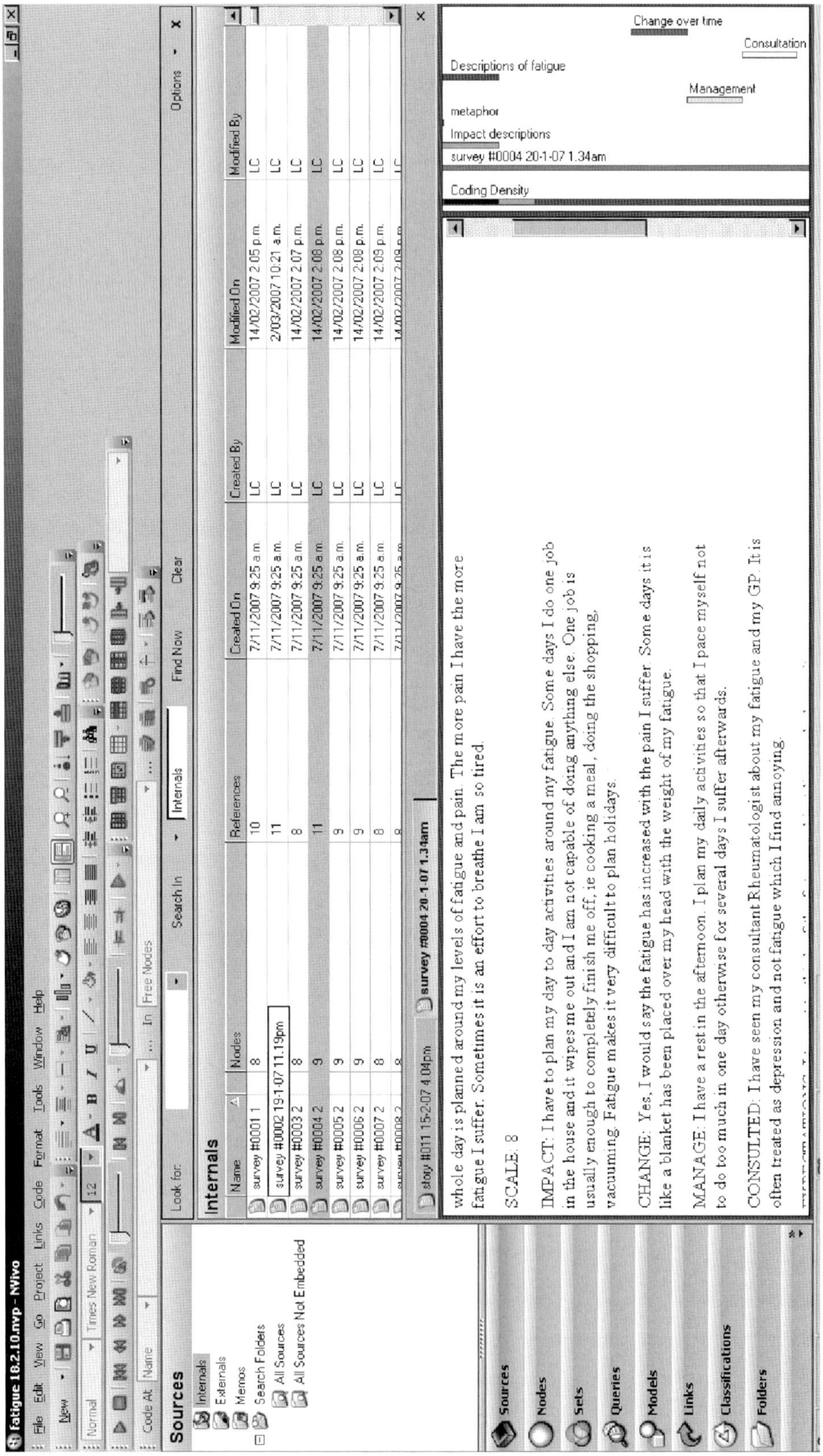

Figure 8.3    NVivo screenshot of an example coding scheme

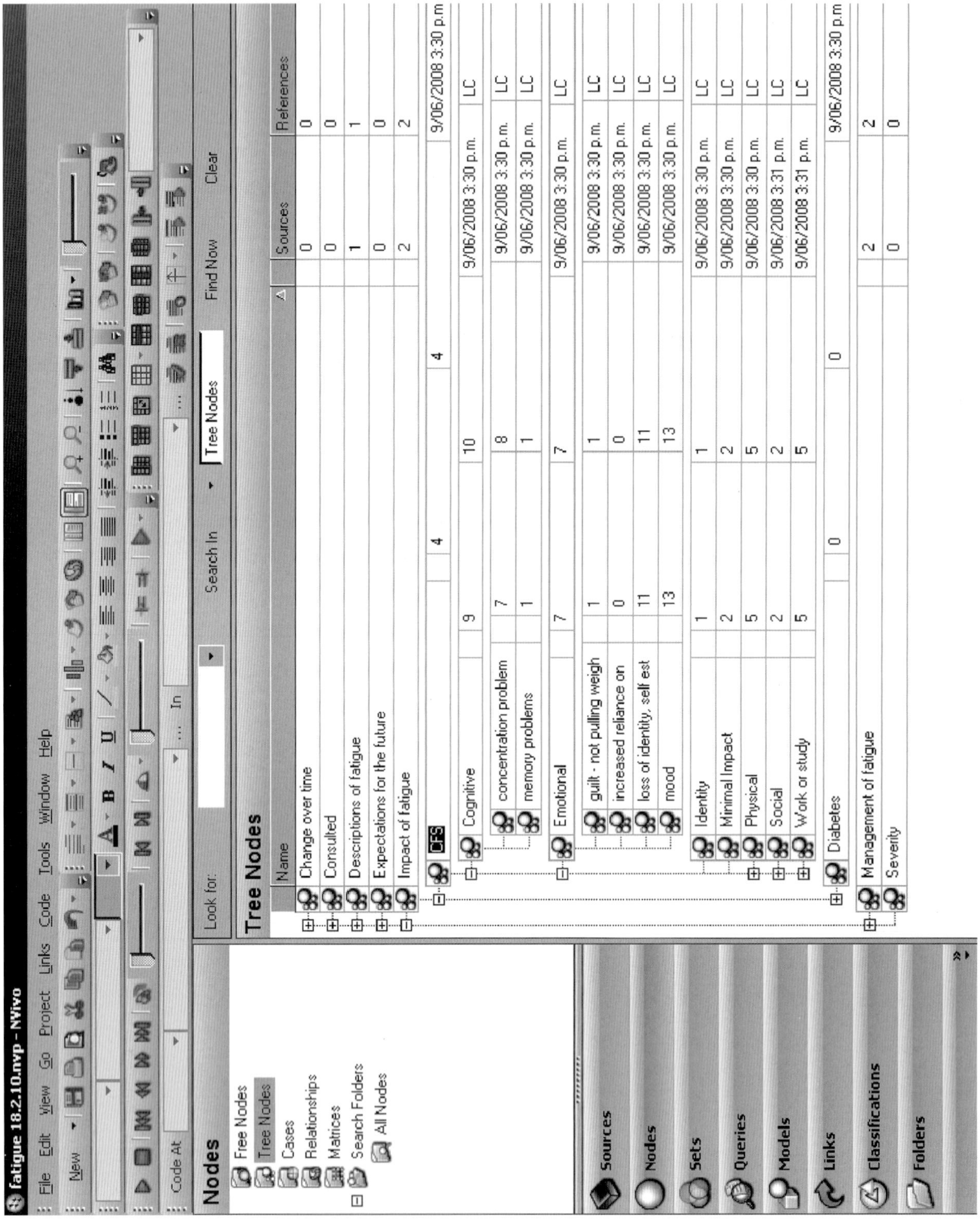

## Developing and testing theory

Software packages can facilitate theoretical modelling by allowing relationships between themes to be explored and displayed. This can take the form of building a hierarchical system or producing a diagrammatic representation. Hutchison and colleagues (2009) created a model in NVivo (Figure 8.4) to summarise conceptual development as analysis progressed in a study on how people successfully change their physical activity habits in order to improve their own personal health and/or well-being.

In deciding whether or not to invest in a software package consider:

- the cost of the software and licence
- the hardware required to run the system
- your level of computer self-efficacy and that of others who may be working with you on the data analysis
- the amount of data for analysis.

Links for further information on qualitative data analysis software packages are given at the end of the chapter.

Figure 8.4   Model showing conceptual development

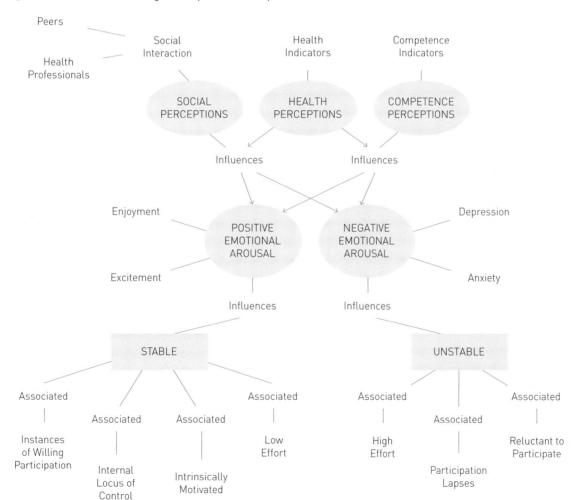

## Implications for evidence-based practice

Traditionally, EBP has been associated with clinical trials, and the gap between research and practice is well documented. Qualitative studies have the ability to help close this gap by creating inductive evidence with a patient-centred focus on which to base practice and also data for further research, for example to inform clinical trials.

It is critical that the data analysis process is clear for the reader so that it can be critiqued and the quality of the study assessed, and also to allow for replication in the future. Analysis should be clearly guided by the methodology; it should follow a process and the considerations around trustworthiness should be set out. These processes will allow for qualitative studies to make a bigger contribution to EBP through inclusion in integrative reviews and policies.

# SUMMARY

- Qualitative data analysis in nursing research is a creative and complex process, but one wholly grounded in the data collected.
- All data collected require a systematic approach to analysis.
- There are a number of approaches to qualitative data analysis and the approach taken for any given study will be determined by the methodology guiding the study.
- The chosen research methodology and method will drive the process of analysis and the choice of approach will be guided by a number of considerations including the research question and data collection method/s.
- The researcher may choose to follow general inductive principles of qualitative research and choose a generic approach such as 'thematic analysis', or else analysis may be embedded in a grounded theory, phenomenological or ethnographic design.
- An important consideration is the development of trustworthiness of the analytic process in order to achieve and demonstrate a thorough, systematic and transparent process to the reader.

PRACTICE EXERCISE 8.1

Ann and her team conduct a phenomenological study among patients who re-present themselves to the emergency department with chest pain within six months. They interview 10 patients at their homes using open-ended questions. They ask participants to tell how they felt when they experienced pain and what they did before coming to the hospital. Following are transcripts of participant A and participant B.

*Participant A*: 'I had this sharp pain on my right shoulder when I was working in the garden. It started at about 4 or 5-ish in the afternoon. I did not think much about it and carried on for another 30 minutes or so. I felt strange so I just stopped what I was doing for a while. The pain just went. Ten minutes later, the pain came back. This time it was quite painful and then it went to my heart. (A pointed her finger underneath the left side of her chest, slightly underneath her breast.) I was frightened and I did not have anyone to talk to. The pain was worse than the pain I had last time when I went to the hospital. I lay down but the pain persisted. I was scared and decided to go to the hospital.'

*Participant B*: 'My work (running a restaurant) is so stressful and busy. I have to make sure that all bills are paid, my workers turn up on time and they look after the clients well. I also have to make sure that my family have what they need. I had this pain, not too painful or anything but it did not go away and that worried me. I put up with it for about an hour or so and then I sweated and the pain moved from my right arm to my left arm. I told my wife and she kept on telling me to go to the hospital. Once I got there, they [healthcare personnel] checked me over and I had to stay in hospital for about a week. My business almost stopped while I was in hospital. This time, I had the same pain and I thought I'd better have it checked rather than leaving it too late. This time I did not talk to anyone, even my wife. I did not want to be [admitted] to the hospital again. I was scared.'

Work through the transcripts and assign codes to those words or sentences you believe are meaningful and related to the focus of the study. Based on your codes, are you able to develop possible common themes from interview transcripts A and B? List two.

Answer: The suggestions below are not exclusive but indicate a potential response. Underlined words relate to how respondents felt. Words highlighted in green relate to what the respondents did before coming into hospital.

*Participant A*: 'I had this sharp pain on my right shoulder when I was working in the garden. It started at about 4 or 5-ish in the afternoon. I did not think much about it (pain) and carried on for another 30 minutes or so. I felt underline{strange} so I just stopped what I was doing for a while. The pain just went. Ten minutes later, the pain came back. This time it was quite painful and then it went to my heart. (A pointed her finger underneath the left side of her chest, slightly underneath her breast.) I was underline{frightened} and I did not have anyone to talk to. The pain was worse than the pain I had last time when I went to the hospital. I lay down but the pain persisted. I was underline{scared} and decided to go to the hospital.'

*Participant B*: 'My work (running a restaurant) is so stressful and busy. I have to make sure that all bills are paid, my workers turn up on time and they look after the clients well. I also have to make sure that my family have what they need. I had this pain, not too painful or anything but it did not go away and that underline{worried} me. I put up with it for about an hour or so and then I sweated and the pain moved from my right arm to left arm. I told my wife and she kept on telling me to go to the hospital. Once I got there, they (healthcare personnel) checked me over and I had to stay in hospital for about a week. My business almost stopped while I was in hospital. This time, I had the same pain and I thought I'd better have it checked rather than leaving it too late. This time I did not talk to anyone, even my wife. I did not want to be (admitted) to the hospital again. I was underline{scared}.'

Although researchers would not create themes from limited data, two 'themes' that are starting to emerge from the above are: fear of the unknown—respondents described feeling scared, frightened and worried; and deferred action—participants adopted a wait-and-see strategy rather than seeking medical advice straightaway.

## PRACTICE EXERCISE 8.2

In the study described in the exercise above, the interviewer also makes notes on the interview (conduct, context, events) and a reflective summary. Discuss why an interviewer might do this and the advantages of this practice.

ANSWER: Notes help to recall non-verbal behaviours, context and events. For example. how participants responded, such as long pauses, talking quickly, looking away, looking at the floor. Whether there were others in the room that may have influenced the interview. Interruptions to the interview. Reflection after the interview helps the researcher to understand how they felt and reacted to the interview and, moving forward, how this might influence the interpretation of the data.

## PRACTICE EXERCISE 8.3

Many adults living with type 2 diabetes find it hard to maintain optimum glycaemic control. A group of researchers are interested in exploring this important area and pose the question, 'what factors influence glycaemic control from the perspective of those living with type 2 diabetes?'

From this scenario on glycaemic control, what qualitative data collection methods could be used to explore this question? List five different sources of data that could be collected and possible approaches to data analysis based on the nature of the data collected through each approach.

ANSWERS:

1. semi-structured interviews analysed through thematic analysis
2. focus group interviews analysed through thematic analysis
3. film or photographs analysed through an open coding approach
4. diary entries using content analysis
5. drawings, using a closed coding approach.

## PRACTICE EXERCISE 8.4

For the two studies outlined below, what methodology would you use, how would you collect the data for each and what would be the key features of the process of analysis?

* A study of nursing culture in the intensive care setting.
* The lived experience of living with multiple sclerosis.

ANSWER: Culture is traditionally explored through an ethnographic approach. Data would be collected through a range of sources such as interviews, observation and field notes to ensure that a breadth of data is gathered. The ethnographic approach the researcher is using will determine the focus of the analysis, but typically this would entail moving backwards and forwards through the data and writing and rewriting the findings. Researchers are active participants in the process of data collection and analysis, and it is necessary to acknowledge their role and influence.

The lived experience is explored through a phenomenological approach. Data would be collected through in-depth interviews. Again, the specific approach chosen would influence the process of analysis but this would typically involve:

* reading to get a narrative sense of the text as a whole, then dividing the text into 'meaning units' that differentiate changes in meaning
* expressing the meanings in more general and transferable ways
* formulating a narrative structure that highlights the common themes across experiences and cases
* illustrating the common themes with quotations and drawing out the variety of experiences within a theme.

## PRACTICE EXERCISE 8.5

Try conducting an interview, transcribing this and coding.

Find a friend, colleague or family member and ask them to take part in an informal interview with you. Choose a topic they feel comfortable with, such as health, illness or service provision. You may wish to use the following question, 'How do you define a healthy lifestyle?' Conduct the interview for 10 minutes, using a broad, open question to start the interview and using more focused questions to explore responses as the interview progresses. Record the interview and transcribe this yourself into a word-processing package. Immediately after the interview write a memo to record your initial response to the interview and your perception of it. The memo can include a summary of the interview, unexpected events such as reaction to questions, or an interruption. The memo will help to prompt your recall when analysing the interview, and facilitates exploration of your position (e.g. beliefs, emotions, viewpoints) during the analysis.

How long did it take to transcribe the interview? Typing skills vary but it is likely to take you considerably longer to transcribe the interview than to conduct it.

Review the questions you asked. Did you lead the interviewee in a particular direction in any way? In hindsight, would you have asked follow-up questions to explore a concept further?

Read through the data several times until you become familiar with it. Then highlight or mark in some way those parts of the text that relate to the question driving the interview (e.g. the definition of a healthy lifestyle) and name these. You have started to identify codes. These are likely to be revised as analysis continues and are the first steps in qualitative data analysis.

# EXAMPLE OF DATA ANALYSIS

This appendix provides an example of data analysis on extracts from interviews with people living with a family member with heart failure (Whitehead 2009). The following responses are in relation to the question 'what impact has living with a family member with heart failure had on your life?'

*Leah:* We've had a few scary times when he cannot get his breath you know you wonder now is this going to be anything but we have the phone number of the hospital, the doctor the heart staff and that there and had a few bad days but on the whole he's improved a wee bit, he wasn't sleeping before, he couldn't lie down in bed or anything. When I got him lying down even trying to get pillows up high can't help him, he can't stand it, he can't stand being too warm. He's sleeping a bit better now so it's really keep my fingers crossed you know.

*Mary:* Well I just worry what's going to happen to him yeah, but now he's got the phone on yeah I'm a bit more peaceful yeah I think like if his breathing is not good at night-time I'm awake you know, if he goes to the toilet I'm instantly awake.

Below, the text that relates to areas that appear significant for the family member have been highlighted.

*Leah:* We've had a few scary times when he cannot get his breath you know you wonder now is this going to be anything but we have the phone number of the hospital, the doctor the heart staff and that there and had a few bad days but on the whole he's improved a wee bit, he wasn't sleeping before, he couldn't lie down in bed or anything. When I got him laying down even trying to get pillows up high can't help him, he can't stand it, he can't stand being too warm. He's sleeping a bit better now so it's really keep my fingers crossed you know.

*Mary:* Well I just worry what's going to happen to him yeah, but now he's got the phone on yeah I'm a bit more peaceful yeah I think like if his breathing is not good at night-time I'm awake you know, if he goes to the toilet I'm instantly awake.

These small excerpts already tell us a lot about the impact of living with someone with heart failure:

The family member can have trouble breathing and this is scary (Leah) and something to be vigilant about, especially at night-time (Mary).

Family members monitor the family member's condition constantly (in these examples through the symptom of breathlessness). Condition alerts them to the possibility of an exacerbation of the condition.

The ability to contact others is important. Both Leah and Mary mention the importance of being able to call someone and for Leah, having direct access to specialists was important.

Sleep disruption is noted by both Leah and Mary. Disrupted sleep for the family member is directly raised by Mary and implied by Leah.

A sense of helplessness and inability to control the illness and the future was expressed several times through the following words: 'you wonder now is this going to be anything', 'can't help him', 'keep my fingers crossed', 'worry what's going to happen to him'.

These findings have been generated from only a small part of the interview with Leah and Mary. The above process should be continued for the entire interview before moving on to analyse the other interviews conducted. During this process you would note similarities between interviews, such as disruption to sleep. You will find that some areas are common to many interviews and these will become themes. The themes are defined by the data, for example disruption to sleep and within this theme (if the data drives this) you may create a number of sub-themes such as causes of sleep disruption (for the person living with heart failure), impact of sleep disruption (for the person living with heart failure, and for the family members).

## FURTHER READING

Baker, T. & Wang, C. (2006). Photovoice: Use of a participatory action research method to explore the chronic pain experience in older adults. *Qualitative Health Research* 16, 1405–13.

Glaser, B. (1978). *Theoretical Sensitivity: Advances in the Methodology of Grounded Theory*. Mill Valley, CA: Sociology Press.

Glaser, B. & Strauss, A. (1967). *The Discovery of Grounded Theory: Strategies for Qualitative Research*. Chicago: Aldine.

Miles, B. M. & Huberman, A. M. (1994). Introduction: Three approaches to qualitative data analysis. In B. M. Miles & A. M. Huberman (eds), *An Expanded Sourcebook: Qualitative Data Analysis*. London: SAGE Publications, pp. 8–12.

## USEFUL WEBSITES

The Computer Assisted Qualitative Data Analysis Networking Project (CAQDAS) provides information on available software packages: <http://caqdas.soc.surrey.ac.uk>

ATLAS.ti: <www.atlasti.com/index.html>

HyperRESEARCH: <www.researchware.com>

NVivo: <www.qsrinternational.com>

## REFERENCES

Anderson, C. & Adamsen, L. (2001). Continuous video recording: A new clinical research tool for studying the nursing care of cancer patients. *Journal of Advanced Nursing* 35, 257–67.

Baker, T. & Wang, C. (2006). Photovoice: Use of a participatory action research method to explore the chronic pain experience in older adults. *Qualitative Health Research* 16, 1405–13.

Ball, M. & Smith, G. (1992). *Analyzing Visual Data*. London: SAGE.

Colaizzi, P. F. (1978). Psychological research as the phenomenologist views it. In R. S. Valle & M. King (eds), *Existential Phenomenological Alternatives for Psychology*. New York: Oxford University Press.

Coyne, I. & Cowley, S. (2006). Using grounded theory to research parent participation. *Journal of Research in Nursing* 11(60), 501–15.

Diem-Wille, G. (2001). A therapeutic perspective: The use of drawings in child psychoanalysis and social science. In T. V. Leeuwen & C. Jewitt (eds), *Handbook of Visual Analysis*. Thousand Oaks, CA: SAGE, pp. 119–33.

Erlandson, D., Harris, E., Skipper, B. & Allen, S. (1993). *Doing Naturalistic Inquiry: A Guide to Methods*. Newbury Park, CA: SAGE.

Fetterman, D. M. (1989). *Ethnography: Step by Step*. Newbury Park, CA: SAGE.

Fetterman, D. M. (1998). *Ethnography: Step-by-Step*, 2nd edn [Applied Social Research Methods Series, vol. 17]. Thousand Oaks, CA: SAGE.

Gadamer, H. (1989). *Truth and Method*, 2nd edn. London: Sheed & Ward.

Gardezi, F., Lingard, L., Espins, L., Whyte, S., Orser, B. & Baker, G. R. (2009). Silence, power and communication in the operating room. *Journal of Advanced Nursing* 65(7), 1390–9.

Gaskins S. & Forte L. (1995). The meaning of hope: Implications for nursing practice and research. *Journal of Gerontological Nursing* 21(3), 17–25.

Geertz, C. (1973). Thick description: Toward an interpretive theory of culture. In *The Interpretation of Cultures: Selected Essays*. New York: Basic Books.

Giorgi, A. (1985). Sketch of a psychological phenomenological method. In A. Giorgi (ed.), *Phenomenology and Psychological Research*. Pittsburgh: Duquesne University Press, pp. 8–22.

Giorgi, A. (1986). A phenomenological analysis of descriptions of conceptions of learning obtained from a phenomenographic perspective. Publications from the Department of Education, Göteborg University, Sweden.

Guillemin, M. (2004). Understanding illness: Using drawings as a research method. *Qualitative Health Research* 14, 272–89.

Heidegger, M. (1996). *Being and Time*, transl. Joan Stambaugh. Albany, NY: State University of New York Press.

Husserl, E. (1970). *The Idea of Phenomenology*. The Hague: Nijhoff.

Hutchison, A., Halley Johnston, L. & Breckon, J. (2009). Using QSR-NVivo to facilitate the development of a grounded theory project: An account of a worked example. *International Journal of Social Research Methodology* 13(4), 283–302.

Krouse, H. (2001). Video modelling to educate patients. *Journal of Advanced Nursing* 33, 748–57.

McCaffery, M. (1983). *Nursing the Patient in Pain*. London: Harper & Row.

Merleau-Ponty, M. (1964). *The Primacy of Perception, and Other Essays on Phenomenological Psychology, the Philosophy of Art, History, and Politics*. Evanston, IL: Northwestern University Press.

Morgan, A. (1993). *Improving Your Students' Learning: Reflections on the Experience of Study*. London: Kogan Page Ltd.

Olsson, P., Jansson, L. & Norberg, A. (1998). Parenthood as talked about in Swedish ante and postnatal midwifery consultations. *Scandinavian Journal of Caring Sciences* 12, 205–14.

Robertson, M. & Boyle J. (1984). Ethnography: Contributions to nursing research. *Journal of Advanced Nursing* 9(1), 43–9.

Seneviratne, C. C., Mather, C. M. & Then, K. L. (2009). Understanding nursing on an acute stroke unit: Perceptions of space, time and interprofessional practice. *Journal of Advanced Nursing* 65(9), 1872–81.

Strauss, A. & Corbin, J. (1990). *Basics of Qualitative Research: Grounded Theory Procedures and Techniques*. London: SAGE.

Strauss, A. & Corbin, J. (1998). *Basics of Qualitative Research: Techniques and Procedures for Developing Grounded Theory*, 2nd edn. Thousand Oaks, CA: SAGE.

Swann, G. (2000). Photography in wound care. *Nursing Times* 96, 9–12.

Thomas, J. (1993). *Doing Critical Ethnography*. London: SAGE.

Van Manen, M. (1994). Pedagogy, virtue, and narrative identity in teaching. *Curriculum Inquiry* 4(2), 135–70.

Whitehead, L. (2004). Enhancing the quality of hermeneutic research: Decision trail. *Journal of Advanced Nursing* 45(5), 512–18.

Whitehead, L. (2009). *Living with Chronic Illness: Exploring the Role of the Family in Supporting Members Living with Heart Failure*. Families Commission, New Zealand.

Wilson, B. & Crowe, M. (2008). Maintaining equilibrium: A theory of job satisfaction for community mental health nurses. *Journal of Psychiatric and Mental Health Nursing* 15(10), 816–22.

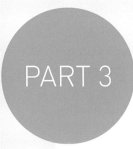

# PART 3

# QUANTITATIVE AND MIXED METHODS RESEARCH

Let us presume that after Ann and Bob have reviewed the literature for a second time, Bob feels that the underlying reason for patients with chest pain re-presenting to the ED is not socio-cultural beliefs but patients' personal demographic factors and the perceived severity of their chest pain. He would also like to generalise his research results to a wider group of patients with chest pain in other healthcare organisations. What is required in such a situation is a change in the research pathway from a qualitative to a quantitative approach to enquiry. The change in focus will also mean a change to the research question. We now bring you to Chapters 9 to 12 which provide in-depth information about quantitative research.

Chapter 9 describes the methods that can be used in selecting participants and deciding on a sample size or participant numbers in order to obtain a representative sample of the participant population to be studied. Chapter 10 will be useful for Bob in deciding which research design will be the most appropriate to answer their new research question. Bob can find information in Chapter 11 useful in selecting data collection tools to gather his needed data. Information technologies such as the internet and personal digital assistants (PDA) as data collection tools and the examples are presented in this chapter. Bob has reviewed these and decided to use a simple pen and paper with structured questionnaire for collecting the data.

The hospital has called for research grant applications. Ann has now decided to use a qualitative research design to explore the experiences of patients with chest pain. Bob on the other hand wants to investigate personal demographic factors impacting on patients' decision to re-present to the emergency department.

Both Ann and Bob have been successful with their respective grant applications. Ann had reviewed each of the different qualitative designs and decided on a phenomenological approach to enquiry which she believes is the most appropriate for her research question concerning a lived experience. Bob decided on a cross-sectional study. Both Ann and Bob have received good support from their colleagues and research team, who have provided constructive feedback throughout the processes of developing a research proposal and collecting data.

As part of her study Ann and her team conducted in-depth interviews with 10 participants. At the completion of the tenth interview, no new information was forthcoming, so Ann decided that no further interviews were required. Bob and his team collected data from 80 patients as planned. Together, Ann and Bob have now gathered a large amount of data that needs to be analysed. In keeping with a phenomenological research design Ann has selected a thematic approach for the analysis of her interviews. Chapter 8 provides a useful guide in selecting an appropriate method of data analysis that is consistent with the qualitative research design of the study. Bob has chosen a quantitative analysis approach, which is consistent with his chosen research design. Chapter 12 provides a comprehensive discussion of the various methods of data analysis used in quantitative research.

If Ann and Bob are not happy in limiting their design to either a qualitative or quantitative approach because they feel that both methods have much to offer to their project, an alternative pathway is open to them—that of taking a mixed methods approach. Chapter 13 discusses the different types of research designs or pathways that can be used in conducting mixed method research as well as issues of method and challenges that Ann and Bob will need to resolve as a result of using two different approaches in the one project.

CHAPTER 9

# SAMPLING IN QUANTITATIVE RESEARCH

Maree Johnson and Sungwon Chang

## CHAPTER LEARNING OBJECTIVES

After reading this chapter you will be able to:

- critically evaluate a sample and the target population
- describe the difference between probability and non-probability sampling approaches
- outline different types of sampling methods in quantitative research studies
- appreciate the factors that influence the sample size.

# Introduction

In the previous chapters you have become familiar with some aspects of the research process, especially in qualitative research. This chapter will focus on sampling methods in quantitative research. Sampling, or the selection of suitable persons to participate in a quantitative study, is often challenging. Sampling has a major impact on the interpretation of the findings, length of the project and the overall costs. Selecting the right sample size and type of participants reduces time and costs for the researcher. Quantitative sampling seeks to achieve the study's specific purpose by selecting the right type and right number of cases for a quantitative study. In this chapter we will explore these issues in sampling for studies using a quantitative method.

# Populations and samples

Let us say that Bob, a nurse and his team would like to explore whether a structured health education program will reduce the number of patients with chest pain re-presenting at an emergency department (ED). They expect that if the health education is effective then it will be applied to patients at other hospitals. Due to limited resources, Bob and his team are unable to conduct this research project with all patients with chest pain that re-present at EDs of all state hospitals. They have to decide how to select patients who will participate in their study to represent all patients with chest pain. The next sections will introduce you to a few concepts relating to population and **sample** in quantitative research.

A population is defined as 'a complete set of persons or objects that possess some common characteristic of interest to the researcher' (Nieswiadomy 2008, p. 188). A sample is a subset of the population. Often nursing and midwifery research involves studying a small number of cases (a sample) rather than the entire group (a population) the investigator is interested in. In quantitative research the usual goal is to produce a representative sample (i.e. similar to the population of interest) in order to generalise the findings to an entire population. **Generalisation** is defined as the 'act of reasoning that involves drawing broad inferences from particular observations' (Polit & Beck 2010a, p. 1451). And Thompson (1999, p. 68) says 'the ability to generalise is almost totally dependent on the adequacy of the sampling'.

This process of selecting cases is not a haphazard matter but is based on scientific principles constituting a sampling theory that guides the sampling method. In addition to sampling theory, the selection of a sample should be considered in light of the research aims, questions or hypotheses, the interventions (if applicable) and the data collection methods. At this point we need to clarify the difference between the **target population** and the **accessible population**.

It is usually difficult or impossible to access the target population (the whole population) of interest due to cost, time and accessibility. Hence researchers tend to define a subset of the population they can more readily sample, called accessible population. This listing of the accessible population is called the **sampling frame** from which the sample will be drawn. Consequently, the results of the research or generalisation from the research only apply to the accessible population and not to the target population. Sampling frames may have features that restrict the inclusion of specific persons or units that you may wish to study. For example, conducting a telephone survey of older people using a telephone listing will result in limited number of older people who did not

**Sample:** A subset of persons or units that carry the same characteristics as the overarching population.

**Generalisation:** The extent to which findings are applicable to another similar sample or population.

**Accessible population:** The collection of all possible observation units that might have been chosen in a sample; the population from which the sample was taken.

**Target population:** The entire group the researcher is interested in and to whom the study results are to be generalised.

**Sampling frame:** A list (e.g. map or other specification) of all the elements in the population from which a sample is to be selected.

have a telephone being recruited. Similarly, the Australian census is unlikely to capture all those persons who are homeless or who are living within some form of temporary shelter (Speirs et al. 2013). The importance of this to the study may be substantial or insignificant depending on the aim of the research.

## THINKING DEEPLY

The sampling frame is a list of elements for your population of interest. Consider the sampling frame below for a study of the incidence of falls in the elderly:

> New South Wales inpatient statistical collection which covers all patients admitted to public hospitals, public psychiatric hospitals, public multipurpose services, private hospitals, private day procedure centres, and sleep disorder centres...

What systematic bias might this sampling frame introduce into the study? What might you do to reduce this bias? Think about those who see general practitioners and those who fall but do not present to any healthcare organisation.

## Probability sampling and non-probability sampling

There are two major approaches to sampling: **probability sampling** and **non-probability sampling**. In probability sampling each case from the population has an equal chance of being selected for the sample and the cases are chosen by a process known as **random selection**. In other words, in probability sampling the researcher identifies, in some way, all the cases in the population, and then allows random chance to determine which ones are to be included in the sample. Because the selection of the sample is determined in a non-systematic and random way, the researcher can assume that the characteristics of the sample approximate the characteristics of the total population. This is the reason why probability sampling is synonymous with random sampling. A casual or haphazard sample does not qualify as a random sample. For example, just taking whoever is available does not constitute random sampling as not everyone who is in the population of interest potentially had the chance to be included. In random sampling, all cases from the population must have an equal chance of being included in the study and hence the method delivers a good representation of the whole population.

All researchers recognise that no matter how hard a researcher tries, it is impossible to select a sample that perfectly duplicates the population. One way to express this lack of perfect fit between the sample and the population is by reporting the **sampling error** (i.e. the difference between the sample value and the population value). Sampling error is 'unavoidable because no sample can ever totally represent the population' (Thompson 1999, p. 68). The use of probability sampling enables inferences to be made to the population with a level of precision that can be determined from statistical theory (Thompson 1999). Minimising sampling error, to no more than 5%, is the goal of any sampling technique.

Non-probability sampling methods are usually cheaper and easier to implement, but usually result in a less accurate and representative sample, as some cases may have little or no chance of being selected. As such, researchers cannot claim representativeness and they are limited in their ability to generalise their research results to the population.

**Probability sampling:** A sampling approach that allows for all participants to have an equal chance of being selected.

**Non-probability sampling:** Occurs where the researcher cannot ensure that each case in the population has been represented in the sample, so that they cannot claim representativeness of the sample.

**Random selection:** A sampling method in which every case has the same opportunity to be selected for the study.

**Sampling error:** Error resulting from taking a sample instead of measuring every unit in the population.

**Sampling bias:** Any influence that produces systematic distortion in the sample, where increasing the sample will increase the bias effect.

Furthermore, non-probability samples may contain sources of bias not known or recognised by the researchers. As there is no assurance that each case has a chance of being included in the sample, it is difficult if not impossible to estimate **sampling bias** (i.e. a sample that is selected in a manner that is systematically different from the population). In spite of this, non-probability sampling is used frequently for practical reasons.

---

## TIPS AND SKILLS

In quantitative research, the probability sampling method is always preferable. But when the total number of cases within a population is unknown or each case in the population cannot be individually identified, non-probability sampling can be used instead. However, when the latter is used, it is important for nurse researchers to describe accurately the details of how samples were selected so that the likely representativeness of the sample can be assessed.

---

Defining the characteristics of the study population is achieved through eligibility (inclusion and exclusion) criteria (Polit & Beck 2010b). In a cluster RCT of stroke patients by Middleton and colleagues (2011), they stated that: 'Patients were eligible if they spoke English, were aged 18 years or older, had had an ischaemic stroke or intracerebral haemorrhage, and presented within 48 h of onset of symptoms' (p. 1699).

## Different sampling approaches in quantitative studies
### Probability sampling approaches

Probability sampling approaches in quantitative studies include simple random sampling, stratified random sampling, cluster sampling, systematic random sampling and randomised controlled trials. Non-probability sampling approaches include convenience sampling, purposive sampling and quota sampling and snowball sampling.

### Simple random sampling

Simple random sampling is defined as an approach in which every case has the same opportunity to be selected for the study. The procedure involves obtaining a complete listing of cases in the population, allocating a number for each case, and generating a set of random numbers. Tools are available to generate random numbers such as add-on modules for Microsoft Excel™ or using a table of random numbers (see Appendix 9.1).

Table 9.1 outlines an example of random sampling using numbers. A nurse investigator needs to select, say, 10 study participants from an outpatient clinic that has 200 patient bookings per week. The nurse initially obtains a listing of all the healthcare record numbers of the patients attending during the defined period of one week. Every healthcare record number is then allocated a number from 1 to 200. Then, using either a random numbers table or random numbers generated by computer software, the following numbers are generated: 2, 3, 77, 23, 45…. The patients (healthcare record numbers) selected at random (using generated numbers) are requested to participate in the study.

**Table 9.1**    Selecting a random sample of 10 study participants from an outpatient listing of 200 patients

| Healthcare Record Number | Name | Numbers allocated by researcher |
| --- | --- | --- |
| R6249 | Frederick Topaz | 1 |
| P2278 | Mary Jacobs | 2* |
| Z4477 | Amanda Chan | 3* |
| T3395 | Steven Jones | 4 |
| C2388 | Samir Fernandez | 5 |
| . . . | | |
| D6785 | Sophie Stavros | 200 |

*Patients selected using random numbers.

## Stratified random sampling

**Stratified random sampling** segments the population according to existing strata (or groupings) (category of nurse, qualifications, current place of work) that are relevant to the research study. The researcher obtains a listing of all cases within the relevant stratum and then selects the sample from within the stratum, so that the sample from each stratum is included. It is important that the cases in a stratum are similar to each other, but cases between strata (or groups) should be as different as possible to one another. This method is usually used if each stratum contains distinctly different types of units or individuals from those in other strata. By using stratified sampling we can ensure that each distinct group within a population is represented in a sample.

**Stratified random sampling:** A sampling method where a similar proportion of cases to the population are selected in each stratum.

## Cluster random sampling

**Cluster random sampling** is often used in studies where the total sample required is much smaller than the available population. It is commonly used to reduce the costs of the project by decreasing the geographic distribution of the sample (Neuman 2010). Here it is important that the clusters (or groups) are similar to one another or the sampling may be biased.

For example, we will assume there are 12 hospitals with operating rooms in Melbourne. Operating room nurses consist of registered nurses, nursing educators and nurse managers. We will randomly select four clusters (or hospitals), and all operating room nurses working in those selected four hospitals become our sample (Figure 9.1).

**Cluster random sampling:** A method where a random selection of a subset of usually geographically dispersed components of the population is made and forms the sample.

Figure 9.1 Cluster random sampling

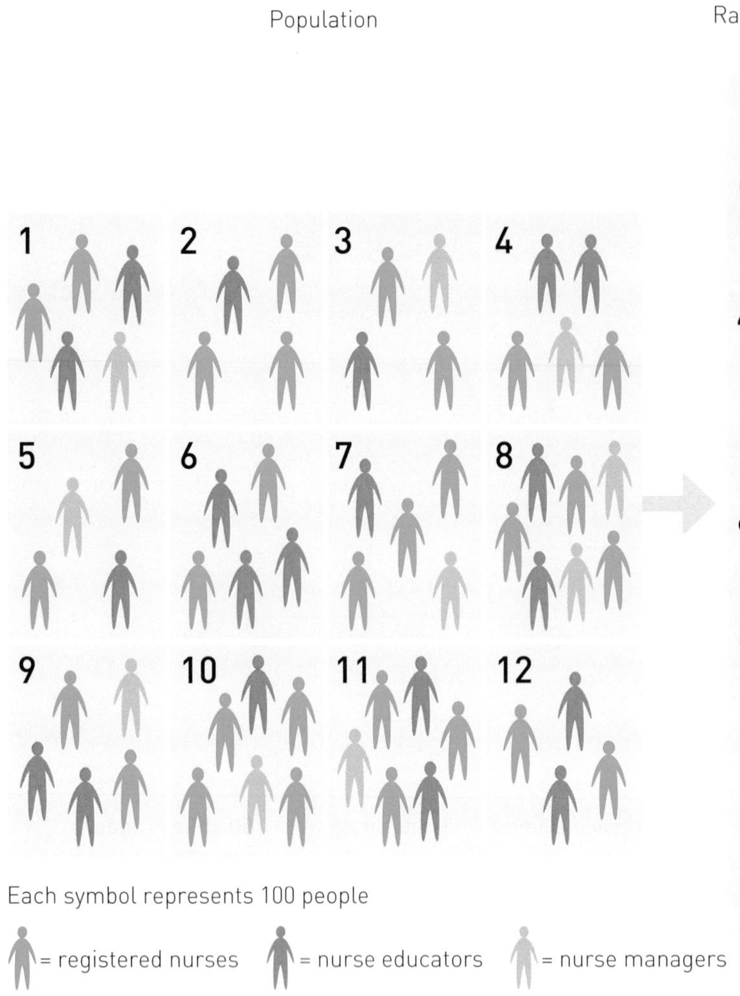
Population
Random Selection of Clusters
Sample (People in the Clusters)
1
2
3
4
5
6
7
8
9
10
11
12
1
4
9
10
Each symbol represents 100 people
= registered nurses
= nurse educators
= nurse managers

Source: Derived from the original figure from Leedy & Ormrod 2005, p. 204

## Systematic sampling

**Systematic sampling:** A method where every *n*th case (set interval) is selected from the list.

**Systematic sampling** is when a population list is used as a sampling frame. It involves dividing the sampling frame into a number of equal-sized intervals, followed by randomly selecting a first element in the first interval and then every *n*th element in each of the intervals in a systematic way for inclusion in the sample. A systematic sample consists of units that are equally spaced in the list with the number of intervals equating to the size of the required sample. For example, a researcher is seeking a sample of 500 patients from a listing of all patients who attended the outpatients clinic ($n$ = 5000) in 2013. Since only 500 patients are required, every tenth patient (or having an interval width of 10; 5000/500 = 10) from the list is selected to result in the required 500 patients. The first selected patient in the list must be randomly selected (referred to as a random start) from the random number table or by computer generation. In this example, the starting point is between 1 and 10, say 4. Units selected would be 4th, 14th, 24th…4994th. The procedure for selecting a systematic random sample is very easy and can be done manually. Byrd and others (2009), for example, used systematic sampling to explore barriers that neonatal intensive care unit nurses face when attempting to optimally manage newborn pain. They used a listing of California registered nurses with current membership in the National Association of Neonatal Nurses to obtain their sample.

The relative merits of the various probability sampling methods are summarised in Table 9.2.

**Table 9.2**  Summary of the various types of probability sampling methods

| Sampling method | When to use it | Advantages | Disadvantages |
|---|---|---|---|
| Simple random sampling | Population is similar to one another on the research variable | No chance of researcher bias as all units in the population have equal chance of being selected<br><br>Does not require extensive prior knowledge of the population<br><br>Ideal for statistical purposes | Requires an accurate list of the whole population, which is hard to achieve, especially in a large population<br><br>Time-consuming |
| Stratified random sampling | Population consists of different distinct groups that may influence the research outcome | Achieves an adequate representation of subgroups, which may not be achieved by simple random or systematic sampling | Required to know the characteristics of the target population in order to identify and select from the strata correctly<br><br>Time-consuming |
| Cluster random sampling | A sampling frame consists of similar clusters (or groups) as sampling units rather than individual units | Less expensive than simple random as it is easier to access units within a cluster than across a cluster | Larger sampling errors than simple or stratified random sampling |
| Systematic sampling | Populations are similar on a research variable | Ensures a high degree of representativeness of the population<br>Easier than simple random sampling as there is no need to use a randomisation process | Ordering of elements in sampling frame may create biases if the system interacts with some hidden pattern in the population<br><br>Less random than simple random sampling |

In many complex studies the use of several sampling strategies is required. For example, Johnson and others (2001) identified a sampling frame of nurses from the annual survey of the Nurses Registration Board of New South Wales (sampling frame). Three types of sampling approaches were used:

> This database was accessed using a specially designed computer program and a series of sampling strategies—(1) all nurses from some specialty groups; (2) systematic sampling, or selecting every third nurse on the list of other specialty groups; and (3) stratified random sampling from other groups—to result in a group of 11621 nurses being available to participate in the…study. (p. 48)

### Randomised controlled trials

Randomised controlled trials or RCTs are the gold standard experimental design for evidence-based practice. RCTs initially use all the available sample within the data collection period (all people attending the emergency department) and then use random selection and random assignment (probability sampling) (Thompson 1999). As noted above, random selection (simple random sampling) refers to the selection of a subset of cases from a listing of all cases using a random numbers table or computer number generation procedures. Random assignment or allocation refers to the assignment of a selected case (or patient) to a specific intervention or control group and is more fully described as a quantitative design (see Chapter 10).

## Non-probability sampling approaches

Non-probability sampling approaches in quantitative studies are similar to those in qualitative studies (see Chapter 5). These include convenience sampling (also referred to as accidental), purposive sampling, network sampling, quota sampling and snowball sampling.

- *Convenience sampling* is an approach where the nurse researcher locates a sample that is 'convenient'. This sample may or may not be representative of the population. This approach is frequently used in nursing research and is appropriate when little is known about the topic.
- *Purposive sampling* is where the researcher recruits participants to the study based on some attribute that the researcher considers to be appropriate. For example, a nurse researcher may wish to obtain information on decision-making in complex wound care. The researcher recruits nurses from the burns units and plastic surgery units as it makes sense to focus on those most directly involved in the management of complex wounds.
- *Quota sampling* is a process where nurse investigators wish to obtain a distribution on a particular characteristic that is important to the study. For example, a nurse investigator may wish to recruit patients with venous leg ulcers with a certain surface area (known to heal at differing rates). By having 10 patients with small wound surface areas (5–500 mm$^2$), 10 patients with medium surface areas (501–2000 mm$^2$) and 10 with large surface areas (2001–5000 mm$^2$), a good distribution of wound areas is included.
- *Snowball sampling* is the final approach and involves the identification of potential study participants through contact with other participants. This approach is often

used where a condition or attribute is rare or sensitive in nature. Hence the best way to obtain a sample is by contacting an initial few cases and asking them about other potential participants.

## THINKING DEEPLY

Below is a fictitious study. Please suggest a sampling approach that you believe is appropriate.

The nurses' and midwives' registering authority of Western Australia has commissioned you to undertake a survey of all nurses and midwives to determine their beliefs about a national recruitment strategy for nurses not actively working in healthcare. Describe how you would ensure that all categories of nurses and midwives could be included in the study. Define the sampling frame and sampling plan or approach and say how you would proceed. Think broadly about sampling frames, for example organisations, media or internet.

As outlined above, there are several sampling methods to choose from and there is no single best method. The correct method of sampling will depend on what the research aims to achieve and the wider population to which the results should relate (Denscombe 2010, p. 54). Gillespie and others (2010) have shown how two different methods of sampling operating room nurses in Australia have led to different results.

## Sampling for surveys

Conducting a large survey requires particular attention to sampling procedures to ensure that an adequate sample is obtained. Three aspects ensure sampling adequacy: the sample frame, the sample size and the specific design of the sampling procedures. Crockett's guide comprehensively outlines considerations for surveys: the resources available (time, money and personnel), accuracy (standard error), the amount of detail needed in the results or number of subgroups, the proportion of the population with the attributes to be measured, the variability of the attributes in the target population, the non-response rate expected and the sample design (Crockett 1989).

Non-response rates are particularly important in estimating the required sample size. Wherever possible, the researcher should locate surveys carried out in similar populations to estimate the likely response rate. Response rates can vary within subgroups—nurse managers may respond to surveys more frequently than clinical nurses, for instance. Response rates of 60% or more are recommended (Badger & Werrett 2005).

## Bias in sampling

Bias is any influence or condition that distorts the data. In sampling, bias can occur when we generalise from the sample to the population. Among the conditions that lead to bias is when the accessible population is not a good representation of the target population. Furthermore, non-responses may also cause bias, especially if the non-respondents differ from the respondents in some way on the characteristics of interest.

## Sample size

After gaining some understanding of sampling, the next step is to find how many people you need to be included as your sample, that is, to determine an appropriate sample size. The size of the sample should be large enough to help answer research questions and to generalise the findings to the underlying population with a high degree of confidence. However, it should be small enough to be efficient and economical.

So how do you find the 'correct' sample size? A range of resources are available to help you find the answer. There are tables that give approximate sample sizes for various situations as well as statistical programs to calculate sample size. There are also websites that can be used for calculating sample size (see Useful websites). But they all generally require some understanding of statistics, and the researcher needs to have decided on several key issues.

To start with, there is a slight difference in the information required to calculate a sample size for surveys (where the main purpose would be to estimate the population characteristics) to, say, clinical trials (where the main purpose is to test for differences between groups) (refer to Chapters 10 and 11).

As seen above, every situation is different and the sample size depends on the nature of the population as well as the type of statistical analysis expected to be used in the study. In general, the following situations require a larger sample size:

- If there is greater variability in population (i.e. there is more diversity in the characteristic of interest).
- If the data analysis is to take place on several subgroups, then a large enough sample size is required at the subgroup level.
- If a high degree of precision is desired in making inference to the population from the sample, you would require a larger sample size. Remember, the larger the sample size the smaller the sampling error (5% or less desired).
- When a less efficient sampling method has been used. For example, cluster sampling is less efficient in representing the population than stratified sampling. Hence you would need a larger sample to generalise to the population with the same degree of confidence.
- If you expect that a low percentage of people will agree to participate in the study, then increase the sample size to ensure the final number in the study is adequate to answer the research question with adequate statistical power (see also Chapter 12).

**THINKING DEEPLY**

Identify one article that used a survey research design. Describe the sampling method. What type was it? Why did the author(s) use this particular type of sampling method? Discuss the issue of generalisability in nursing and midwifery research. Do you believe samples drawn from populations are really representative of the populations from which they were drawn? Why or why not?

## TIPS AND SKILLS

When reading a quantitative study, take a few moments to think about the sampling design used. Consider if the matters below have been addressed.

1  Is the target or accessible population identified and described? Are eligibility criteria specified? To whom do the authors generalise the result?
2  Are the sample selection procedures clearly described? What type of sampling plan was used?
3  How adequate is the sampling plan in terms of yielding a representative sample?
4  Did some factor other than the sampling plan affect the representativeness of the sample (e.g. a low response rate)?
5  Are possible sample biases identified?
6  Is the sample size large enough? Was the sample size justified on the basis of a power analysis or other rationale?

## Implications for evidence-based practice

When reviewing a research study, evidence-based practitioners should carefully read the description of the sample provided by the nurse or midwife reported in the study. Any sample estimations provided in the study will inform the reader as to the adequacy of the sample used to test the study hypothesis, particularly where the effectiveness of an intervention is being tested.

# SUMMARY

- Sampling is a critical element of the research process.
- Researchers study a sample that is a subset of the total population.
- In quantitative sampling the aim is to get a sample that is representative of the population, so the findings of the sample can be applied (or generalised) to the population.
- Attention to sampling within the design process can result in considerable cost and time savings for researchers.
- Probability sampling approaches are preferred but often non-probability approaches are more feasible.
- Sample size estimation is critical and should be considered in relation to the study design.

## PRACTICE EXERCISE 9.1

What is the main reason for using probability sampling?

ANSWER: It is important to use probability sampling when you want to produce representative samples to understand the characteristics of a population based on study of a sample (i.e. to directly generalise from your sample to your population).

## PRACTICE EXERCISE 9.2

You are going to investigate the factors impacting on nursing work in New South Wales, including satisfaction of nurses with their work. Consider the three different sampling approaches below. Identify the sampling procedure and sampling frame in each approach. Discuss advantages and disadvantages of each approach.

a Take a random sample of 500 nurses from the list obtained from Nurses and Midwives Board NSW of all registered nurses.

ANSWER: The sampling procedure here is a simple random sampling. The population we wish to sample is nurses working in New South Wales. In this approach, we assume the sampling frame (the list from the Nurses and Midwives Board NSW) would be very close to the population (all nurses working in New South Wales) and the sampling units are the population units. The main advantage of this procedure is that there is a high degree of representativeness in the sample. However, it is conditional in that the sampling frame would be similar to the population.

b Take a random sample of 200 nurses from each area of practice (such as emergency and medical/surgical departments) as obtained from the Board.

ANSWER: This is an example of stratified random sampling. This approach would be appropriate if there is a belief that the areas of nursing practice would impact upon work satisfaction (i.e. the topic of the study). The strata here are different areas of nursing practice. Hence the list from the Nurses and Midwives Board NSW sampling frame (registered nurses) will be prepared separately for each area of practice (e.g. emergency, medical/surgical). Stratified sampling ensures a high degree of representativeness. For the example here, all areas of practice will be represented in the final sample. The main disadvantage is that it is time-consuming.

c   Pick a random number, K, between 1 and 100. Starting with the kth nurse on the list from the Board, select every 50th nurse on the list.

ANSWER: This is an example of systematic sampling. The sampling frame is the same as in simple random sampling. The main advantage is that you can achieve a high degree of representativeness without using a table of random numbers. The disadvantage is that it is less representative than a simple random sampling.

## PRACTICE EXERCISE 9.3

A midwifery-initiated oral health screening tool and assessment process is to be trialled in the antenatal clinic at Christchurch Hospital. The actual study participants are 400 randomly selected pregnant women (200 in the treatment group and 200 in the control group) who will be randomly allocated to either the treatment group or the control group. The treatment group is women who will receive a set of oral health screening items and a free oral assessment by an oral hygienist. The control group is women who receive an oral health promotion brochure and a delayed treatment, similar to the treatment group at a later stage in the study.

Answer the following for each of these studies:

i   What type of sampling approach was used?

ANSWER: Probability sampling. Randomisation and random allocation.

ii   Was this approach appropriate for the study? If so, why? If not so, why?

ANSWER: Yes. Appropriate as every woman has an opportunity to participate in the study and there is no evidence of systematic bias being introduced.

iii   Will the findings derived from this sample be likely to be generalisable to either the population or to other groups? Why?

ANSWER: Most likely the findings could be generalisable to other New Zealand women of similar criteria to those in this study. Random selection and random allocation have taken place in this study. Therefore there is a good chance that the sample will be representative of the population. In addition, random allocation will ensure that the result of the study is generalisable to the population.

## PRACTICE EXERCISE 9.4

How can sampling volunteers cause bias in a sample?

ANSWER: Volunteers may differ systematically on some important characteristic compared with the whole population. In some cases volunteers will try harder than conscripts on any measure of performance in order to make the treatment appear effective.

## PRACTICE EXERCISE 9.5

For each of the sampling types below, decide first whether the type would be appropriate for quantitative or qualitative research or both, and second, whether the type represents probability or non-probability or both approaches. Present your answer as a table.

| Type | Probability/non-probability (Answers) |
| --- | --- |
| 1. Simple random sample | Probability |
| 2. Quota | Non-probability |
| 3. Cluster random sample | Probability |
| 4. Systematic sample | Probability |
| 5. Purposive sample | Non-probability |
| 6. Convenience sample | Non-probability |

# APPENDIX 9.1
# A RANDOM NUMBERS TABLE

Guide to using a random numbers table

A random numbers table is used to select random numbers. First, the researcher applies a number to each unit in the sampling frame. Next, consider the size of the accessible population in your sampling frame. If, for example, the population is 100 cases, only two-digit numbers (01–99) are considered. Determine the starting point randomly (i.e. close your eyes and randomly select anywhere in the table). Then start with the upper left-hand digits in the designated block and work downward through the numbers in the table.

In an example in this chapter, 'a nurse investigator needed to select, say, 10 study participants from an outpatient clinic that has 200 patient bookings per week'. Hence we will need up to three-digit numbers less than 200. Say the starting point was column C, row 15 (612155). The first three-digit number is 612. As the population is 200, there is no one with a number allocation of 612 in your list. Hence this number is skipped. Then go to the next three-digit number <155> and there is a person with that number. Person 155 on the list is selected. Going down the list the next three-digit number is 36, also on the listing. Continue to select three-digit numbers until you have all 10 values between 001 and 200.

**Random numbers table**

| 1 | 2 | 3 | 4 | 5 | 6 | 7 | 8 | 9 | 10 |
|---|---|---|---|---|---|---|---|---|---|
| 45280 | 67711 | 73860 | 2295 | 43548 | 46348 | 64506 | 83473 | 73456 | 30067 |
| 17913 | 23253 | 7231 | 55297 | 84542 | 70251 | 39680 | 4836 | 9368 | 48889 |
| 22185 | 10436 | 45684 | 39939 | 83733 | 25794 | 73051 | 57838 | 50361 | 72792 |
| 58097 | 2700 | 15777 | 29662 | 88005 | 12977 | 11504 | 42480 | 49552 | 54893 |
| 99091 | 53161 | 90950 | 51025 | 97359 | 31799 | 81596 | 32203 | 53825 | 42075 |
| 71724 | 8704 | 24322 | 4027 | 64911 | 55702 | 56770 | 53566 | 63179 | 34339 |
| 49293 | 75997 | 95887 | 62774 | 62111 | 37544 | 37803 | 90141 | 6568 | 30730 |
| 68779 | 70656 | 11909 | 14708 | 32867 | 78392 | 41816 | 98427 | 28594 | 91209 |
| 91614 | 75592 | 23658 | 79460 | 38612 | 8041 | 99755 | 77728 | 17249 | 98686 |
| 90546 | 78796 | 14045 | 8300 | 52093 | 94155 | 41412 | 52757 | 33471 | 45625 |
| 17854 | 65920 | 21722 | 80874 | 76860 | 42016 | 19990 | 59511 | 40948 | 23195 |
| 21058 | 56307 | 50562 | 94355 | 62975 | 83674 | 95019 | 87542 | 9972 | 42680 |
| 68720 | 39880 | 26399 | 40285 | 98628 | 50157 | 22126 | 53102 | 60175 | 65515 |
| 12109 | 36271 | 63784 | 28131 | 61647 | 34540 | 42421 | 92219 | 69383 | 64447 |
| 34135 | 70192 | 8904 | 45884 | 34944 | 14649 | 75533 | 92882 | 93950 | 90746 |
| 22790 | 77669 | 86474 | 13177 | 33067 | 73397 | 99291 | 74724 | 48425 | 764 |
| 31740 | 24263 | 46693 | 79401 | 7836 | 49089 | 25331 | 43489 | 89014 | 78997 |
| 86878 | 85405 | 16381 | 23454 | 28794 | 12772 | 60838 | 90082 | 75792 | 45221 |
| 24926 | 71261 | 5700 | 55498 | 6104 | 27726 | 15977 | 51225 | 18922 | 62715 |
| 60234 | 96291 | 35003 | 71983 | 61043 | 40748 | 1632 | 18981 | 20049 | 16845 |
| 3768 | 12572 | 39275 | 59166 | 99495 | 25390 | 823 | 74524 | 26862 | 69847 |

| 1 | 2 | 3 | 4 | 5 | 6 | 7 | 8 | 9 | 10 |
|---|---|---|---|---|---|---|---|---|---|
| 5500 | 33935 | 75188 | 51429 | 69588 | 15113 | 5095 | 61706 | 65315 | 27931 |
| 38871 | 86937 | 16181 | 1891 | 71319 | 36476 | 41007 | 80528 | 35407 | 44212 |
| 77324 | 45021 | 88814 | 57434 | 78133 | 89478 | 82001 | 4432 | 37139 | 65574 |
| 47416 | 61302 | 93087 | 44616 | 43144 | 74119 | 54634 | 59975 | 43953 | 92019 |
| 84801 | 22590 | 82664 | 28999 | 63438 | 86678 | 63843 | 58906 | 47157 | 82405 |
| 3363 | 40344 | 55961 | 35667 | 96550 | 87341 | 88410 | 85205 | 94818 | 65979 |
| 80933 | 7636 | 27526 | 94414 | 93750 | 69183 | 42884 | 95223 | 38207 | 62370 |
| 82606 | 98223 | 77928 | 38812 | 29603 | 30671 | 27467 | 37080 | 8241 | 21317 |
| 49898 | 69788 | 36676 | 36012 | 11445 | 11704 | 64043 | 80469 | 4632 | 58702 |
| 44557 | 85810 | 88610 | 6768 | 52293 | 15718 | 72329 | 2496 | 65111 | 77265 |
| 49493 | 97559 | 53361 | 12513 | 81942 | 73656 | 51630 | 91151 | 72588 | 54834 |
| 52698 | 87946 | 82201 | 25994 | 68056 | 15313 | 26658 | 19181 | 41612 | 47762 |
| 359 | 71520 | 58038 | 71924 | 30267 | 55239 | 53766 | 84742 | 91814 | 97155 |
| 43748 | 41353 | 95423 | 59770 | 93287 | 66179 | 74060 | 23858 | 74465 | 96087 |
| 35608 | 39217 | 1832 | 40544 | 50966 | 66584 | 46289 | 7173 | 24522 | 25590 |
| 10377 | 14909 | 54430 | 9309 | 18113 | 44816 | 38148 | 5036 | 30931 | 79806 |
| 26458 | 97618 | 84137 | 98023 | 56366 | 81337 | 79865 | 10840 | 80269 | 83069 |
| 67451 | 21522 | 85869 | 19385 | 92278 | 159 | 49957 | 564 | 47821 | 6972 |
| 66642 | 77065 | 92682 | 72388 | 33271 | 50620 | 51689 | 48484 | 76660 | 20454 |
| 70915 | 64247 | 31135 | 57029 | 5904 | 6163 | 58502 | 74928 | 52498 | 66383 |
| 76197 | 17449 | 1227 | 46752 | 36735 | 93346 | 96955 | 18518 | 89882 | 54229 |
| 81133 | 29199 | 2959 | 68115 | 46089 | 85610 | 67047 | 2900 | 35203 | 66988 |
| 84337 | 19586 | 89073 | 9772 | 21117 | 13640 | 36071 | 9568 | 96491 | 56566 |
| 22386 | 31999 | 24726 | 76256 | 48225 | 79201 | 86273 | 68315 | 14245 | 29862 |
| 80065 | 32403 | 87746 | 60638 | 68520 | 18317 | 95482 | 20249 | 81537 | 1427 |
| 17045 | 48021 | 28535 | 33876 | 58443 | 38408 | 57375 | 47357 | 3968 | 72992 |
| 37339 | 60579 | 37744 | 32808 | 13840 | 44153 | 13581 | 78737 | 83269 | 27063 |
| 70452 | 61243 | 62311 | 59107 | 76601 | 57634 | 99696 | 46953 | 31335 | 64852 |
| 67652 | 43085 | 16786 | 69124 | 48830 | 89678 | 3564 | 61906 | 59570 | 52034 |

## FURTHER READING

Bland, M. (2000). *An Introduction to Medical Statistics*. Oxford: Oxford University Press.

Casey, D. & Devane, D. (2010). Midwifery basics: Understanding research (3): Sampling. *Practising Midwife* 13, 40–3.

Daniel, J. (2012). *Sampling Essentials: Practical Guidelines for Making Sampling Choices*. Thousand Oaks, CA: SAGE Publications.

Dattalo, P. (2008). *Determining Sample Size: Balancing Power, Precision, and Practicality*. New York: Oxford University Press.

Lohr, S. L. (2008). Coverage and sampling. In J. Hox., E. De Leeuw & D. A. Dillman (eds), *The International Handbook of Survey Methodology*. New York: Lawrence Erlbaum Associates, pp. 97–112.

Sydor, A. (2013). Conducting research into hidden or hard-to-reach populations. *Nurse Researcher* 20(3), 33–7.

## USEFUL WEBSITES

A program that can be used for random selection and random assignment can be found on the following sites: <www.randomizer.org><www.random.org>

Another site that provides a program for random assignment:<www.graphpad.com/quickcalcs /randomize1.cfm>

Here is a sample size calculator for surveys: <www.surveysystem.com/sscalc.htm>

The following two sites have a free G-Power Program to determine sample size needed: <www.ats.ucla. edu/stat/gpower><hedwig.mgh.harvard.edu/sample_size/size.html#ssize>

## REFERENCES

Badger, F. & Werrett, J. (2005). Room for improvement? Reporting response rates and recruitment in nursing research in the past decade: Methodological issues in nursing research. *Journal of Advanced Nursing* 51(5), 502–10.

Byrd, P. J., Gonzales, I. & Parsons, V. (2009). Newborn intensive care units: A pilot survey of NICU nurses. *Advances in Neonatal Care* 9(6), 299–306.

Crockett, R. A. (1989). *An Introduction to Sample Surveys: A Users Guide*. Catalogue No. 12020.2. Canberra: Australian Bureau of Statistics.

Denscombe, M. (2010). *The Good Research Guide for Small-scale Research Projects*, 4th edn. Maidenhead, UK: Open University Press.

Gillespie, B. M., Chaboyer, W. & Wallis, M. (2010). Sampling from one nursing specialty group using two different approaches. *Journal of Advanced Perioperative Care* 4(2), 78–85.

Johnson, M., Marsden, J., Day, E. & Chang, S. (2001). Nursing skill assessment within populations: Scale developing and testing. *Contemporary Nurse* 10, 46–57.

Leedy, P. D. & Ormrod, J. E. (2005). *Practical Research: Planning and Design*, 8th edn. Upper Saddle River, NJ: Prentice Hall.

Middleton, S., McElduff, P., Ward, J., Grimshaw, J. M., Dale, S., D'Este, C., Drury, P., Griffiths, R., Cheung, N. W., Quinn, C., Evans, M., Cadilhac, D., Levi, C., on behalf of the QASC Trialists Group (2011). Implementation of evidence-based treatment protocols to manage fever, hyperglycaemia, and swallowing dysfunction in acute stroke (QASC): A cluster randomised controlled trial. *Lancet* 378 (9804), 1699–706.

Neuman, W. L. (2010). *Social Research Methods: Qualitative and Quantitative Approaches*, 7th edn. Boston: Pearson/Allyn & Bacon.

Nieswiadomy, R. M. (2008). *Foundations of Nursing Research*, 5th edn. New Jersey: Pearson Education.

Polit, D. F. & Beck, T. C. (2010a). Generalization in quantitative and qualitative research: Myths and strategies. *International Journal of Nursing Studies* 47(11), 1451–8.

Polit, D. F. & Beck, T. C. (2010b). *Essentials of Nursing Research. Appraising Evidence for Nursing Practice*. Baltimore: Lippincott Williams & Wilkins.

Speirs, V., Johnson, M. & Jirojwong, S. (2013). A systematic review of interventions for homeless women. *Journal of Clinical Nursing* 22(7–8), 1080–93.

Thompson, C. (1999). If you could just provide me with a sample: Examining sampling in qualitative and quantitative research papers. *Evidence-Based Nursing* 2(3), 68–70.

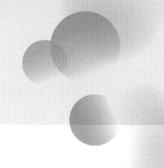

# CHAPTER 10

# QUANTITATIVE RESEARCH DESIGN

Sansnee Jirojwong and Karen Pepper

## KEY TERMS

quantitative data
extraneous variable
causality
bias
validity
experimental
  research design
randomised
  controlled trial
quasi-experimental
  research design
non-experimental
  research design
internal validity of
  research design
external validity of
  research design
placebo effect
double-blind
  strategy
crossover study
descriptive study
epidemiology
cohort study
case control study
cross-sectional
  study

## CHAPTER LEARNING OBJECTIVES

By the end of this chapter you will be able to:

- define quantitative research
- understand the major characteristics of quantitative research designs
- list and describe characteristics of commonly used types of quantitative research designs
- explain terms frequently used in the design of quantitative research and apply the terms in a research scenario
- understand the strengths and weaknesses of each quantitative research design
- discuss the implications of quantitative research for evidence-based nursing and midwifery.

## Introduction

Nurses and midwives are in the unique situation of being frequently in contact with patients for relatively long periods during their care, so they are often in a position where they can see patterns of cause and effect in which certain events or interventions appear to improve—or worsen—health outcomes for patients. If these observations are carried out in a systematic way, they can potentially be used to discover the causes of health problems, or to prove whether a treatment is truly effective.

For example, it is now standard practice to wash our hands frequently to reduce cross-infection from one patient to the other. This is because many studies have identified the cause (washing hands) and effect (reduction of cross-infection among patients) relationship through a number of observations and systematic investigations (Gould et al. 2007). In the early 19th century, Ignaz Semmelweis, a physician at an obstetric clinic, observed that medical students and obstetricians often did not properly wash their hands while caring for women after birth, and this was followed by postpartum infection and deaths.

Consequently, he ordered students and obstetricians to wash their hands before examining patients and this led to the reduction of postpartum infection (Noakes et al. 2008; Rea & Upshur 2001).

Florence Nightingale similarly observed that increased cleanliness reduced deaths among soldiers during the Crimean War (Meyer & Bishop 2007); later this led to strict rules of environmental cleanliness to reduce infection among patients.

In order to draw such conclusions with confidence, however, researchers must choose an appropriate research design that provides a systematic framework in which to collect and analyse their observations. Often this will include collecting quantitative information, such as the number of infections occurring after different types of care. This chapter will help readers to understand the general concepts of quantitative research design. Different quantitative research designs and their implications for nursing and midwifery care will be described. When possible, we will use research studies on hand washing and infection as illustrative examples of different quantitative research designs.

## What is quantitative research design?

Like all forms of health research, quantitative research designs are intended to provide a framework for collecting and interpreting observations in order to answer a research question. What distinguishes quantitative research designs from the qualitative designs discussed in earlier chapters is that these observations will involve the collection and analysis of **quantitative data**—that is, data in the form of numbers or measurements. For example, Semmelweis observed the number of women who died of postpartum infections both before and after strict hand-washing practices were implemented, and found that the number of deaths decreased after hand-washing was introduced (Noakes et al. 2008; Rea & Upshur 2001).

The events that researchers observe, and in some cases measure, are called *variables*. Variables are qualities, properties or characteristics of persons, things or situations that can change or vary. In research, variables are characterised by degrees, amounts and differences. They are also concepts of various levels of abstraction concisely defined to facilitate their measurement or manipulation within a study (Burns & Grove 2009).

There are three types of variables: independent, dependent and extraneous. A *dependent variable* is the outcome variable that is hypothesised to depend on or be

> **Quantitative data:** These can be either categorical or numerical; statistical methods are directly linked to the type of data investigated.

caused by another variable, the independent variable. An *independent variable* is thought to cause or influence the dependent variable. In an experimental study that explores cause and effect between two or more variables, an independent variable is a 'cause' that is manipulated by researchers, and the dependent variable is the presumed 'effect'. An **extraneous variable** is any other variable that is present that may plausibly also affect the dependent variable.

**Extraneous variable:** Any variable apart from the independent variable that may plausibly also affect the dependent variable.

**Causality:** A relationship of cause and effect. It has a minimum of three conditions: a strong relationship between the proposed cause and effect; the proposed cause must precede the effect in time; and the proposed cause must be present whenever the effect occurs.

**Bias:** Any influence that produces distortion in the results of the study.

**Validity:** The degree to which a measurement instrument measures what it is intended to measure.

Quantitative research aims to describe and examine relationships, and where possible, to determine **causality** between variables. Quantitative research incorporates logical *deductive reasoning* as the researcher examines phenomena in selected situations in order to make generalisations (Polit & Beck 2004). In Semmelweis's case, he was able to deduce from his observations that hand-washing reduced maternal mortality rates in his own unit, and that a strict hand-washing regime should therefore be recommended to prevent postpartum mortality more generally (Noakes et al. 2008; Rea & Upshur 2001).

Quantitative research can be used in different settings (health units, communities, geographical areas) and with various population groups (sick people, well people, people of different age or gender, and ethnic groups). A rigorous and controlled design is required to answer a research question (LoBiondo-Wood & Haber 2010). Steps used in the research process need to be clearly defined and strictly adhered to (see Chapter 3). Logical deductive reasoning is important to the development of quantitative research. Different steps in the investigation need to be logically linked together. Strengths, potential errors and weaknesses of every step including measurement, sampling, statistical analysis and generalisation need to be explored, and their impact on the study results has to be explained by researchers.

Quantitative research requires careful control. Researchers should maintain objectivity, and not let value judgments influence the study. If this does not happen, **bias** occurs and can detrimentally affect the **validity** of the research. Researchers use techniques of control to identify and limit the phenomenon or problem to be researched. For example, they attempt to limit the effects of outside variables not being studied. They also use measurement instruments to precisely measure the variables under investigation and produce numerical data. Statistical analyses can then be conducted to reduce and organise data, to describe groups and to identify differences between groups. Control of such aspects of the research provides findings that accurately represent the reality of the sample being studied, so the findings can be generalised. Generalisation involves the application of trends or general tendencies to a population that is identified by studying a sample of that population.

This chapter will be devoted to examining some of the most common types of quantitative research designs that are used in nursing and midwifery, and in health research more generally. We will be looking at the kinds of research questions that are best answered by each type of quantitative research design, and will also consider the strengths and weaknesses of each type of design. Chapter 11 will discuss measurement and other aspects of quantitative data collection in more detail, and Chapter 12 will explain how statistics can be used to analyse the data collected in quantitative research.

## Quantitative research and causality

For nurses, midwives and other health practitioners, our main interest in research lies in the evidence it provides about what causes health problems in the first place, and what interventions can be reliably used to treat or prevent these problems. In both cases this means that we are going to be particularly interested in research designs that can prove causation; specifically, that a suspected 'cause' really does cause a health problem, and that a proposed treatment really does cause the health problem to get better.

Certain types of quantitative research designs—**experimental designs**, or **randomised controlled trials**—are particularly good for demonstrating these types of causal relationships. Other types of quantitative designs can show that there is a relationship of some kind between health variables, without proving that the relationship is definitely a causal one. We need to be aware of the difference between experimental quantitative research designs versus **quasi-experimental** and **non-experimental quantitative designs**, as this will affect how confident we can be in applying the results of such research to our professional practice.

So what are the characteristics of research designs that prove causation? Typically, such designs require the researchers to observe and measure events across populations, locations or conditions, to see if the observed events vary in a consistent way across those conditions. In other words, the researcher *manipulates the independent variable(s)* in order to see if this has a systematic effect on the dependent variable.

In addition, such research designs typically require researchers to observe and measure events across *time*. In order to prove a cause-and-effect relationship, you must show that the 'cause' occurs before the 'effect', and that the occurrence of the 'cause' is consistently followed by 'effect' (and that if the 'cause' doesn't occur, then the 'effect' doesn't occur either).

You can see a rough version of these principles at work in Semmelweis's case. Initially, he observed that the number of postpartum maternal deaths was higher in Clinic 1, which was staffed only by doctors and their students who were dissecting diseased dead bodies on site as well as attending women in labour, compared with Clinic 2, which was staffed entirely by midwives who only attended live women in labour. This pattern of events across the two groups led Semmelweis to conclude that something about the doctors and students was causing the higher number of deaths, and he suspected that the relatively dirty hands of the doctors and students may have been to blame. (Note that no one knew anything about bacteria at this point in history!) However, this observation by itself is not enough to prove a causal connection between dirty hands and infection. So his next step was to manipulate the cleanliness of the practitioners' hands to see if this had an effect on death rates. He did this by observing the numbers of postpartum maternal deaths both before and after implementing strict hand-washing among the doctors and students (i.e. across time), and found the number was reduced after the hand-washing regime was implemented, allowing him to conclude that the dirty hands were indeed the culprit and that hand-washing caused a reduction in maternal mortality (Noakes et al. 2008; Rea & Upshur 2001).

Since Semmelweis's time, health researchers have developed increasingly more sophisticated research designs to maximise the ability of researchers to find consistent relationships between the variables they are investigating, and to verify if those relationships are causal. In addition, the results of a research project should be applicable to the general population. In order to achieve these aims, a research design should ideally have both *internal* and *external validity*.

## Internal validity

**Internal validity** is the methodological rigour of a study, where any potential biases are minimised. It is also the ability to tell that the independent variable has actually made the difference or changed the dependent variable. The researchers' ability to identify and

**Experimental research design:** A research design used to test cause-and-effect relationships between variables. Research participants are randomly assigned to either an intervention group or a control group.

**Randomised controlled trial:** A study in which similar people are randomly allocated to two (or more) groups to test a specific treatment. The experimental group receives the treatment to be tested. Another group, the comparison or control group, receives an alternative treatment, a dummy treatment (placebo) or no treatment at all.

**Quasi-experimental research design:** Research in which the researchers manipulate an independent variable in order to evaluate the change of a dependent variable.

**Non-experimental research design:** Research in which researchers collect data without introducing any manipulation or change.

**Internal validity of research design:**
A property of research design that reflects the extent to which a causal conclusion based on a study is warranted, or that can exclude other factors as alternative explanations of the observed association between the variables under investigation.

control potential threats to internal validity will influence the credibility of the research results, and their subsequent usefulness for applications in clinical settings. In practical terms, this means that researchers must ensure they select appropriate measurement tools and measurement procedures so that observations are accurate, maintain a consistency of observations among those who collect the data, and ensure that participants are included in the study without any prejudice.

The following is a summary of the main threats to internal validity that researchers must try to identify and control when designing a quantitative research project.

### History

History refers to an event that may have an effect on the dependent variable, either inside or outside the study setting or location. For example, a researcher may want to research the efficacy of a staff education program in increasing the frequency of hand-washing among nurses. However, if she implements her education program at the same time that there is an outbreak of Severe Acute Respiratory Syndrome (SARS) infections, it will be difficult to tell if any increase in nurses' hand-washing is due to the education program or due to the nurses' increased caution inspired by the SARS outbreak. (In this example, the SARS outbreak would act as an extraneous or confounding variable.)

### Maturation

Maturation can be physical, biological and developmental processes that a participant has experienced and that might influence the study directly and indirectly. For example, a study of health conditions in older patients conducted over a prolonged period is likely to be influenced by untoward conditions that occur in older age, that is, the physical maturation of the participants.

### Testing

The responses of participants who undertake the same test or a similar test may be influenced by the test itself. For example, a researcher might want to check the effectiveness of a staff education program on proper hand hygiene techniques by using a quiz to test nursing staff on their knowledge of these techniques both before and after the education program. Participants may have a better score because the test is repeated, not because of any actual change in their knowledge.

### Instrumentation

Instrumentation for measuring the study variables can be a major threat to quantitative research if an inappropriate instrument is chosen. Using an inappropriate measurement will give results that do not reflect what the study variable intended to measure. For example, in a research project that aims to increase hand-washing rates among nurses, it may be better if the researchers measure hand-washing rates by observing and noting down each instance of hand-washing themselves rather than relying on the number of hand-washings reported by the nurses themselves, which may be distorted by nurses being too busy to remember to report, or exaggerating their rate of hand-washing to make a good impression.

### Mortality

Mortality or attrition is the loss of participants between two or more points of the study, and includes those who do not complete follow-up measurements, who are often referred to as participants who are 'lost to follow-up' or 'drop-outs'. Where possible, the characteristics of people who drop out need to be compared to those who remain in the study as the former may have dropped out because some effects of the intervention could have had an impact on the overall outcomes of the study if they had remained.

For example, a researcher might want to check the long-term effectiveness of a staff education program on proper hand hygiene techniques by testing nursing staff on their knowledge of these techniques both immediately after and six months after the education program. It is likely that not all the original sample of nurses will return for testing again after six months, and it is plausible that those who return will be the ones who were most enthusiastic about the education program. The test results of this group in the later test may therefore be misleadingly high.

### Selection bias

Selection bias refers to bias introduced when selecting participants. Researchers may select a particular group that does not represent the whole study population. Recruitment methods should try to reach all potential participants to take part in the study. Self-selection that contributes to selection bias needs to be assessed or monitored. An example is the use of telephone interviews, which will exclude households with silent phone numbers or no landline phones. Similarly, personal observation studies of nurses during day shift will exclude nurses who mainly work during other shifts. Selection bias can influence the ability to draw conclusions or to allow generalisation of the study results to the population. Selection bias also refers to the selection of patients that may do better with the intervention proposed than others. By selecting such patients it is more likely that the intervention will be found effective.

## External validity

**External validity** is the same as 'generalisability', the ability to apply the results of the study to wider populations and locations. We can understand external validity by asking the question, 'To what extent can the results of this study be applied outside the study group and location?'

One factor that can ensure the external validity of a research project is to make sure that the sample selected to participate are representative of the population of interest. Appropriate sampling techniques were discussed in Chapter 9.

Matters that affect internal validity will also influence external validity. Three major threats to external validity are the interaction effect of selection, the reactive effects of being studied and the interaction effect of testing (Schneider et al. 2007).

> **External validity of research design:** The extent to which the results of a study can be generalised to other situations and to other people.

### Interaction effect of selection

One or more factors that influence the validity of selection of the study sample, including selection bias, mortality and maturation, can also affect the external validity.

### Reactive effects of being studied

When participants' responses are distorted by their awareness that they are being observed (known as the *Hawthorne effect*), it will limit the researcher's ability to apply the results to wider populations.

### Reactive or interaction effect of testing

Researchers also need to know the impact of testing and history on their study. The use of previous testing may influence the researcher's ability to generalise the study results to wider populations. For example, if a study is investigating improvements in nurses' knowledge of infection control and requires participants to complete the same test questionnaire several times, their scores may increase simply due to previous exposure to the test.

## Choosing a quantitative research design

In order to select a suitable quantitative research design, it is important for researchers to review the nature of the research question they wish to investigate. Chapter 3 discusses various steps required when conducting a research project. The next few sections will focus on important issues related to designing a quantitative research for a particular study. Researchers need to ask themselves the following questions:

1  *What is the purpose of the research?* In some cases researchers will simply want to describe variables or groups within their environment. For example, a study by Mamhidir and colleagues (2010) wanted to find out the current level of knowledge that primary healthcare personnel including district nurses and nurse assistants had about multidrug-resistant bacteria and preventive hygiene measures such as hand-washing. In other cases, researchers may want to examine relationships between two or more variables, or to examine causality between variables. For example, a study by KuKanich and colleagues (2013) wanted to see if the introduction of a gel sanitiser and an informational poster would cause an increase in the frequency of hand-washing by staff in two outpatient healthcare clinics.

2  *Will a treatment or the manipulation of an intervention occur?* If so, the researcher must then also ask, how will the treatment be controlled by the researcher? How many groups are to be included in the study? What sample selection method will be used to obtain the samples to be treated and observed? What strategies will be used for the comparison of variables or groups? For example, the study by Mamhidir and others (2010) simply observed and compared the existing levels of knowledge about hand hygiene in different groups of healthcare workers. However, the study by KuKanich and her colleagues (2013) actively introduced an intervention (gel sanitisers and posters) to see if this improved hand hygiene among clinic staff.

3  *What data will be collected, and when?* Specifically, by what method will the variables be observed and measured, and how many times will they be observed? Have possible extraneous variables been identified? If so, will information about them be collected? Will there be any strategy used to control for extraneous variables? In the study by Mamhidir and others (2010), data were collected by asking staff to complete a scored questionnaire about hand hygiene knowledge on a single occasion. In the study by KuKanich and colleagues (2013), the researchers recorded how many times clinic staff washed their hands both before and after the gel sanitiser and posters were introduced.

Researchers who conduct quantitative research also need to consider various practical matters such as cost and maintaining sufficient sample size throughout the study period. Timelines have to be adhered to, and strategies planned for participant recruitment and follow-up (see details in Chapter 3). If the study is expected to take a long time to complete, administrative and management issues need to be attended to at the beginning. These include having a protocol and manual for the project team (MacLennan 2009).

# Types of quantitative research designs

We use two major criteria in the categorisation of quantitative research designs. The first is the *time* when the information is collected on the occurrence of the phenomenon being studied. The second is the degree to which the researchers *manipulate the independent variable* in order to explore whether or not there will be a *change in the independent variable*. In this section we describe three major designs: experimental design, quasi-experimental design and non-experimental design. Commonly used variations of each design will be described. There is a proliferation of research designs, and readers are advised to consult advanced research textbooks to explore details of designs not included in this book.

We begin by describing experimental research designs, in which the manipulation of independent variables across groups, conditions and time are carefully controlled, and then proceed to describe quasi-experimental and non-experimental designs in which these elements are less tightly controlled or even absent.

## Experimental design

Over the past few decades, scientifically tested interventions have been used to improve the health status of individuals in both clinical and community settings. Examples include immunisations to prevent infectious diseases and hand-washing by nursing and other health staff in clinical settings to reduce infection (Beaglehole & Bonita 2004). The effectiveness of these and many other health interventions have been tested and proved by experimental research.

Experimental research involves manipulating one or more independent variables, and then observing subsequent changes in a dependent variable. In nursing and midwifery research, this typically means introducing one or more health interventions and then observing the outcomes. Experimental designs also involve observing and measuring the dependent variable repeatedly *over time*, such as before and after an intervention, to show how the independent variable changes the dependent variable.

The experimental design is the most powerful quantitative design in health research, because it is the only design that allows us to demonstrate that a genuine cause-and-effect relationship exists between the independent and dependent variables. Threats to the validity of research results are controlled by randomisation, the use of control (or comparison) groups, and the active manipulation of the treatments or interventions by the researcher (Burns & Grove 2009).

### Experimental design or randomised controlled trial

An experimental design, also often called a randomised controlled trial or randomised clinical trial or RCT, has three major characteristics: randomisation, use of a control group and manipulation of interventions.

What does *randomisation* mean? It means that the researcher selects participants from the study population and assigns each participant randomly to either an intervention group or a control group. This helps to prevent the threat to internal validity known as selection bias, because it ensures that the characteristics of the participants in the intervention and control groups will be similar before the intervention occurs, so that any differences observed between the groups after the intervention can be attributed to the effects of the intervention. If you don't assign participants randomly (for example, if you allowed your participants to choose which group they wanted to be in), then you risk having groups that are already different from each other from the outset, and you won't be able to tell whether any differences found between the intervention and control groups after the intervention are due to the intervention or due to these original differences. This would be random selection.

Once the groups are formed, the intervention group then receives the intervention or treatment being tested by the experiment. The *control group* does not receive the intervention, but instead receives either a **placebo** treatment, an existing routine treatment or no treatment at all. The role of the control group is to serve as a comparison for the intervention group. Because everything about the control group is the same as the intervention group apart from the intervention, this allows us to control for the influence of extraneous variables which are likely to affect the control and intervention groups equally. This helps protect against other threats to internal validity such as history, maturation and testing effects.

These different treatments, which are *actively manipulated* by the researcher, constitute the independent variable of the experiment. Any differences in observed outcomes between the groups are likely to be caused by the manipulation, assuming that both the control group and the intervention group are similar in all aspects except the independent variable.

Table 10.1 shows the basic structure of a typical experimental (RCT) design. The following symbols are used to represent elements of the design: R represents randomisation to an intervention group, X represents the receipt of the intervention and O is the measurement of outcomes. The numbers 1, 2, 3 and so on represent the time data was collected (Polit & Beck 2004).

**Placebo effect:** The reported response or change in the dependent variable by an individual who does not receive an intervention or receives an inert intervention.

**Table 10.1**   Major characteristics of an experimental design or randomised controlled trial

| Group | Data collection | | Data collection |
| --- | --- | --- | --- |
| | Before Intervention | Intervention | After Intervention |
| Intervention: *Random selection (R)* | O1 | X | O2 |
| Control: *Random selection (R)* | O1 | None | O2 |

For example, White and others (2001) conducted an RCT to assess whether an alcohol-free, instant hand sanitiser containing surfactants, allantoin and benzalkonium chloride (SAB) could reduce illness-related absenteeism in elementary school students when regular soap-and-water hand-washing was not readily available. In this example, the hand sanitiser treatment that will be manipulated by the researchers is the independent variable, while the measured rates of student absenteeism is the dependent variable that is expected to be affected by the independent variable.

First, the researchers randomly assigned 32 school classrooms to either the control group (16 classes) or the intervention group (16 classes). The classes in the intervention group then received SAB sanitiser to use, while the control group was given a similar-looking but inactive placebo solution. This random assignment makes it unlikely that there would be some sort of consistent difference between the classes in the two groups apart from the intervention. For example, if the researchers had just installed the SAB sanitiser non-randomly in all 16 classes in one school and the placebo in all 16 classes at another school, then it would be difficult to tell whether any subsequent differences in student absenteeism between the groups was due to the SAB sanitiser, or due to some other factor that differed between the schools. In this case, the school that the participating students attended would become an extraneous variable that confounded the interpretation of the results.

A **double-blind strategy** was used, so individual students did not know which of the two treatments they were using, and the researchers who collected data did not know what treatment each student was using. (Double-blind strategies are used wherever possible so that the behaviour or responses of individual participants are not influenced by the knowledge that they are or are not receiving the treatment being tested by the RCT. In this example, the students in the control group may not have bothered to use the placebo solution at all if they knew it was fake.)

In this study, a comparison of the outcomes between the two groups showed that students using the SAB sanitiser were 33% less likely to be absent due to illness than those using the placebo. Thanks to the use of randomisation, the use of a control group, and the active manipulation of the independent variable, the researchers were able to maximise the internal validity of the research design, and conclude that use of the SAB sanitiser *caused* a reduction in illnesses in the students.

**Double-blind strategy:** A method of studying a drug or a procedure in which both the participants and researchers are kept unaware of who is actually getting which specific procedure.

## •.THINKING DEEPLY

### Design an experimental research project

Now that you know the main elements of experimental (RCT) research design, try designing an experimental (RCT) research project yourself.

*The research question:* Imagine that you are testing a new in-service program that is supposed to increase the frequency of hand-washing among all healthcare workers in long-term care units. The program involves putting posters around the unit to prompt staff hand-washing, and installing many dispensing points for hand-washing gel. A number of long-term care units are willing to be participants in your research project. Now design a research project that will allow you to conclude that this new in-service program causes an increase in the frequency of hand-washing. You'll need to consider the following issues:

1  How will you form your intervention and control groups?
2  What is the independent variable (i.e. the intervention)? What will you do to the intervention group, and what will you do to the control group?
3  Could you use a double-blind strategy in your project, as White and colleagues (2001) did in their project? Why, or why not?
4  What is the dependent variable (i.e. the measured outcome)? How will you make these observations/measurements? How many times will you need to make observations, and when will you make them?
5  If the intervention works, what pattern of results do you expect to see?

(Hint: Use Table 10.4 and the study above by White et al. (2001) as a model for your design.)

### Factorial design

A factorial design is a more complex variation on the basic experimental design that is used when researchers want to manipulate two or more independent variables simultaneously. Several hypotheses can be tested at the same time.

As an example, consider a research project that aims to investigate patient recovery from surgery by providing two types of intervention: instruction in coping activities, and information relating to the recovery from surgery. Table 10.2 shows this factorial design, where participants in Group A will receive instruction in coping activities and a description of typical sensations experienced after surgery. Group B will receive instruction in coping activities and a description of typical events experienced after surgery. Group C will receive instruction in coping activities without any information relating to recovery from surgery. Group D will not receive instruction in coping activities but will receive information on the typical sensations experienced after surgery. Group E will not receive instruction in coping activities but receive information on the typical events experienced after surgery. Group F will not receive any type of intervention and serves as a control group (Johnson et al. 1978). As in all experimental designs, participants are assigned to groups randomly prior to receiving their group's designated interventions. The pattern of results would tell researchers whether receiving instruction in coping activities improved patient recovery, whether the type of information given about recovery affected recovery, and whether combining instruction in coping activities with types of information given about recovery had any added effect on patient recovery.

**Table 10.2**   Example of factorial design

| | | Instruction in coping activities (randomly allocated) | |
| --- | --- | --- | --- |
| | | Receive | Not receive |
| Information given relating to recovery from surgery (randomly allocated) | Description of typical sensation | Group A | Group D |
| | Description of typical events | Group B | Group E |
| | No information | Group C | Group F |

**Crossover study:** A study that administers more than one treatment sequentially to each participant so that comparison can be made of the effects of different treatments on a dependent variable for the same participant.

### Crossover design

Another variant of experimental design is **crossover design**, also known as counterbalanced design. Each participant will serve as participant in both intervention and control groups. They are randomly allocated to the sequence of receiving an intervention and being a control (see Table 10.3). This design will allow a participant to act as their own control and therefore reduce biases between the intervention and control conditions. The three criteria for experimental designs (randomisation, manipulation and control) are met.

**Table 10.3**   Major characteristics of crossover design

|  | Time 1 | Time 2 |
| --- | --- | --- |
| Group 1 *(randomly allocated)* | Receives intervention treatment | Receives control treatment |
| Group 2 *(randomly allocated)* | Receives control treatment | Receives intervention treatment |

## Implications for evidence-based practice

**USING THE RESULTS OF EXPERIMENTAL RESEARCH IN CLINICAL HEALTH PRACTICE**

For the end-users of health research, such as nurses, midwives and other health practitioners, the results of experimental research designs are supposed to be the best way of assuring themselves that a given health treatment has been proved to be safe and effective before it is put into practice in the field. However, this relies on the researchers having used a properly designed and internally and externally valid experimental research procedure to produce these results.

In recent years, a set of documents called the Consolidated Standards for Reporting Trials (or 'CONSORT Statement' for short) has been developed as a detailed set of guidelines for properly designing experimental (RCT) research projects, and for publishing and assessing their results (Moher et al. 2010; Schulz et al. 2010).

The CONSORT Statement is a checklist and associated flow diagram setting out 25 important research design elements that health researchers should include in the published reports of their experimental (RCT) research projects (see Appendix 10.1 CONSORT 2010 Checklist of Information to Include when Reporting a Randomised Trial). This checklist is also useful to health practitioners such as nurses and midwives who may need to read such reports, as it allows them to check that a research project has met the criteria needed to prove a cause-and-effect relationship between health variables.

## TIPS AND SKILLS

Experimental research (RCT) reports are rather complex and technical documents, and can be difficult to interpret for the inexperienced reader. When reading such reports you might find it helpful to use a copy of the CONSORT Statement checklist as a guide to interpretation (Moher et al. 2010; Schulz et al. 2010).

The CONSORT Statement checklist, flow diagram and additional information explaining how to use them can be found on the CONSORT Group's website <www .consort-statement.org/consort-statement>.

## Quasi-experimental research designs

In both quasi-experimental research and experimental research, one or more independent variables are manipulated by the researcher to assess their causal relationship with a dependent variable. Both types of research also typically involve observing and measuring a dependent variable more than once, in order to see how that dependent variable changes over time.

However, quasi-experimental research differs from experimental design in that it lacks randomised assignment of participants to intervention groups, or lacks a comparison or control group. This is often due to practical or ethical problems in assigning participants at random to treatment groups, or in withholding treatments for participants in control groups.

This lack of randomisation or control means that quasi-experimental designs are more vulnerable to problems with their internal validity. Researchers must be much more cautious about inferring causal relationships between independent and dependent variables in quasi-experimental studies than they would in experimental studies, as they cannot be sure that the outcomes they are observing are produced purely by manipulation of the independent variable rather than the effect of some inadequately controlled extraneous variable.

Specific types of quasi-experimental research designs and their characteristics will be described in the following section. The following symbols will be used to represent time of intervention and data collection:

- $O1$ = Measurement of outcome (dependent variable) at Time 1
- $O2, O3, \ldots On$ = Measurement of outcome variable at Time 1, 2, 3 to $n$th time
- X = Intervention (independent variable).

## Non-equivalent control group design

There is no randomisation in selecting either a control group or an intervention group (see Table 10.4). Reasons for absence of randomisation may include the administrative or ethical implications of randomisation, or the potential for information relating to the intervention being transferred from one group to the other (LoBiondo-Wood & Haber 2010).

**Table 10.4** Characteristics of non-equivalent control group design

| Intervention group (not randomly allocated) | O1 X O2 |
|---|---|
| Control group (not randomly allocated) | O1    O2 |

## After-only non-equivalent control group design

No data are collected prior to an intervention. Data including the outcome variable (dependent variable) of both control and intervention groups are collected only after the intervention is introduced (see Table 10.5). If there is a difference between both groups in the outcome variable, researchers may tentatively assume that this is caused by the intervention.

**Table 10.5** Major characteristics of after-only non-equivalent control group design

| Intervention group (not randomly allocated) | X O1 |
|---|---|
| Control group (not randomly allocated) | O1 |

### Pre-test-post-test design

Pre-test-post-test design is also called a one-group, before-after design (LoBiondo-Wood & Haber 2010). There is no randomisation or control group. Data are collected before and after the intervention (see Table 10.6). Changes of outcome or dependent variable are assumed to be caused by the intervention.

**Table 10.6**   Major characteristics of pre-test-post-test design

| Intervention group | 01 X 02 |
| --- | --- |

### Time series design

Compared to the pre-test-post-test design, a time series design allows researchers to monitor changes in the dependent variable over a long period. Data are collected a few times before and also after the intervention (see Table 10.7). This design is useful in assessing the influence of time on the outcome variable. Like the pre-test-post-test design, this design does not have randomisation or a control group.

**Table 10.7**   Major characteristics of time series design

| Intervention group | 01  02  03 X 04  05  06 |
| --- | --- |

## Non-experimental research designs

Non-experimental designs are used to describe a health-related phenomenon in a more or less natural setting. There is no attempt to manipulate any study variable or to identify a cause-and-effect relationship between variables, therefore no causation can be concluded from non-experimental research.

As with quasi-experimental designs, non-experimental designs are often used when it is not possible for practical or ethical reasons to randomly assign participants to treatments, or to manipulate treatments. A good example can be found in the long history of research that aimed to show that smoking caused lung cancer (Wingo et al. 1999). For practical and ethical reasons you cannot easily demonstrate this by running an experimental (RCT) design, as it would require randomly assigning participants to smoking ('intervention') and non-smoking ('control') groups, and then insisting that the participants do this for several decades while the researchers observe which group ends up with the greatest numbers of lung cancer cases! For this reason much of the early research on this topic was non-experimental in nature, at least on human subjects. This research strongly indicated that there was a strong statistical relationship between smoking and lung cancer, but without technically proving that this relationship was causal. Unfortunately, this allowed critics such as tobacco manufacturers to argue for many years that there was 'no proof' that smoking caused lung cancer.

Despite these shortcomings, non-experimental research can be particularly useful when researchers want to investigate and describe a new health phenomenon. As with the early studies on smoking and lung cancer, data from non-experimental research can be used to identify apparent patterns between the health variables of interest, and this information can be used to develop more complex future studies on these variables.

Descriptive research design, comparative design and correlation design are frequently used examples of non-experimental designs and are discussed below.

### Descriptive research design

In this type of research, investigators describe phenomena using descriptive statistics such as frequency, number and percentage. They use interviews, observation and questionnaires or checklists to collect data. Descriptive designs usually involve making observations and measurements of participants on a single occasion, rather than comparing observations across time. An example of descriptive research is the study discussed earlier by Mamhidir and colleagues (2010) that used a questionnaire to collect data on healthcare workers' current level of knowledge about multidrug-resistant bacteria and preventive hand hygiene.

**Descriptive study:**
This aims to accurately describe characteristics of persons, places, situations or groups, and the frequency with which certain phenomena occur.

**Descriptive studies** are usually conducted when little is known about the health phenomenon under investigation. For example, the earliest studies of new diseases like HIV/AIDS in the 1980s and SARS in the 2000s were descriptive studies that described individuals who had the disease and their characteristics. The time, place and environment where the disease occurred were systematically investigated (Centers for Disease Control 1982; Friis & Sellers 2004; Heymann & Rodier 2004; Kunanusont et al. 1988). Once these characteristics were identified, researchers could then start to develop hypotheses about the likely sources of these ailments, and the type of populations they were likely to affect. These hypotheses were then able to be investigated further using more complex correlational, quasi-experimental and experimental studies.

A descriptive study can involve observing one or many variables, but as there is no attempt to assess causality, the study variables are generally not defined as dependent or independent variables. Bias can be reduced by careful explanation of conceptual and operational definitions of the variables (Burns & Grove 2009), appropriate sample selection and size, valid and reliable measurement of the phenomena, and data collection procedures that achieve some environmental control.

### Comparative design

Comparative design is used when the study aims to assess the differences between the study variables. An audit is a good example of a comparative design. Hospital or residential care audits have been used to monitor the quality of health services. Variables such as the actual length of hospital stay or waiting times are compared against the standard set by health departments. Statistical analysis can then be used to assess whether there is a significant difference between the actual data and the expected standard time period.

### Correlation study design

Correlation study design is used to assess a relationship between one or more independent variables and a dependent variable. When there is a change in an independent variable, researchers are interested to observe whether the dependent variable will also change consistently. Note that in correlational studies, both independent and dependent variables will be quantitative variables.

Correlation designs typically involve the researcher collecting single observations of each variable from a single sample of participants, and then statistically analysing the data to see if there is any systematic relationship in that data between the variables.

If it appears that there is a relationship between the variables, the existence of a positive or negative correlation needs to be explored. A positive correlation exists if the changes of both the independent and dependent variable are in the same direction (Figure 10.1). In other words, an increased value of the independent variable is related to an increased value of the dependent variable, and vice versa. A negative correlation means that the change in the dependent variable is occurring in the opposite direction to that of the independent variable (Figure 10.2). In other words, an increased value of the independent variable is related to a decreased value of the dependent variable.

For example, if researchers found that heavier mothers tended to give birth to babies with higher birth weights (and lighter mothers tended to give birth to babies with lower birth weights), this would represent a positive correlation between maternal weight and baby weight. Similarly, if researchers found that pregnant women with higher measured levels of psychological stress tended to give birth to babies with lower birth weights (and vice versa), this would represent a negative correlation between maternal stress levels and baby weight.

The results of correlational research must be interpreted with caution. Correlation by itself does not prove that one variable causes the other; it merely shows that there is a relationship between the variables. When a correlational relationship is found between two variables, it is possible that Variable A has caused Variable B, or that Variable B has caused Variable A, or that a third variable has caused both A and B. In our second example, the relationship between higher maternal stress and lower baby birth weight does not prove that maternal stress causes the baby to be smaller. It's possible that a third factor, such as physical illness during pregnancy, may have caused both the stress and the lower baby weight.

Figure 10.1  Positive correlation between independent and dependent variables

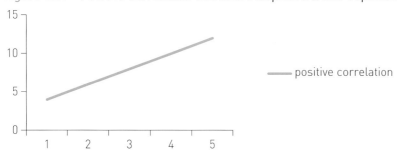

Figure 10.2  Negative correlation between independent and dependent variables

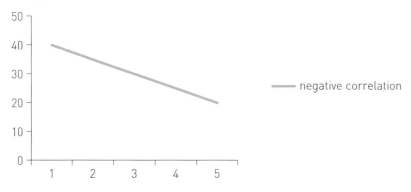

## THINKING DEEPLY

### Design a non-experimental research project

Now that you know the main elements of non-experimental research design, try designing a non-experimental research project yourself.

*The research question:* Hand dermatitis is a common problem affecting nurses and other health professionals, with symptoms that include skin redness, dryness, itchiness and soreness. The commonness of this condition is often blamed on the need for such professionals to wash their hands frequently (Ozyazicioglu et al. 2010). Imagine that you are a researcher who wants to find out if there really is a relationship between the frequency of hand-washing and the measured severity of hand dermatitis symptoms in nurses.

Now design a non-experimental research project that will allow you to find out if there is such a relationship. You'll need to consider the following:

1 Which non-experimental design will you use?
2 What are the variables you will need to observe and measure?
3 How will you make these observations/measurements? Who will you observe, and how many times will you do it?
4 If the hypothesis that there's a relationship between hand-washing and hand dermatitis turns out to be true, what pattern of results do you expect to see?
5 If your data do show a relationship between hand-washing and hand dermatitis, can you then conclude that the hand-washing is causing the dermatitis?

## TIPS AND SKILLS

Quasi-experimental and non-experimental quantitative research designs can show that there is a relationship between health variables, but remember that if you want to be certain that there is a *cause-and-effect* relationship, you need to use an experimental design. Wherever possible, new health interventions should be tested using experimental research (RCTs) to make sure they really work before they are put into practice more generally.

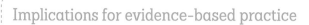

### Implications for evidence-based practice

#### USING QUASI-EXPERIMENTAL AND NON-EXPERIMENTAL RESEARCH IN CLINICAL HEALTH PRACTICE

Despite their limitations, quasi-experimental and non-experimental researches provide much useful information for health practitioners, including information that can be used to guide clinical practice. They are particularly suited for gathering information about existing situations, so that we can identify potential emerging health problems, or shortfalls in existing health practices. Once these are identified, we can then use more strictly controlled experimental designs to verify the causes of these health problems, or to test the efficacy of improved treatments or practices.

Although health research designs were not fully formalised in the early 19th century, Semmelweis's observations and actions regarding the relationship between healthcare workers' hand-washing and postpartum maternal mortality in an obstetric clinic fit the pattern of what we would now call applied non-experimental and quasi-experimental research. Semmelweis's initial observations about the apparent links between doctors with dirty hands and increased postpartum maternal mortality is an early example of descriptive research. His subsequent implementation of a strict hand-washing regime, with the observation of maternal mortality rates before and after the introduction of hand-washing, is an example of what we would now call quasi-experimental design (Noakes et al. 2008; Rea & Upshur 2001). (Of course this means that, strictly speaking, Semmelweis didn't *prove* that the hand-washing caused the observed decrease in maternal mortality, although his results strongly suggested that this was the case. However, modern experimental research, such as the examples discussed in this chapter, have since proved the causal links between hand-washing and infection control, which is why frequent hand-washing is standard practice in healthcare settings today.)

## Epidemiological research designs

We hear the results of research projects through the media. Researchers need to use plain language to further explain their project. An example is the language used during an ABC Health Report program, where a group of cancer researchers discussed screening mammography and its chance of over-diagnosis of breast cancer in Australia (Werner 2014). Many of these projects are epidemiological research.

Next we will briefly present some frequently used epidemiological research designs. It is worth noting that the quantitative research designs described in this chapter are not exhaustive.

**Epidemiology** is the study of the frequency, distribution and determinants of health states and events in the community, and the evaluation of interventions aimed at improving health throughout the community. Epidemiological research may investigate the efficacy of an intervention, the cause of a health problem, or the magnitude of a health problem in the community. It does this by identifying health risk factors and relating them to health outcomes.

Historically, epidemiology was concerned with the patterns in the spread and population characteristics of acute-onset and short-latency problems such as infectious diseases. John Snow, the founder of epidemiology, was able to pinpoint the origin of an outbreak of cholera in London in 1854 by observing the geographic patterns in illness. He noted that the number of cases of cholera were greatest in an area of London supplied by one particular public water pump, and concluded that tainted water from this pump was the probable source of the outbreak. He confirmed this conclusion by having the pump disabled, and subsequently observing a rapid decrease in new cholera infections (Snow 1855). More recently, the increasing importance of chronic disease has seen epidemiologists turn to observing patterns of disease over longer periods in order to determine how and why these diseases develop.

**Epidemiology:** The study of the frequency, distribution and determinants of health states and events in the community, and the evaluation of interventions aimed at improving health throughout the community.

**Cohort study:** A study
in which a group free of
illness is observed for
exposure to risk factors
that are hypothesised
to increase or decrease
the chance of getting
the illness. The study
group will be followed up
through time in order to
compare the frequency of
the illness of groups who
have different levels of
exposure.

**Case control study:**
A study that compares a
group of well individuals
with a group of individuals
who have the illness
or health condition of
interest. The two groups
are compared with
respect to past exposure
to risk factors.

**Cross-sectional study:**
A study based on
observation of a
phenomenon at a single
time for the purpose of
inferring trends over
time.

### Cohort study

A **cohort study** is used when participants are categorised according to the level of their exposure to health risk factors, and then followed through a period of time to observe the occurrence of a disease. For example, one such study investigated whether clostridium difficile bacterial infection in hospitalised patients led to higher subsequent mortality rates. It followed a group of such patients for 180 days, along with a control group of patients who had not been infected while hospitalised, and then observed that the group exposed to the bacterial infection in hospital had a higher number of deaths during that time than the group who had not been exposed to the infection (Mitchell et al. 2013).

### Case control study

A **case control study** identifies existing groups of subjects who either have a disease or health condition ('cases') or do not have that condition ('controls'). The history of their previous exposure to risk factors is retrospectively collected from all participants. Comparison is made by the researchers about the difference in the proportions of people in each group who were previously exposed to risk factors. For example, Sopena and colleagues (2013) investigated the factors that might be linked to an increased risk of general hospital ward patients contracting pneumonia while in hospital by comparing the recent health histories of a group of patients with hospital-acquired pneumonia with a group of similar patients without pneumonia. They found that the pneumonia-infected group was more likely than the non-infected group to have a recent history of malnutrition, chronic renal failure, anaemia, depression of consciousness, recent hospitalisation and thoracic surgery, so it was concluded that these conditions increase the risk of acquiring pneumonia while in hospital. This is an example of retrospective research, which involves the collection and analysis of data relating to past events. Researchers need to be aware of potential biases such as recall bias and the quality of record if information is collected retrospectively.

### Cross-sectional design

**Cross-sectional design** aims to describe a phenomenon among a stratified study group that contains individuals who represent different stages of development, trends or patterns (Burns & Grove 2009). Data are collected from participants at a single point in time, then analysed in relation to the strata that the participants represent within the study group. An example is a study by Smith and Leggat (2005) that investigated needle-stick and sharp injuries among nursing students of different years within their course, and found that third-year students suffered the highest rates of injury.

### Longitudinal design

Longitudinal design (or a prospective study design) is used to follow up a group of participants whose data are collected at different times over a long period in order to assess temporal changes in the study variables. The term 'longitudinal design' may be used to describe a cohort study or an experimental study. An example is a longitudinal study by Karlsson and others (2000) assessing quality of life among surgical patients before and after coronary artery bypass surgery.

### Surveillance

Surveillance is the term applied to research when there is continuous analysis, interpretation and feedback of systematically collected data (Porta & Last 2008). Methods used to collect data emphasise practicality, uniformity and rapidity rather than accuracy and completeness. Information can be used to assess the trend of the studied variables according to time, place and persons. Change can be observed or anticipated and appropriate action (including investigative or control measures) can be taken (Porta & Last 2008). An example is Australian food-borne disease surveillance (Food Standards Australia New Zealand 2013). The quality of data recording and reporting is a major problem when using surveillance data.

## Evaluation studies

Evaluation studies have a broader scope than traditional research designs (see details in Dunt 2009; Dykeman & Cruttenden 2009). In order to improve health outcomes, a healthcare team can introduce changes by implementing a program. Evaluation of this program can be conducted at the beginning of the program, at an early stage, at the end or throughout the course of the program. The scope of the intervention and its context need to be considered when deciding which research designs to use. The scope may include government policies and media campaigns. The context can be the underlying reason for conducting an evaluation.

### Implications for evidence-based practice

**USING EPIDEMIOLOGICAL RESEARCH IN CLINICAL HEALTH PRACTICE**

Epidemiological research tends to focus on the broader influence of social and physical factors on the health of the community, rather than assessing the efficacy of treatments on individuals. At first glance, this may make it seem less directly relevant than other forms of health research to those working one-to-one with patients on the clinical side of healthcare, such as nurses and midwives. However, the results of such research can give us useful insights into the broader social and physical conditions that can either impair or improve the health of our patients, or that can put certain sections of the community—and therefore certain types of individual patients—at greater risk of developing certain health problems.

Epidemiological studies can also alert us to health problems that are becoming more common in the community, so that healthcare providers can prepare to service these increased needs.

# SUMMARY

- Quantitative health research designs differ from qualitative designs in that they involve the observation and analysis of quantitative variables—that is, data in the form of numbers or measurements.
- Experimental research designs (or randomised controlled trials) are considered to be the best way of proving a causal relationship between health variables. They maximise the internal and external validity of the research through the use of randomisation, control groups and the manipulation of independent variables.
- Quasi-experimental research designs have some of the features of experimental designs but do not have all three features of randomisation, control and variable manipulation, so researchers must be more cautious about drawing causal inferences from their results.
- Non-experimental research designs lack randomisation, control and variable manipulation, so while their results may show relationships between health variables they cannot be used to prove that this relationship is a causal one. However, these designs are useful for gathering information about existing health situations and new health problems, which may then be further investigated using more complex or stringent research designs.
- Epidemiological research gives us insights into the social and physical conditions that can influence the health of patients and the general community by investigating the frequency, distribution and determinants of health states and events in the community, and by evaluating interventions that are aimed at improving health throughout the community.

## PRACTICE EXERCISE 10.1

Imagine that you are a researcher who wants to investigate whether type 2 diabetes patients who receive health education from their peers will control their blood sugar levels better than type 2 diabetes patients who receive education from regular sources. Choose the most suitable research design to answer this question, and explain why you chose it.

ANSWER: An experimental design is most suitable, because you can randomly assign diabetes patients to either 'peer education' or 'regular source education' treatment groups, and then observe which treatment group produces the best blood sugar control results after the treatment.

## PRACTICE EXERCISE 10.2

Researchers want to find out if there is a relationship between the number of home visits by a midwife to new mothers who have postpartum depression, and the mothers' measured amount of self-confidence in the mothering role. Choose the most appropriate research design to answer this question, and explain why you chose it.

ANSWER: A correlation design is most suitable, because the researchers are examining the relationship between two measurable variables.

## PRACTICE EXERCISE 10.3

If the researchers in Practice exercise 10.2 do find that there is a relationship between a higher number of midwife visits and a higher level of self-confidence in the new mothers, does this mean that increasing midwife visits will cause an increase in self-confidence in depressed new mothers?

ANSWER: No, we can't assume that increasing midwife visits will cause an increase in the mothers' self-confidence, because this is a non-experimental design and can only show that some sort of relationship exists between the two observed variables. It does not prove that changing one variable will cause the other variable to change too.

## PRACTICE EXERCISE 10.4

A midwifery researcher suspects that there may be a link between smoking and premature births. Two groups of women, one of women who have given birth to babies prematurely and the other of women who have given birth at full-term, were asked to recall whether or not they had smoked during their pregnancy. Based on this information, which research design should the researcher use to find out whether cigarette smoking influences premature birth?

ANSWER: A case control study would be a suitable design, because the researcher will be comparing the past risk factors of existing groups that either have the health problem ('cases') or don't have the health problem ('controls').

## PRACTICE EXERCISE 10.5

Imagine that the midwifery researcher in Practice exercise 10.4 now wants to run an experimental (RCT) research project to prove that the link between maternal smoking and premature birth is a causal one. Would it be possible, both practically and ethically, to design and run such a research project?

ANSWER: In purely practical terms, it would be possible to run an experimental (RCT) design in which you would randomly assign newly pregnant women to two groups, and then manipulate whether they smoked during pregnancy or not. The 'intervention' group would be ordered to smoke throughout their pregnancy, and the 'control' group would be ordered not to smoke at all. The researcher would then observe which group had the greater number of premature births. Of course, you couldn't actually run such a project for ethical reasons—you can't order randomly chosen people to engage (or not engage) in a risky activity like smoking!

## APPENDIX 10.1
## CONSORT 2010 CHECKLIST OF INFORMATION TO INCLUDE WHEN REPORTING A RANDOMISED TRIAL

| Section/Topic | Item No | Checklist item | Reported on page No |
|---|---|---|---|
| **Title and abstract** | | | |
| | 1a | Identification as a randomised trial in the title | |
| | 1b | Structured summary of trial design, methods, results, and conclusions (for specific guidance see CONSORT for abstracts) | |
| **Introduction** | | | |
| Background and objectives | 2a | Scientific background and explanation of rationale | |
| | 2b | Specific objectives or hypotheses | |
| **Methods** | | | |
| Trial design | 3a | Description of trial design (such as parallel, factorial) including allocation ratio | |
| | 3b | Important changes to methods after trial commencement (such as eligibility criteria), with reasons | |
| Participants | 4a | Eligibility criteria for participants | |
| | 4b | Settings and locations where the data were collected | |
| Interventions | 5 | The interventions for each group with sufficient details to allow replication, including how and when they were actually administered | |
| Outcomes | 6a | Completely defined pre-specified primary and secondary outcome measures, including how and when they were assessed | |
| | 6b | Any changes to trial outcomes after the trial commenced, with reasons | |
| Sample size | 7a | How sample size was determined | |
| | 7b | When applicable, explanation of any interim analyses and stopping guidelines | |
| Randomisation: | | | |
| Sequence generation | 8a | Method used to generate the random allocation sequence | |
| | 8b | Type of randomisation; details of any restriction (such as blocking and block size) | |

| Section/Topic | Item No | Checklist item | Reported on page No |
|---|---|---|---|
| Allocation concealment mechanism | 9 | Mechanism used to implement the random allocation sequence (such as sequentially numbered containers), describing any steps taken to conceal the sequence until interventions were assigned | |
| Implementation | 10 | Who generated the random allocation sequence, who enrolled participants, and who assigned participants to interventions | |
| Blinding | 11a | If done, who was blinded after assignment to interventions (for example, participants, care providers, those assessing outcomes) and how | |
| | 11b | If relevant, description of the similarity of interventions | |
| Statistical methods | 12a | Statistical methods used to compare groups for primary and secondary outcomes | |
| | 12b | Methods for additional analyses, such as subgroup analyses and adjusted analyses | |
| **Results** | | | |
| Participant flow (a diagram is strongly recommended) | 13a | For each group, the numbers of participants who were randomly assigned, received intended treatment, and were analysed for the primary outcome | |
| | 13b | For each group, losses and exclusions after randomisation, together with reasons | |
| Recruitment | 14a | Dates defining the periods of recruitment and follow-up | |
| | 14b | Why the trial ended or was stopped | |
| Baseline data | 15 | A table showing baseline demographic and clinical characteristics for each group | |
| Numbers analysed | 16 | For each group, number of participants (denominator) included in each analysis and whether the analysis was by original assigned groups | |
| Outcomes and estimation | 17a | For each primary and secondary outcome, results for each group, and the estimated effect size and its precision (such as 95% confidence interval) | |
| | 17b | For binary outcomes, presentation of both absolute and relative effect sizes is recommended | |
| Ancillary analyses | 18 | Results of any other analyses performed, including subgroup analyses and adjusted analyses, distinguishing pre-specified from exploratory | |

*(Continued)*

*(Continued)*

| Section/Topic | Item No | Checklist item | Reported on page No |
|---|---|---|---|
| Harms | 19 | All important harms or unintended effects in each group (for specific guidance see CONSORT for harms) | |
| **Discussion** | | | |
| Limitations | 20 | Trial limitations, addressing sources of potential bias, imprecision, and, if relevant, multiplicity of analyses | |
| Generalisability | 21 | Generalisability (external validity, applicability) of the trial findings | |
| Interpretation | 22 | Interpretation consistent with results, balancing benefits and harms, and considering other relevant evidence | |
| **Other information** | | | |
| Registration | 23 | Registration number and name of trial registry | |
| Protocol | 24 | Where the full trial protocol can be accessed, if available | |
| Funding | 25 | Sources of funding and other support (such as supply of drugs), role of funders | |

Source: Consolidated Standards of Reporting Trials (CONSORT) Group (2010) The CONSORT 2010 checklist. <www.consort-statement.org/consort-statement>

## FURTHER READING

Craig, J. V. & Smyth, R. L. (2011). *Evidence-Based Practice Manual for Nurses*, 3rd edn. Edinburgh: Churchill Livingstone.

Gordis, L. (2009). *Epidemiology*, 4th edn. Philadelphia: Elsevier/Saunders.

Portney, L. G. & Watkins, M. P. (2009). *Foundations of Clinical Research: Applications to Practice*, 3rd edn. New Jersey: Pearson.

Rothman, K. J., Gallacher, J. E. J. & Hatch, E. E. (2013). Why representativeness should be avoided. *International Journal of Epidemiology* 42(4), 1012–14.

## USEFUL WEBSITES

CONSORT Statement website

<www.consort-statement.org>

The official website of the CONSORT group, including details of the Consolidated Standards for Reporting Trials (CONSORT) statement, which is a checklist to help researchers report their research designs and results in a complete and systematic way.

## REFERENCES

Beaglehole, R. & Bonita, R. (2004). *Public Health at the Crossroads: Achievements and Prospects*. Cambridge: Cambridge University Press.

Burns, N. & Grove, S. K. (2009). *The Practice of Nursing Research: Appraisal, Synthesis, and Generation of Evidence*. St Louis, MI: Saunders Elsevier.

Centers for Disease Control. (1982). A cluster of Kaposi's sarcoma and Pneumocystis carinii pneumonia among homosexual male residents of Los Angeles and Orange Counties, California. *Morbidity and Mortality Weekly Report* 31(23), 305–7.

Dunt, D. (2009). Levels of project evaluation and evaluation study designs. In S. Jirojwong & P. Liamputtong (eds), *Population Health, Communities and Health Promotion*. Melbourne: Oxford University Press, pp. 267–83.

Dykeman, M. & Cruttenden, K. (2009). Frameworks of project evaluation. In S. Jirojwong & P. Liamputtong (eds), *Population Health, Communities and Health Promotion*. Melbourne: Oxford University Press, pp. 253–64.

Food Standards Australia New Zealand. (2013). *Monitoring and Surveillance*. <www.foodstandards.gov.au/science/monitoring/Pages/default.aspx>.

Friis, R. H. & Sellers, T. A. (2004). *Epidemiology for Public Health Practice*. Sudbury, MA: Jones & Bartlett.

Gould, D. J., Chudleigh, J. H., Moralejo, D. & Drey, N. (2007). Interventions to improve hand hygiene compliance in patient care. *Cochrane Database Systematic Review* 18(2), CD005186.

Heymann, D. L. & Rodier, G. (2004). Global surveillance, national surveillance, and SARS: Emerging infectious diseases. *Medscape* 10 February.

Johnson, J. E., Rice, V. H., Fuller, S. S. & Endress, M. P. (1978). Sensory information, instruction in a coping strategy, and recovery from surgery. *Research in Nursing & Health* 1(1), 4–17.

Karlsson, I., Berglin, E. & Larsson, P. A. (2000). Sense of coherence: Quality of life before and after coronary artery bypass surgery—a longitudinal study. *Journal of Advanced Nursing* 31(6), 1383–92.

KuKanich, K. S., Kaur, R., Freeman, L. C. & Powell, D. A. (2013). Evaluation of a hand hygiene campaign in outpatient health care clinic. *American Journal of Nursing* 113(3), 36–42.

Kunanusont, C., Wangroonsarb, Y., Wattanasri, S., Kunasol, P., Wasi, C. & Limpakanjanarat, K. (1988). Surveillance of Acquired Immune Deficiency Syndrome in Thailand through July, 1987. Paper presented at the Regional Scientific meeting International Epidemiology Association, 24–30 January 1988, Pattaya, Thailand.

LoBiondo-Wood, G. & Haber, J. (eds) (2010). *Nursing Research: Methods and Critical Appraisal for Evidence-Based Practice*, 7th edn. St Louis, MO: Mosby Elsevier.

MacLennan, R. (2009). Project planning: Projects and protocols. In S. Jirojwong & P. Liamputtong (eds), *Population Health, Communities and Health Promotion*. Melbourne: Oxford University Press, pp. 123–33.

Mamhidir, A., Lindberg, M., Larsson, R., Flackman, B. & Engstrom, M. (2010). Deficient knowledge of multidrug-resistant bacteria and preventive hygiene measures among primary healthcare personnel. *Journal of Advanced Nursing* 76(4), 756–62.

Meyer, B. C. & Bishop, D. S. (2007). Florence Nightingale: Nineteenth century apostle of quality. *Journal of Management History* 13(3), 240–54.

Mitchell, B. G., Gardner, A. & Hiller, J. E. (2013). Mortality and clostridium difficile infection in an Australian setting. *Journal of Advanced Nursing* 69(10), 2162–71.

Moher, D., Hopewell, S., Schulz, K. F., Montori, V., Gøtzsche, P. C., Devereaux, P. J., Elbourne, D., Egger, M. & Altman, D. G. for the CONSORT Group. (2010). CONSORT 2010 Explanation and Elaboration: Updated guidelines for reporting parallel group randomised trial. *British Medical Journal* 2010;340:c869.

Noakes, T. D., Borresen, J., Hew-Butler, T., Lambert, M. I. & Jordan, E. (2008). Semmelweis and the aetiology of puerperal sepsis 160 years on: An historical review. *Epidemiology & Infection* 136, 1–9.

Ozyazicioglu, N., Surenler, S. & Tanreiverdi, G. (2010). Hand dermatitis among paediatric nurses. *Journal of Clinical Nursing* 19, 1597–603.

Polit, D. F. & Beck, C. T. (2004). *Nursing Research: Principles and Methods*. Philadelphia: Lippincott, Williams & Wilkins.

Porta, M. & Last, J. M. (ed.) (2008). *A Dictionary of Epidemiology*, 5th edn. New York: Oxford University Press.

Rea, E. & Upshur, R. (2001). Semmelweis revisited: The ethics of infection prevention among health care workers (Commentary). *Canadian Medical Association Journal* 164(10), 1447–8.

Schneider, Z., Elliott, D., Whitehead, D., LoBiondo-Wood, G. & Haber, J. (eds) (2007). *Nursing and Midwifery Research: Methods and Critical Appraisal for Evidence-based Practice*. Sydney: Mosby.

Schulz, K. F., Altman, D. G., Moher, D. for the CONSORT Group. (2010). CONSORT 2010 Statement: Updated guidelines for reporting parallel group randomised trials. *British Medical Journal* 2010;340:c332.

Smith, D. R. & Leggat, P. A. (2005). Needlestick and sharps injuries among nursing students. *Journal of Advanced Nursing* 51(5), 449–55.

Snow, J. (1855). *On the Mode of Communication of Cholera*, 2nd edn. London: John Churchill.

Sopena, N., Heras, E., Casas, I., Bechini, J., Guasch, I., Pedro-Botet, M. L., Roure, S. & Sabria, M. (2013). Risk factors for hospital-acquired pneumonia outside the intensive care unit: A case-control study. *American Journal of Infection Control* 42(1), 38–42.

Werner, J. (2014). Breast cancer in Australia: Screening mammography and over-diagnosis, ABC Radio National: Health Report, 13 January 2014. <www.abc.net.au/radionational/programs/healthreport/breast-cancer-in-australia-28part-129/5140204>.

White, C. G., Shinder, F. S., Shinder, A. L. & Dyer, D. L. (2001). Reduction of illness absenteeism in elementary schools using an alcohol-free instant hand sanitizer. *Journal of School Nursing* 17(5), 258–65.

Wingo, P. A., Ries, L. A. G., Giovino, G. A., Miller, D. S., Rosenberg, H. M., Shopland, D. R., Thun, M. J. & Edwards, B. K. (1999). Annual report to the nation on the status of cancer, 1973–1996, with a special section on lung cancer and tobacco smoking. *Journal of the National Cancer Institute* 91(8), 675–90.

CHAPTER 11

# DATA COLLECTION: QUANTITATIVE RESEARCH

Jan Taylor and Jamie Ranse

## CHAPTER LEARNING OBJECTIVES

By the end of this chapter you will be able to:

- analyse the usefulness of different data collection methods
- create a simple questionnaire
- choose an existing instrument or scale to be used in research
- judge the validity and reliability of a scale or instrument
- describe the use of mobile devices and social media to collect research data.

# Introduction

Most of us have provided information to various organisations for their research purposes. Some of us complete a satisfaction form before we check out from a hotel. Every five years, we complete a census form conducted by the Australian Government. We may be approached at an airport or a supermarket by a research assistant who is collecting information for marketing purposes. Information about our use of cancer screening is stored by the Department of Health and Ageing and then analysed and used to report to the wider public. Particular attention to the methods used in data collection ensures the quality and **reliability** of the research. This chapter will explore various methods used to collect data in quantitative research.

**Reliability:** The degree of consistency or dependability with which an instrument measures the attribute it is intended to measure.

# Data collection methods

## Surveys

A survey is a system for collecting self-report information. Surveys can be divided into two broad categories: questionnaires and interviews.

### Questionnaires

Questionnaires are one of the most commonly used data collection methods in nursing and midwifery research. They can be used to measure knowledge, behaviours and perceptions as well as for gathering factual information about respondents (Nieswiadomy 2012). Questionnaires contain different types of questions including closed-ended, open-ended, checklist and rating scales. General characteristics of each type of question will be briefly described and examples of the questions are presented in Box 11.1.

### Types of questions

The following types of questions may be used in a questionnaire:

- *Closed-ended question*: Respondents choose an answer from a given set of alternatives. The dichotomous question (yes/no, male/female) is one example. When using closed-ended questions, the alternatives need to cover all the possible answers or be collectively exhaustive and mutually exclusive, that is, with no overlap between the categories. When unsure that all possible alternatives are covered, the researcher can have an additional category of 'other'.
- *Open-ended question*: An open-ended question allows respondents to answer the question in their own words with sufficient space provided for the answer.
- *Checklist*: A checklist is a list of behaviours, characteristics or information in which the researcher is interested. The participants select possible answers from the list. Some questions allow more than one response. For example, Jirojwong and MacLennan (2004) explored what actions rural Australians take when they are seriously sick. A list of five options ranging from doing nothing to going to a hospital were presented to respondents, who could choose more than one answer.
- *Rating scale*: A rating scale is more useful when the behaviour or characteristic requires precise measurement rather than merely being present or not. Examples of rating scales include the Likert scale, visual analogue and semantic differential.

- The **Likert scale** is used to measure attitudes and beliefs. Respondents indicate their position on a continuum ranging from strongly agree to strongly disagree. In the classic Likert scale the number of possible responses ranges from five to seven.
- A **visual analogue scale** (VAS) is a straight line, 100 mm in length, with anchors representing the extremes of the particular concept being measured. Participants record the intensity of their feelings by placing a cross on the line and scores are calculated by measuring from the lowest extreme point to this cross. The VAS is used to measure concepts such as pain and anxiety.
- The **semantic differential scale** asks respondents to indicate their position or attitude to a concept using two adjectives at opposite ends of a continuum. The number of positions on the scale ranges from five to nine.

**Likert scale:** Used to measure attitudes and beliefs. The degree of agreement or disagreement to a statement of a question is assigned a numerical value.

**Visual analogue scale:** A straight line, 100 mm in length, with anchors representing the extremes of the particular concept being measured.

**Semantic differential scale:** A scale designed to ask respondents their position or attitude to a concept using two adjectives at opposite ends of a continuum.

## Box 11.1

### EXAMPLES OF QUESTIONS

**Fixed response**

Closed-ended questions: the dichotomous question (yes/no) is one example.
'Do you usually speak English at home?'

1   Yes, I usually speak English at home
2   No, another language (Please specify) _____

The question is collectively exhaustive and mutually exclusive.
'During the last week, approximately how many hours of sleep have you usually been getting each night?' (Please circle one number only).

1   0–4 hours
2   5–6 hours
3   7–8 hours
4   More than 8 hours

The use of 'other' category
'How are you feeding your baby at present?' (Please circle one number only).

1   Breastfeeding only
2   Breastfeeding plus some formula
3   Formula only
4   Other (Please specify) _____

*Open-ended questio*ns allow respondents to answer the question in their own words.
'Overall, what do you think is contributing to and/or causing the fatigue you have experienced in the past week?' _____

_____

_____

**Checklists**

A checklist is a list of information in which the researcher is interested. The participant checks the appropriate answer.
'What method/s of pain relief have you been using in the past 24 hours?' (Please circle ALL that apply; you may circle more than one).

1  Tablets such as panadol (or similar drug)
2  Injections of Pethidine (or similar drug)
3  Patient Controlled Analgesia (PCA)
4  Other. (Please specify) _____
5  None, I have not required any analgesia

**Rating scale questions**

Likert Scale: Creedy and associates (2008) examined midwives' breastfeeding knowledge. One of the tools they used was the Newborn Feeding Ability Questionnaire. This questionnaire contained 21 questions with a five-point Likert scale. Question 1 is set out below.

A normal full-term infant is born with instinctive reflex ability to breastfeed effectively.

1 strongly disagree, 2 disagree, 3 not sure, 4 agree, 5 strongly agree.

Visual Analogue Scale: Here pain is ranked on a VAS scale with 0 representing no pain and 10 representing the worst pain possible.

No Pain                          Worst Pain Possible

(0)                             (10)

|_____|

Semantic differential scale: Taylor and Johnson (2013) used the Support Behaviour Inventory which utilises a semantic differential scale to measure women's satisfaction with a variety of social support behaviours provided by their partner in the first six months after birth. One of the questions is set out below.

My partner helps me out when I am in a spot:

Very unsatisfied_____ Very satisfied

1_____2_____ 3_____ 4_____ 5_____6

*Administering a questionnaire*

Questionnaires can be administered by various methods including the post, the internet and via an interview. Researchers need to carefully choose the most appropriate method to reach the target study group and design the questionnaire to maximise the response rate as a low response rate will introduce bias and reduce the power of the study.

*Postal questionnaires*

It is recommended that you search the literature and databases for an existing questionnaire that you could use. If you cannot locate a suitable one you can develop your own. Producing a questionnaire from the beginning is a complex task and beyond the scope of this chapter, but we will cover some basic principles.

*Before starting*

Write down the study goals and only develop questions that directly relate to the goals, not just because the information would be interesting. Locate some examples of questionnaires or specific items by searching databases identified in Useful websites at the end of this chapter. Alternatively, approach a researcher who has used a questionnaire and ask for a copy. Researchers usually respond positively to this request. You may locate two or three questionnaires and assess their applicability to your research. You may want to assess their layout, their language and their ease to complete. Compare them and make a note of the features you like for future reference. Now, decide on the information you need to answer the research goals (demographic, outcome and/or explanatory variables). The next step is to develop the questions that will ensure you have the information you need.

When developing the questions, consider the following:

- Use simple everyday language.
- Keep your intended respondents in mind. Will they understand the wording?
- Develop one or more questions for each variable you have identified.
- Check that each question only deals with one matter. For example, 'I am confident in assessing and swabbing infected wounds' should be 'I am confident in assessing infected wounds' and 'I am confident in swabbing infected wounds'.
- Make sure there are no leading questions or double negatives. For example, 'Don't you think the government should fund home births?'
- Give clear and unambiguous instructions for completing the questions.
- Each different type of question should have instructions on how to complete it.

When sequencing the questions:

- Group questions together logically.
- Sequence all the questions related to each variable/topic together.
- Precede each new topic with a descriptive statement to alert the respondent to the change in topic. An example is 'Now I am interested in how you…'
- Start with demographic questions such as age, education.
- Place sensitive questions towards the end of the questionnaire when respondents may be more comfortable in answering them.
- Questions asking for personal details or sensitive information such as income may also be better placed towards the end of the questionnaire.

*Formatting the questionnaire*

It is important to consider the appearance of a questionnaire as this may influence the response rate. Suggestions for formatting include:

- Use an easy-to-read font with a 10–12 point size.
- Ensure there is enough space between questions.
- Make sure the instructions for completing questions, the questions and the spaces for responses are on the same page.
- Leave a space for general comments at the end of the questionnaire.
- Aim to keep the questionnaire as short as possible. Longer questionnaires are usually associated with a poorer response rate (Kitchenham & Pfleeger 2002).

Pilot-testing is critical and may entail more than one testing. First, ask experts in both the content area and questionnaire design to review your questionnaire and then revise it. Second, pilot-test with a group of between 60 and 100 persons with similar characteristics to those who will participate in your study. Take the opportunity to seek information on the clarity of the instructions, wording of questions, general layout, as well as completion time. Revise the questionnaire with suggestions from experts and the responses from participants.

Finally, give your questionnaire a short, meaningful title, and include a covering letter outlining the purpose of the research, who you are, your contact details and why the respondents' participation will be valuable, instructions for returning the questionnaire and expected return date. Mail your questionnaire together with a reply-paid envelope to the potential participants (Houser 2009; Nieswiadomy 2012).

### Advantages and disadvantages

Postal questionnaires are a very cost-effective way of collecting data from large numbers of participants who may be spread across a wide geographic area. They allow anonymity, which can encourage participation when sensitive topics are being explored. A significant problem of surveys is the low response rates. Response rates of 25% to 30% for mailed questionnaires are common. A response rate lower than 50% places the representativeness of the sample in question (Burns 2000). Another disadvantage of questionnaires is their inability to clarify questions and probe responses. This may result in missed questions or inaccurate responses. Finally, questionnaires may not be appropriate for some groups such as participants from CALD backgrounds. Careful attention to detail and an understanding of the processes involved in developing a questionnaire are of immense value to the novice researcher. While developing questionnaires can be complex, Thom (2007) argues that simple self-designed questionnaires can be used to collect information quickly and effectively to inform nursing and midwifery practice.

### Web-based questionnaires

The internet has increasingly become a well-recognised tool for use in everyday activities. In 2001, approximately 35% of Australian households had internet access. In 2010–11, approximately 79% of persons over 15 years of age had access to the internet in Australia (Australian Bureau of Statistics 2012). In the healthcare environment, adequate access to the internet is accepted as a necessity. With an increase in internet availability and access to nurses and midwives, research using the internet is increasing. However, it is important to consider the participants' experience, researcher implications and general advantages and disadvantages of this approach.

The experience of potential participants may directly reflect the success of the research project. They are commonly notified via email of an invitation to participate in an internet-based research project. The initial email invitation should be motivational and easy to read (Dillman et al. 1998). A hyperlink will direct the participant to a unique, specifically designed survey. Occasionally, the web-based survey site may be password-protected to prevent non-invitees from completing the survey. If this is the case, the original email should contain a username and password. While web-based surveys can be developed and distributed with ease, institutions and associations should be strategic in the number distributed as oversaturation of particular populations may result in decreased participation.

Social networking websites such as Facebook and MySpace are increasing in popularity and provide access to potential research participants. These Web 2.0 applications are interactive and have the capacity to generate web-based polls, surveys and other data collection methods. Additionally, these social networking sites commonly allow users to select networks or groups with whom they wish to be affiliated. The Australian College of Nursing is one example of an organisation that has groups on Facebook, which users can join. These methods of participant recruitment may be of particular interest to social researchers.

When contemplating a web-based survey, a number of matters should be considered, such as the use of hybrid approaches, strategies to increase responses, design principles and protection of participants.

Some participant populations may not have regular access to the internet and may prefer a traditional mail survey approach. In these circumstances, the researcher should consider a hybrid approach, where participants receive a paper copy of the survey and are provided with an internet site where they can choose either (Duffy 2002). Various stand-alone software packages exist that will assist the researcher in designing and collating their survey. There are software programs that combine data collected from online and postal surveys. An example is the Remark software packages. The Remark OMR (optical mark recognition) software scans and collates paper-based surveys, while the Remark Web Survey assists with developing, distributing and collating web-based surveys.

Various strategies can be applied to increase the response rate of web-based surveys, such as pre-notification of the survey, personalising messages, using simple formatting and strategically reminding participants (Perkins 2011).

Morris and colleagues (2004) explored trends in nursing education. The researchers emailed deans of schools of nursing and midwifery to complete an online survey. It was on the second email to non-responders that most participants completed the survey.

The design principles outlined in Box 11.2 need to be considered when using the internet. They will assist in promoting a user-friendly survey and enhance a favourable response rate. Many web-based survey tools are available, including SurveyMonkey <www.surveymonkey.com>. Depending on the survey tool, the input from the participant may be delivered to the researcher in varying appearances. The researchers may receive an email of individual responses, or alternatively they may access an internet site that contains a contemporaneous collation of the responses.

## Box 11.2

### WEB-BASED SURVEY DESIGN PRINCIPLES

- Have a motivational introductory screen.
- Focus on ease of reading.
- Start with an easy question.
- Use a similar format to that of a paper-based survey.
- Keep questions to one screen and avoid the need to scroll.
- Allow participants to skip questions and return at a later time.
- Avoid advanced and/or specialist programming.
- Be cautious when using problematic question types, such as open-ended and 'tick all that apply'.

Source: Adapted from Dillman et al. 1998

An important part of an online design is testing the environment or piloting. Having someone who has previously designed a web-based survey may assist novice researchers in designing, building and testing the survey appropriately.

Data collected should be stored on a password-protected individual computer, rather than on public-accessible computers (Gill et al. 2013). The researcher should establish their survey on their institution's server in preference to a free online survey site such as SurveyMonkey. Storage data on free online survey internet sites may have some degree of accessibility to other people than the researchers. Some human research ethics committees may prefer that researchers do not use free online surveys. Anonymity and confidentiality, security, self-determination and authenticity, full disclosure and fair treatment of participants' data entry need to be considered (Buchanan & Zimmer 2013).

A recent government survey found that nearly half of all Australian adults owned a smartphone (Australian Communications and Media Authority 2013). This level of usage creates another viable method for conducting online survey research. Stapleton (2013) outlined that when adjusting a survey for mobile survey takers, the following should be considered:

- Smartphones have varying screen sizes, so use a simple survey design with few visual distractions.
- If using a logo, keep the image small as these take longer to download.
- Keep the survey short. Asking too many questions has the potential to negatively influence survey completions.
- Use vertical rather than horizontal radio buttons as the input type for questions. Horizontal radio buttons require respondents to scroll across to see all options. This can lead to participants choosing the response most easily visible.
- Avoid the use of the dropdown response format as that can be handled in a variety of ways on the range of smartphones.
- Screens for smartphones are small, so be concise with labels and instructions.
- Reduce the amount of typing required by the participant. Use open-ended questions wisely. Consider if you could ask the same question using a multiple response format.

Finally, consider accessing a service offering software that optimises your survey. This software detects the mobile phone requesting the survey download and provides it specifically for that mobile phone browser and operating system. Stapleton (2013) demonstrated lower non-completion rates among respondents receiving an optimised version of the survey. SurveyMonkey is one service that offers this option.

### Advantages and disadvantages

A web-based survey is cheaper than telephone and postal surveys as it does not require postage or a hard copy of a survey form (Hardigan et al. 2012). The main costs associated with online surveys are incurred at the beginning of the data collection process, with the establishment and uploading of the survey. Some internet sites offer free surveys, which may suffice for the novice researcher with a small budget and sample size. Cost savings occur during data collection and data entry. The researcher will usually receive responses in a usable format such as an Excel spreadsheet. Further, the time lag between distributing a web-based survey and the researcher receiving it back is shorter than for other types of survey. One month is a reasonable time for the distribution and collection of the web information (Stewart 2003).

It is important to know the response rate. Depending on the distribution strategy of web-based surveys, a response rate may be difficult to ascertain, particularly surveys accessible to all internet users. In web-based surveys for specific populations, such as a workplace, all employees should be included so that the denominator is known. Response rates in the literature from web-based surveys have been less than those from traditional methods, with response rates of 20% to 30% being reported (Hart et al. 2009).

The potential populations' characteristics that may affect their accessibility to a web-based survey have to be considered (Courtney & Craven 2005). On the other hand, web-based surveys may provide access to populations that are otherwise difficult to reach (Ahern 2005), such as research across continents or with geographically diverse populations.

In summary, the web provides a rapid approach to designing, developing and delivering a survey. Questionnaires can be distributed and the responses can be collected in a timely manner. Although researchers have an initial cost outlay in the design stage, this method reduces the cost of production of hard copy of the questionnaire, postage and data entry.

## Interviews

### Structured interviews

Structured interviews use an interview schedule to collect data and can be administered face to face or over the telephone. Participants respond to a set of questions where the questions and the possible answers are predetermined, similar to a questionnaire. The structured interview is most appropriate when you are collecting factual data from participants in a study.

Participants need to know what is required of them when taking part in the study. Interviews should be scheduled at a time suitable for both the interviewer and the interviewee, and they should know the length of time required of them. An interview should be carried out in a quiet private area so the interviewee is able to speak freely without being overheard. Choosing an area where the interviewee feels comfortable is also essential (Doody & Noonan 2013).

Matters to consider include developing questions, pilot-testing the interview schedule, training interviewers and recording responses. Developing interview questions is similar to the process of designing a questionnaire. Questions are generally closed-ended with a range of possible predetermined responses (Polit & Beck 2012). The interview schedule has to be piloted using participants with similar characteristics to those who will be included in the study. Problems with the questions, the sequence of questions and the proposed method of recording the responses are assessed during this pilot stage.

To ensure consistency in interviewing, the interviewer has to ask the same questions in the same sequence using the same manner and tone of voice. If more than one interviewer is collecting data, they need to be trained and a protocol needs to be drawn up (MacLennan 2009) so that the same set of procedures is followed with each participant. Training includes having the interviewers rehearse the interview and the use of role play, with each interviewer playing the part of the interviewer as well as the interviewee (Nieswiadomy 2012). Data from interviews is recorded on data collection sheets, tape-recorded or videotaped with the participants' consent.

White (2003) used the following process to explore the extent to which 40 Australian intensive care nurses from seven metropolitan intensive care units considered brain death a meaningful concept of death. A structured one-hour interview consisted of 38 items which had been previously reviewed for their applicability for the study by an expert panel. Interviews were conducted adjacent to the participant's place of work and were audiotaped with their consent. Responses were also entered into a record of interview sheet. Interviewer reliability was determined by having an observer present during the early interviews (White 2003).

### Advantages and disadvantages

This type of data collection allows the interviewer to clarify any questions that are unclear. Researchers can control who participates as it is clear who is being interviewed—unlike mailed questionnaires where someone other than the intended participant may complete it (Polit & Beck 2012). However, structured interviews are costly in time and money. Other expenses such as travel and venue hire add to the costs. In summary, while costly, structured interviews are more personal, gain a higher response rate and result in fewer missing responses.

### Telephone interviewing

Despite a downward trend in the numbers of households with fixed telephone lines, mobile phone ownership has increased (Australian Communications and Media Authority 2011). This availability of telecommunications means that telephone interviews are a viable method for use in clinical research.

Participants need to understand their commitment, which includes timing of calls, number of calls needed to complete the study, estimated length of time of each call and the types of questions. Participants should have access to a toll-free number should they wish to reschedule a call, ask questions or raise concerns. This information is usually provided during the consent process (Musselwhite et al. 2007).

Telephone interviews are generally not designed to last longer than 20 minutes. They are best suited to research with a specific focus rather than a general topic. Computer-assisted telephone interviewing (CATI) has made the process of telephone interviewing easier and quicker. CATI is a software program that allows the questions to be displayed on a computer screen (Polit & Beck 2012) and the interviewer codes the respondent's answers directly into the computer file. It facilitates data collection and improves the quality of data as there is less opportunity for data entry errors. The technique is suitable for large surveys.

### Advantages and disadvantages

Telephone interviews are less costly than face-to-face interviews. The data can be collected quickly and easily across states and time zones, giving access to populations that are otherwise hard to reach. They provide a degree of anonymity that may encourage participation in research where sensitive topics are being explored, such as illicit drug use. However, it may be more difficult to ensure a representative sample as only potential respondents with telephones can be reached. Whether or not this is a problem depends on the purpose of your study. When a potential respondent is not available, call-backs may be time-consuming.

In summary, telephone interviewing is most useful in research with a specific focus, but it may be more difficult to obtain a representative sample. Telephone interactions have the potential to be impersonal, so it is important to build rapport with the interviewee (Smith 2005).

## Observation

Observation is a data collection technique in which the researcher directly observes behaviour with the express aim of describing it. It can be classified as either *participant observation*, when the observer interacts with the people and the activities being observed, or *non-participant observation*, when the observer views the activities without interacting with the people being observed. It is this latter kind that is discussed here.

There are two types of non-participant observation. **Overt non-participant observation** involves observation by the researcher with the full knowledge of the participant. The participant is aware of being observed, knows what will be observed and who will observe them. **Covert non-participant observation** involves observation where the participant is not aware that they are being observed (Nieswiadomy 2012). In general, covert observation is not considered ethical as it violates the principle of informed consent (Watson et al. 2010). See also Chapter 7 on overt and covert observation.

A number of steps are needed when using non-participant observation. They include identifying who and what is to be observed and having clear and objective definitions of the behaviour, action or event. As before, the categories for observation need to cover all the possible behaviours (collectively exhaustive) as well as ensuring no overlap between the categories (mutually exclusive). The categories then form the basis for constructing the data collection instrument (Polit & Beck 2012). Researchers need to check whether or not an existing checklist or rating scale is available. The process of locating and choosing an existing scale is covered in the following section.

In structured observation the researcher is aiming for objectivity. However, total objectivity is not possible because the process of observing is susceptible to bias. The observers' knowledge, experiences and values all contribute to how events may be interpreted and recorded. Researchers need to be mindful of the tendency to rate a participant's observed behaviour more highly because of a positive overall impression of that participant (the Halo effect). The use of a structured data collection tool may reduce these subjective elements of observation.

Participants may change their behaviour when they know they are being observed (the **Hawthorne effect**). Nieswiadomy (2012) suggests that although people initially change their behaviour if they know they are being observed, over time they revert to their usual behaviour. Aiming to make observation as unobtrusive as possible is one way to manage this problem. If there is more than one observer, training is essential (see also 'Structured interviews' above). Interrater reliability, that is, the degree to which two or more observers allocate the same score to an observation, is essential.

Video-recording and audio-recording methods can be used where the events are too rapid or too complex for pen and paper. The data can be collected at the time of the action or event and analysed later. These methods permit the researcher to play and replay the data, ensuring accuracy of coding and analysis (Watson et al. 2010).

Gerdtz and Bucknall (2001) used structured observation to describe triage nurses' decision-making in an adult emergency department in an Australian tertiary hospital. A single observer collected data using a 20-item instrument adapted for the study. Before use, the reliability of the instrument was tested using two independent observers who recorded 10 occasions of triage with 94.6% agreement. The authors acknowledged that the Hawthorne effect may have influenced the results but argue that the observed behaviours reflect what the nurses believed were their best performance.

**Non-participant observation (overt):** Observation of participants (with their full knowledge) by a researcher who does not take an active part in the situation.

**Non-participant observation (covert):** Observation of participants where they are not aware of being observed.

**Hawthorne effect:** A phenomenon in which participants improve or modify their behaviour as a result of being part of an experiment or research study.

Structured observational methods collect data about what participants do rather than relying on their verbal accounts of their own behaviour, which may or may not be accurate. They are very useful when it is difficult for participants to give answers or to give reliable answers—for example, pre-verbal children and older persons with impaired communication skills (Polit & Beck 2012).

It is challenging to be both a researcher and a midwife or nurse, particularly if an event that places an individual at risk occurs during observation. In these circumstances the welfare of the individual takes precedence and the researcher's role is abandoned for the clinician's role. Observing in the clinical setting is time-consuming as time is required for the behaviours or events to occur. Ensuring sufficient participants may also be difficult, as many people do not want to be observed. The use of audio- and video-recording methods can be expensive as they require specialist equipment (Watson et al. 2010). In summary, structured observation is a useful data collection method for nursing and midwifery research. The structured observation needs checklists and this is not suitable where there is limited understanding of the topic.

Table 11.1 summarises the advantages and disadvantages of various data collection methods in terms of time, cost, response rate and access to potential respondents.

## Choosing an existing instrument or scale

A range of instruments can be used to collect quantitative data. We will explore issues relating to the use of existing instruments or scales, the personal digital assistant, personal computers and laptops. A **psychometric scale** is a set of written questions or statements designed to measure a particular concept, for example anxiety or self-esteem. The questions or statements in the scale are called items (Macnee & McCabe 2008). A number of ways can be used to locate a validated scale. A review of the literature on the topic may identify an already existing scale. Another source is a compendium of research tools. These texts summarise the characteristics of scales that have been used in nursing and midwifery research including the name, the variables measured, the population, reliability and validity data and where to access the scale. The book *Instruments for Clinical Health-Care Research* (Frank-Stromborg & Olsen 2004) contains reviews of clinical scales that measure concepts such as body image, fatigue and sleep.

### Data collection instruments

Another source of research tools is the Mental Measurement Yearbook available via the OVID interface. This database covers more than 4000 commercially available tests in categories such as personality and sensory motor assessment. The Health and Psychosocial Instruments (HAPI) database is also available via OVID. HAPI contains a variety of measurement instruments in various formats including questionnaires, interview schedules, scales and checklists. Many scales are copyrighted and the researcher will need to obtain written permission to use the tool. Some cases will involve a cost. As previously stated, developers of these research instruments are generally delighted but they may stipulate that the scale is not to be altered in any way. Some scales are available in the public domain and permission to use them is not required.

There are a number of factors that should be considered when selecting a scale for use. It is essential to ensure that the scale you use measures what you want to measure in your study. For example, if you want to measure resilience it is essential that the

**Psychometric scale:** A set of written questions or statements designed to measure a particular concept such as anxiety or stress.

**Table 11.1** Advantages and disadvantages of different data collection methods

| | Questionnaires | | Interviews Observation | | |
|---|---|---|---|---|---|
| | Mail | Web-based | Face-to-face | Telephone | Structured observation |
| Cost | Provides large amounts of structured data at a relatively low cost | Cheaper in comparison to traditional methods. Main cost occurs during the development phase | More costly than mailed questionnaires | Less costly than face-to-face interviews. More costly than mailed questionnaires | Can be costly if the behaviours to be observed occur infrequently |
| Time | Additional time required for sending reminders and repeat questionnaires to non-responders | Decreased data collection period as there is no lag time for postal delivery | More time-consuming | Allows data to be collected quickly and relatively easily. Call-backs may be time-consuming | Immersion in the field requires considerable time commitment |
| Response | Typically low response rates | Harder to track accurate response rates. May not accurately represent the desired population | Higher response than mailed questionnaires | More difficult to get a representative sample | More difficult to get a representative sample |
| Accessibility | Provides access to populations spread over a wide geographic area. Those who respond to the survey may be different from those who did not, thus biasing the findings | Provides access to hard-to-reach populations. Provides access to larger number of potential participants. Assumes potential participants have access to the internet | | Provides access to hard-to-reach populations | Provides access to populations who are not able to answer questions: pre-verbal children and older persons with impaired communication skills |
| Other | Allows anonymity, which can encourage participation when sensitive topics are being explored. Less suitable for some groups (e.g. participants from culturally and linguistically diverse backgrounds) | Anonymity of participants is easier to maintain. Some online surveys lack flexibility and have limitations in the number and type of data entry fields that are available | Permits clarification of questions | Allows anonymity, which can encourage participation when sensitive topics are being explored. Lack of visual cues may inhibit flow of interview | The presence of the observer may influence the situation |

instrument you choose measures resilience, not some other concept such as coping. Selecting a reliable and valid scale is also important. Frank-Stromborg and Olsen (2004) argue that there is a strong relationship between the amount of psychometric information provided by the developer and the quality of a scale. Where the commonly expected measures of reliability and validity are missing it should be assumed that the quality of the scale is not supported. Understanding what are the most appropriate measures for demonstrating quality and how to interpret these statistics will be covered in the next section.

The feasibility of using the scale also needs to be assessed. If you were interested in measuring fatigue in a group of women undergoing chemotherapy for metastatic breast cancer, a brief and simple instrument to measure their fatigue is required, so that it does not contribute to the fatigue the women experience. Some scales are costly to purchase and require particular expertise in scoring or administering. Unless you have access to these resources and expertise, it may be easier to choose another scale. In some scales the wording may not be relevant for the current population and substitution of some words may be necessary, for example, substituting 'nappy' for 'diaper' in a scale originally developed in the USA, for use with Australian parents. In summary, many factors should be considered when evaluating a scale, and whether or not the scale is the most appropriate for the study often calls for judgment (Frank-Stromborg & Olsen 2004).

## Quality of existing instruments

Quality is an important consideration when selecting a scale for use in research. Frank-Stromborg and Olsen (2004) describe a good scale as valid and reliable. It measures what it is supposed to measure (validity) and it measures the concept consistently across settings and groups of participants (reliability).

Reliability is the degree of consistency or dependability with which a scale measures a concept (Polit & Beck 2012). Three types of reliability will be considered: equivalence, homogeneity and stability.

**Equivalence** involves comparing the degree to which two raters measuring the same event obtain the same results (Burns & Grove 2012). This is also referred to as **interrater reliability**. Exploring interrater reliability is an essential step if the researcher intends to use an observational scale. Cohen's kappa statistic is used to examine the agreement between two raters observing the same event simultaneously and rating it independently. The value of Cohen's kappa ranges from −1.0 (perfect disagreement) to 1.0 (perfect agreement). Values of 0.41 to 0.60 indicate fair agreement, 0.61 to 0.8 indicate moderate agreement, while levels above 0.8 indicate good agreement (Frank-Stromborg & Olsen 2004).

Equivalence also refers to the degree to which two different forms of a particular scale are able to produce similar results when completed by the same participant/s on different occasions (Burns & Grove 2012). In practice there are few scales that have alternative forms, so this type of reliability can seldom be assessed.

**Homogeneity or internal consistency** is the extent to which all items in the scale measure the same variable (Burns & Grove 2012). The most commonly used test of consistency for an instrument with a Likert-scaled response format is the Cronbach's alpha coefficient. The value for the coefficient should range between 0.00 and 1.00. The higher the coefficient the more the measure is internally consistent. A reliability coefficient of >0.70 is considered acceptable for a newly developed instrument with values of between 0.8 and 0.94 desirable. Values >0.95 indicate redundancy in the scale;

**Equivalence or interrater reliability:** This means comparing the degree to which two raters measuring the same event obtain the same results.

**Homogeneity or internal consistency:** The extent (strength of association) to which all items in the scale measure the same concept or construct. The most commonly used test of consistency is the Cronbach's alpha coefficient.

that is, some items on the scale are measuring the same question in a different form (Gillespie & Chayboyer 2013). The Kuder-Richardson (KR20) coefficient is the same as Cronbach's alpha and is used when the items on the scale are dichotomous (yes/no).

**Stability or test-retest reliability** refers to the ability of a scale to produce the same or similar results with the same group of participants on two (or more) occasions. The two sets of scores are compared using a correlation coefficient. Reliability coefficients (r) range from 0.0 to 1.0 and a high correlation between the scores supports the stability of the measure. Test-retest reliability assumes that the concept or variable being measured has not changed during the measurement period (Burns & Grove 2012).

## Validity of existing instruments

The validity of a scale refers to the extent to which it measures what it is supposed to measure. If a researcher wishes to measure self-esteem in a group of adolescents, a scale that truly measures self-esteem and not some other construct such as resilience is needed. Three types of validity are considered: content, criterion and construct.

**Content validity** refers to the extent to which the items or questions reflect the concept being measured. It is subjective and usually based on prior research and expert opinion (Burns & Grove 2012).

**Criterion validity** is used to evaluate whether or not a scale measures what it is supposed to measure by comparing it with another measure known to be valid. Criterion validity can be subdivided into two types: concurrent and predictive. If a researcher wished to test whether or not a newly developed 10-item scale measured fatigue, they could ask participants to complete the scale and at the same time (concurrently) ask them to rate their fatigue on a visual analogue scale measuring 0–10. If the scores from the scale closely match the scores from the visual analogue, the researcher could conclude that there is some evidence for the concurrent validity of the scale. Predictive validity refers to the ability of a scale to predict a future occurrence (Burns & Grove 2012).

**Construct validity** is the extent to which the instrument measures what it is supposed to measure (Macnee & McCabe 2008). Construct validity is established over time with an accumulation of evidence. Methods to establish construct validity include convergent, divergent and multitrait-multimethod.

The *convergent approach* involves the use of two instruments that are supposed to measure the same variable or construct (two measures of depression). Participants are asked to complete both measures and then a correlation analysis is used to assess whether the scores change in the same direction. If one goes up, the other should go up. The *divergent approach* uses measures that are theoretically opposite (fatigue and vitality) and examines the correlation between them, which should be negative. The *multitrait-multimethod approach* is based on the premise that different measures of the same construct should produce similar results while measures of different constructs should produce dissimilar results (Gillespie & Chayboyer 2013). Statistical methods such as factor analysis can also be used to measure construct validity. Factor analysis identifies and groups together items in a scale that measure the same underlying attribute. For further reading on the use of factor analysis to demonstrate construct validity, see Polit and Beck (2012).

## Mobile devices and social media

Innovative ways to engage potential participants should be considered by all researchers, to ensure maximal participation. The emergence of mobile devices with access to the internet means that researcher can have ready access to information and databases to

**Stability or test-retest reliability:** The ability of a scale to produce the same or similar results with the same group of participants on two (or more) occasions.

**Content validity:** The extent to which items on a scale reflect the concept being measured.

**Criterion validity:** Used to evaluate whether or not a scale measures what it is supposed to measure by comparing it with another measure known to be valid.

**Construct validity:** The extent to which a scale measures the underlying construct.

## TIPS AND SKILLS

A number of standard questions such as the SF-36 Health Survey are used across population groups. They have to be translated and back-translated to a language that is widely used. Their reliability and validity have to be checked so they are culturally sensitive and acceptable to the studied groups.

### Implications for evidence-based practice

Evidence-based practice has become an expected standard in healthcare. The evidence from any research will only be as good as the data from which it was drawn. The method chosen to generate the data is therefore a crucial component. There are a variety of data collection methods commonly used in quantitative research, and choosing the right one for the research question, the problem, the design, and the accuracy and consistency of results is at the centre of successful data collection.

assist in the collection of data. Various types of mobile devices exist, historically personal digital assistants (PDA) and now tablet personal computers (tablet PC), such as the Apple iPad, have been used for most types of data collection (Bobula et al. 2004; Fahey & Ranse 2010) and observation of practice.

### Personal digital assistant (PDA)

A PDA is a small hand-held device which was used to store the owner's personal information. These devices were popular in the 2000s as an emerging technology. Today they are replaced by other mobile devices such as smartphones and tablet PCs. In research, PDAs had primarily been used for data collection and capture. PDAs were convenient because the researcher could enter real-time information into an electronic form (Figure 11.1). Once data is entered into the PDA, it is synchronised with a personal computer and imported into a database, removing the need for paper forms and later transcription (Guadagno et al. 2004).

Fahey and Ranse (2010) used PDAs at a large agricultural show in Australia to collect information about the types of advice, clinical interventions and activities that healthcare professionals undertook.

Guadagno and associates (2004) used hand-held devices in four emergency departments to conduct a multicentre study on elder neglect. Information collected from participants included an individual interview and a physical examination. Once data had been entered by the data collectors at the various sites, the data were transferred to a central location via a telephone line.

### Tablet personal computers

Since the introduction of PDA technology, the mobile device market has increased in competitiveness. As such, this has given rise to new technology such as the smartphone and tablet PC. Collecting data using these devices has many advantages. Tablet PCs can be connected to the internet to allow for real-time back-up of collected data. Some tablet PCs do not require specialised programs to create data collection forms or to collect data.

Figure 11.1   Examples of PDA screens used to collect data

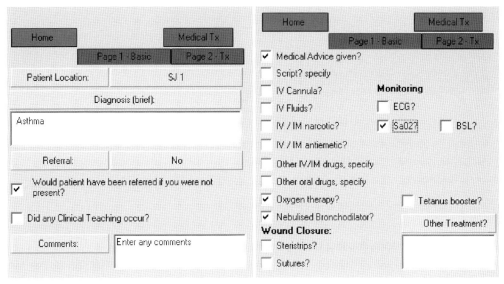

Source: Fahey & Ranse 2010

Microsoft programs such as Excel and Access will function to their normal capacity, reducing the need for specialised knowledge of information technology. Additionally, several mobile devices can be used simultaneously that synchronise collectively. This synchronisation will then create a single database.

Applications (or apps) are developed for many purposes. As such, apps can be developed for research and data collection purposes. Researchers can build and develop their own app to meet their research needs. Mostly these are inexpensive, but the use of apps relies on the acceptance of the users, adequate testing of the technology before use and a back-up strategy in the event of equipment failure (Guadagno et al. 2004).

If designing an app to create a data collection tool for use with a mobile device, a computer software program is needed. Such software programs are available online, and include Pendragon Software <www.pendragon-software.com> and HanDBase <www.handbase.com>. In some instances, forms can be generated using Microsoft Access or similar programs and then transferred from the researchers' app, which is hosted on a tablet PC, to a personal computer which can access the entered data.

Mobile devices do not restrict researchers to single-centre studies; in fact they allow for the use of multiple mobile devices, which have the ability to link their data.

## Social media

Social media platforms, such as Twitter <twitter.com>, Facebook <facebook.com>, LinkedIn <linkedin.com. au> and YouTube <youtube.com> have an increasing uptake among nurses and midwives. These platforms are used for a variety of reasons, such as social networking, the provision of health messages to the public, ability to communicate within a political forum, or conversing during and following a conference (Kaplan & Haenlein 2010). Social media can also be used as a recruitment strategy for data collection purposes. Social media lend themselves to being used as an effective purposive or snowballing sampling strategy. Additionally, Facebook has a 'polling' feature where researchers can ask questions that are then shared among friends, work colleagues and wider social networks.

# SUMMARY

- The methods used to collect quantitative data are a crucial element in determining the quality of the research. There are a number of quantitative methods that may be used and the task for the beginning researcher is to choose a method or methods that are consistent with the purpose of the research and the chosen design.
- Each data collection method has its own characteristics that researchers need to be aware of. For example, using internet-based data collection is not suitable for people who are not capable in information technology. If the data collection methods are not appropriate then the research findings can be challenged.

## PRACTICE EXERCISE 11.1

The SF-36 Health and Well-Being is a standard questionnaire which can be used to assess an individual's general well-being. There are 36 questions, which evaluate physical and mental health. One of the questions is shown below.

In general, would you say your health is:

Excellent   Very Good   Good   Fair   Poor

*Two* team members will collect data by the personal face-to-face interviewing method. They have tested the questionnaire by asking 10 patients admitted to the hospital with chest pain as their chief complaint. They have found that interrater reliability of the questions ranges between 0.80 and 0.95. Does this confirm that the questionnaire has reliability? Explain.

Source: J. E. Ware (2010). SF-36® health survey update.
<www.sf-6.org/tools/sf36.shtml>

## PRACTICE EXERCISE 11.2

Create a survey using SurveyMonkey. To do this exercise, readers will need to be at a computer with active internet access.

1   In your desired internet browser, go to <www.surveymonkey.com>.
2   Click on 'Join now for free!'
3   Enter your details to obtain a username and password.
4   Plan what you would like to ask your respondents and list the variables.
5   Once you have logged on using your username and password, click on 'create survey'.
6   Design a survey with 10 questions:
    (a)   the first five should relate to participant demographics, such as age, gender, sex, postcode, income, highest level of education, religion
    (b)   the next five questions should explore a topic of interest to you.
7   Once your survey is complete, send it to five colleagues.

## PRACTICE EXERCISE 11.3

a   You are a member of a team of researchers investigating the factors influencing increased turnover rates among nurses and midwives working in a large community health centre. The team is aware of research that links emotional exhaustion, a component of burnout, with decreased job satisfaction and seeking employment elsewhere (voluntary turnover). You have been asked to locate a scale to measure emotional exhaustion, and a search of the databases of available instruments identifies an existing scale that could be used. Outline the steps you would take in deciding whether or not this instrument is suitable for your study.

b Below are two fictitious studies that use a structured telephone interview to collect data. What factors do you need to consider when using the telephone for collecting data? The research has ethics approval and potential participants have consented to take part in the study.

*STUDY A*

The maternity unit where you work has recently revised the discharge information given to women following birth. The topics include breastfeeding, infant care and behaviour, physical changes and self-care, emotional changes, resuming sexual activity, and community supports and services. Information is provided in hard copy and online. You have been asked to evaluate women's satisfaction with the information using a rating scale ranging from very satisfied to very dissatisfied for each topic. You decide to collect the data using a structured telephone interview four weeks after the birth.

*STUDY B*

The medical ward in the country hospital where you work has recently developed a structured discharge information program for patients in rural areas living with a chronic illness. The program includes information about managing chronic illness as well as links to sources and websites that deal with particular illnesses. The information is provided in hard copy and online. You have been asked to evaluate client satisfaction with the information using a rating scale ranging from very satisfied to very dissatisfied for each topic. You decide to collect the data using a structured telephone interview four weeks after discharge from hospital.

## FURTHER READING

Frank-Stromborg, M. & Olsen, S. (2004). *Instruments for Clinical Health-Care Research*. Boston: Jones & Bartlett.

Polit, D. & Beck, C. (2012). Developing and testing self-report scales. In D. Polit & C. Beck (eds), *Nursing Research: Generating and Assessing Evidence for Nursing Practice*. Philadelphia: Lippincott Williams & Wilkins, pp. 351–78.

Walonick, D. (2004). Survival Statistics StatPac Inc. <www.statpac.com/surveys>.

## USEFUL WEBSITES

<http://freeonlinesurveys.com>

Free online surveys; provides a service to develop, distribute and collate free online surveys.

<http://handbase.com>

HanDBase, a software platform that allows for the development of form and the collection of data on a hand-held device, such as a personal digital assistant.

<www.ovid.com/site/catalog/DataBase/866.jsp>

Health and Psychosocial Instruments (HAPI) contains a variety of measurement instruments suitable for use in nursing and midwifery research including questionnaires, interview schedules, scales and checklists.

<www.kwiksurveys.com>

Kwik surveys provide a service to develop, distribute and collate free online surveys.

<www.ovid.com/site/catalog/DataBase/120.jsp>

Mental Measurement Yearbook covers more than 4000 commercially available tests in categories such as personality, developmental, behavioural and sensory motor assessment.

<www.pendragon-software.com>

Pendragon Software, a software platform that assists the researcher in development of forms and the collection of data on a hand-held device, such as a PDA.

<www.gravic.com/remark>

Remark has a number of products that will assist with data collection and analysis.

<www.surveymonkey.com>

SurveyMonkey is a service to develop, distribute and collate free online surveys. The most popular web-based survey.

## REFERENCES

Ahern, N. (2005). Using the internet to conduct research. *Nurse Researcher* 13(2), 55–70.

Australian Bureau of Statistics. (2012). *Household Use of Information Technology, 2010–2011*. (publication no. 8146.0). Canberra: Australian Government.

Australian Communications and Media Authority (2011). *Converging Communications Channels: Preferences and Behaviours of Australian Communication Users*. Canberra: Australian Government.

Australian Communications and Media Authority (2013). *Smartphone Tablets: Take-up and Use in Australia*. Canberra: Australian Government.

Bobula, J., Anderson, L., Riesch, S., Canty-Mitchell, J., Duncan, A., Kaiser-Krueger, H., Brown, R. & Angresano, N. (2004). Enhancing survey data collection among youth and adults: Use of handheld and laptop computers. *Computers, Informatics, Nursing* 22(5), 255–65.

Buchanan, E. & Zimmer, M. (2013). Internet research ethics. *The Stanford Encyclopedia of Philosophy*. <http://plato.stanford.edu/archives/fall2013/entries/ethics>.

Burns, N. & Grove, S. (2012). *The Practice of Nursing Research: Appraisal, Synthesis, and Generation of Evidence*. St Louis, MI: Elsevier.

Burns, R. (2000). *Introduction to Research Methods*. Sydney: Longman.

Courtney, K. L. & Craven, C. K. (2005). Factors to weigh when considering electronic data collection. *Canadian Journal of Nursing Research* 37(3), 150–9.

Creedy, D., Cantrill, R. & Cooke, M. (2008). Assessing midwives' breastfeeding knowledge: Properties of the Newborn Feeding Ability questionnaire and Breastfeeding Initiation Practices scale. *International Breastfeeding Journal* 3, 7.

Dillman, D. A., Tortora, R. D. & Bowker, D. (1998). Principles for constructing web-surveys. SESRC Technical Report 98-50, Pullman, Washington. <www.sesrc.wsu.edu/dillman/papers/websurveyppr.pdf>.

Doody, O. & Noonan, M. (2013). Preparing and conducting interviews to collect data. *Nurse Researcher* 20(3), 28–32.

Duffy, M. E. (2002). Methodological issues in web-based research. *Journal of Nursing Scholarship* 34(1), 83–8.

Fahey, D. & Ranse, J. (2010). The role of medical officers at mass gathering events. Unpublished research.

Frank-Stromborg, M. & Olsen, S. (2004). *Instruments for Clinical Health-Care Research*. Boston: Jones & Bartlett.

Gerdtz, M. F. & Bucknall, T. K. (2001). Triage nurses' clinical decision making. An observational study of urgency assessment. *Journal of Advanced Nursing* 35(4), 550–61.

Gill, F., Leslie, G., Grech, C. & Latour, J. (2013). Using a web-based survey tool to undertake a Delphi study: Application for nurse education research. *Nurse Education Today* 33(11), 1322–8.

Gillespie, B. & Chayboyer, W. (2013). Assessing measuring instruments. In Z. Schneider, D. Whitehead, G. LoBiondo-Wood & J. Haber (eds), *Nursing and Midwifery Research: Methods and Appraisal for Evidence-based Practice*. Sydney: Elsevier.

Guadagno, L., Vandeweerd, C., Stevens, D., Abraham, I., Paveza, G. J. & Fulmer, T. (2004). Using PDAs for data collection. *Applied Nursing Research* 17(4), 283–91.

Hardigan, P., Succar, C. & Fleisher, J. (2012). An analysis of response rate and economic costs between mail and web-based surveys among practicing dentists: A randomised trial. *Journal of Community Health* 37(2), 383–94.

Hart, A., Brennan, C., Sym, D. & Larson, E. (2009). The impact of personalised prenotification on response rates to an electronic survey. *Western Journal of Nursing Research* 31(1), 17–23.

Houser, J. (2009). *Nursing Research: Reading, Using and Creating Evidence*. Boston: Jones & Bartlett.

Jirojwong, S. & MacLennan, R. (2004). Do people in rural and remote Queensland delay using health services to manage the episodes of incapacity? *Health and Social Care in the Community* 12(3), 233–42.

Kaplan, A. & Haenlein, M. (2010). Users of the world, unite! The challenges and opportunities of social media. *Business Horizons* 53(1), 59–68.

Kitchenham, B. & Pfleeger, S. (2002). Principles of survey research: part 3: Constructing a survey instrument. *ACM SIGSOFT Software Engineering Notes* 27, 20–4.

MacLennan, R. (2009). Project planning: Projects and protocols. In S. Jirojwong & P. Liamputtong (eds), *Population Health, Communities and Health Promotion*. Melbourne: Oxford University Press, pp. 123–33.

Macnee, C. & McCabe, S. (2008). *Understanding Nursing Research: Reading and Using Research in Evidence-Based Practice*. Philadelphia: Lippincott Williams & Wilkins.

Morris, D. L., Fenton, M. V. & Mercer, Z. B. (2004). Identification of national trends in nursing education through the use of an online survey. *Nursing Outlook* 52(5), 248–54.

Musselwhite, K., Cuff, L., McGregor, L. & King, K. M. (2007). The telephone interview is an effective method of data collection in clinical nursing research: A discussion paper. *International Journal of Nursing Studies* 44, 1064–70.

Nieswiadomy, R. M. (2012). *Foundations of Nursing Research*. New Jersey: Prentice Hall.

Perkins, R. (2011). Using research based practices to increase response rates of web-based surveys. Educause review online. <www.educause.edu>.

Polit, D. & Beck, C. (2012). *Nursing Research: Generating and Assessing Evidence for Nursing Practice*, 8th edn. Philadelphia: Lippincott Williams & Wilkins.

Smith, E. (2005). Telephone interviewing in healthcare research: A summary of the evidence. *Nurse Researcher* 12(3), 32–41.

Stapleton, C. (2013). The smartphone way to collect survey data. *Survey Practice* 6(2). <www .surveypractice.org>.

Stewart, S. (2003). Casting the net: Using the internet for survey research. *British Journal of Midwifery* 11(9), 543–5.

Taylor, J. & Johnson, M. (2013). The role of anxiety and other factors in predicting postnatal fatigue: From birth to 6 months. *Midwifery* 29(5), 526–34.

Thom, B. (2007). Role of the simple self-designed questionnaire in nursing research. *Journal of Pediatric Oncology Nursing* 24(6), 350–5.

Watson, H., Booth, J. & Whyte, R. (2010). Observation. In K. Gerrish & A. Lacey (eds), *The Research Process in Nursing*. UK: Wiley-Blackwell, pp. 382–93.

White, G. (2003). Intensive care nurses' perceptions of brain death. *Australian Critical Care* 16(1), 7–14.

# CHAPTER 12

# QUANTITATIVE DATA ANALYSIS

Petra Buettner, Reinhold Muller and Monika Buhrer-Skinner

## CHAPTER LEARNING OBJECTIVES

By the end of this chapter you will be able to:

- understand how to describe quantitative data
- describe the main functions of inferential statistics
- interpret a confidence interval
- explain statistical hypothesis testing and the uncertainties involved
- interpret a p-value
- choose the correct statistical test relating two characteristics
- understand some concepts of multivariable procedures.

### KEY TERMS

statistic
parameter
p-value
inferential statistics
research hypothesis
measures of central
  tendency
confidence interval
statistical
  hypothesis test
alpha error (Type I
  error)
beta error (Type II
  error)
confounding
  variable
multivariable
  procedures

# Introduction

Nurses and midwives working in the clinical, education or management sectors are called upon to provide information or data about how effective nursing is in improving patient outcomes. Quantitative data analysis using statistics is able to provide the necessary information to demonstrate the effectiveness of nursing and midwifery interventions.

As in all areas of research, there are many new terms and formulae associated with statistics. This chapter introduces the nurse or midwife to topics important in quantitative data analysis that are relevant to practice, education and management. Many other aspects of complex statistics are beyond the scope of this chapter and further reading is suggested where appropriate.

# Why statistics?

**Statistic:** The number or data that describe a sample.

In our modern world we are inundated with **statistics** to an unprecedented degree. Often we do not hear information of the whole study population (or **parameter**) (see also Chapter 9). Statistics are used in the media to provide information, for example on economics, employment and road accidents, and in opinion polls and surveys. Health professionals are even more likely to be confronted with statistics than the general public: the books and publications we are all required to read to remain on top of our profession are often jam-packed with statistics.

**Parameter:** The number or data that describe a population.

For example, a study conducted by researchers based at Curtin University investigated compassion fatigue and compassion satisfaction and their associations with anxiety, depression and stress in registered nurses working in a tertiary hospital (Hegney et al. 2013). The study found that higher anxiety levels were correlated with nurses who were younger, worked full-time and without a postgraduate qualification. Twenty per cent of participating nurses had elevated levels of compassion fatigue and 7.6% had a very distressed profile. In September 2013 the *British Medical Journal* reported the results of a cluster randomised controlled trial based in general practices in Victoria (Blackberry et al. 2013). The study compared a goal-focused telephone coaching by practice nurses with usual primary care in its effectiveness at improving glycaemic control in patients with type 2 diabetes. The study concluded that the addition of a goal-focused coaching role onto the ongoing generalist role of a practice nurse without prescribing rights was found to be ineffective (p=0.84).

**p-value:** The result of a statistical hypothesis test. The p-value gives the probability of obtaining in a sample a difference as large as the actually observed one (or an even larger one) if in reality (i.e. in the wider population) there is no such difference. Thus the p-value is the probability that an observed difference is attributable to chance alone. The smaller the p-value, the less likely that an observed difference occurred by chance alone. If the p-value is less than a set alpha error (usually less than 0.05), then the result of the statistical hypothesis test is called statistically significant.

These examples show that, broadly speaking, statistics provide us with (1) numbers, and numbers are an unambiguous language understood by everybody in the same way, and (2) tools to measure the uncertainty or random error involved when inferring from a sample to the wider target population. This uncertainty is expressed in the **p-value**, which seems to be ubiquitous in research papers and which we will introduce later. The ability to assess the uncertainties involved when deducing from a sample to the wider population is the main reason for the ongoing triumph of statistics in the health sciences.

## Implications for evidence-based practice

The use of appropriate statistical procedures to analyse quantitative data is essential to confirming or refuting research hypotheses posed by nursing or midwifery researchers. The quality of a study and its results is partly judged by the use of adequate statistical methods. Incorrect statistical methods may lead to wrong or misinterpreted research results.

Let us begin by introducing a study conducted by nurses in Queensland. Edwards and others (2009) described a randomised controlled trial of quality of life in a community nursing intervention for patients with chronic leg ulcers. Overall, 67 patients with venous leg ulcers were randomly allocated to either the Lindsay Leg Club® model of care or the traditional community nursing model. The study showed that patients who received care under the Leg Club® model demonstrated significantly improved outcomes in quality of life, morale, self-esteem, healing, pain and functional ability. The authors concluded that this model of care should be evaluated further and should eventually be implemented by community health organisations involved in the care of this group of patients. We will refer back to this example throughout this chapter.

## Descriptive versus comparative statistics

Statistics allow us to address descriptive as well as comparative quantitative research questions. Descriptive statistics will deal with the sample data and describe these data in a comprehensive way. Comparative or **inferential statistics** will be used with the aim of detecting differences between groups. For example, inferential statistics would be used for comparing the results from the group of patients treated under the Lindsay Leg Club® model of care with results from the traditional community nursing model.

All quantitative research should start by formulating a **research hypothesis**—the scientific question the study will be designed to answer with statistical confidence. A research hypothesis includes a precise quantitative statement about the hypothesised result.

**Inferential statistics:** Applied during the study design to estimate the appropriate sample size according to the specified research hypothesis and during the analysis to confirm or reject the research hypothesis.

**Research hypothesis:** A precise statement about the research question the study will be designed to answer. It must be plausible and falsifiable.

---

### Box 12.1

RESEARCH HYPOTHESIS

A quantitative research hypothesis is a precise statement about the question the study will be designed to answer. It must be plausible and falsifiable. The research hypothesis should clearly state study factor and outcome variables and should give a quantitative statement about the expected result of the study. A hypothesis is 'falsifiable' if it can be proved to be wrong.

Example: In the Lindsay Leg Club® model study introduced above, the authors investigated whether participants receiving care under the Leg Club® model would show improved quality of life in comparison with participants receiving individual home care. In this study, quality of life was measured with Spitzer's quality of life index (Spitzer et al. 1981) for chronically ill patients, described by mean value and standard deviation. This scale has a range from 0 = poor quality of life to 10 = excellent quality of life.

A possible quantitative research hypothesis for this study is:

The mean value of the quality of life score in the group receiving the Lindsay Leg Club® intervention will be improved by 1 unit (mean value change from 8 to 9), while the quality of life score for the control group remains unchanged (mean value unchanged at 8).

Comment: In this research hypothesis the study factors are intervention and control, while the outcome is quality of life. The hypothesis is precise as it provides

*(Continued)*

*(Continued)*

a quantitative statement of expected results (it gives the mean values) and it is therefore falsifiable. If the study shows the expected improvement in the quality of life of 1 unit or even more in the intervention group compared to the control, then the hypothesis will be supported; if not it is falsified!

Source: Adapted from Edwards et al. 2009

## Descriptive statistics

### Types of quantitative data

We frequently read or hear information based on descriptive statistics. They are presented in various forms such as percentages or averages. Visually, they are presented in graphs. All quantitative research collects quantitative data, that is, information on characteristics that can be measured, classified and subsequently coded into numbers. These characteristics are usually called variables (e.g. age, gender, concurrent adenoidectomy, number of siblings, quality of life) and the information collected is called the data. Data are described using appropriate statistical methods. The correct choice of a statistical method, however, depends on the type(s) of variable(s) collected.

We need to differentiate two major types of variables: categorical and numerical variables (Table 12.1) and this constitutes the first step in finding 'the' correct statistical procedure for a given data set and a given research question (Altman 1991).

Categorical variables have defined categories (variable gender: categories female/male; variable type of nurse: categories registered/enrolled) and the codes given to these categories in statistical analysis are arbitrary; for example, gender codes could be 1 = male and 2 = female, or vice versa, or any other dichotomous code combination. Categorical data can be further classified as being either nominal or ordinal. In an ordinal categorical variable the categories follow a natural order such as pain being reported as

**Table 12.1** Types of quantitative variables

| Categorical | | Numerical | |
|---|---|---|---|
| **Nominal** | **Ordinal** | **Discrete** | **Continuous** |
| No order of categories | Ordered categories | Integer measurements | Real number measurements |
| Examples: | | | |
| Gender | Level of education | Number of children | Reaction time |
| Blood group | Developmental stages of a child | Number of partners | Age |
| Category of nurse | TNM staging of tumours | Number of hospital beds | Height |

low, moderate and high, while this is not the case in nominal variables (e.g. gender: either male or female; blood group: O, A, B or AB).

In contrast, the observed numbers in numerical variables have an intrinsic meaning (e.g. age: 16 years). Numerical variables therefore retain quantitative information on measurements. They can be further classified into discrete or continuous. Discrete numerical variables are usually natural counts and can only take on whole numbers (e.g. number of children: 0, 1, 2, 3…), while continuous data are measurements that can take on any value within a meaningful range. The values are limited only by our ability to measure precisely (e.g. weight: 45.789 kg; height: 145.2 cm).

Please note: Continuous variables are often modified to become discrete or even categorical, but the reverse process is not possible. For example, age of a person might be 18 years, 9 months, 16 days…but we say this person is 18 years old ('age at last birthday'), hence creating a discrete variable from a continuous one. As a rule, always collect quantitative information as precisely as possible. Categorisation can easily be achieved later during data analysis.

## Description of quantitative data

All researchers are required to describe their data by applying descriptive statistics. Basic description of the data allows us to assess their sample and whether the conclusions reached by the research will also apply to our patients. Descriptive statistics are needed for all quantitative research questions. They constitute the core component of descriptive research and the base for further comparative statistical analyses in comparative research. Correct descriptive statistics summarise the collected data in a meaningful way and are—as all statistics—dependent on the type of variables (Table 12.2).

Descriptive statistics for categorical variables usually only describe the number of people in each category (= absolute frequency) and the percentages of each category (= relative frequency). Numerical variables are summarised using a measure of central tendency together with a measure of dispersion.

The most frequently used **measures of central tendency** are the arithmetic mean and the median. These measures point to the centre of the distribution of the numerical data. The arithmetic mean by definition is the sum of the values measured divided by the number of values, while the median is the value in the middle of the ordered observations (= 50%-quantile). Please see examples for calculating mean and median in Box 12.2.

**Measures of central tendency:** A summary phrase in descriptive statistics for numerical data that describe the centre of the distribution. The most frequently used measures of central tendency are the arithmetic mean and the median.

**Table 12.2** Decision table for descriptive statistics and univariate graphical display

| Type of variable | | |
|---|---|---|
| **Categorical** Nominal or ordinal | **Numerical** Discrete or continuous | |
| | Data convex and symmetrical | Data skewed or too few observations to judge |

*(Continued)*

*(Continued)*

| Descriptive statistics | | |
|---|---|---|
| Measures of central tendency and dispersion | | |
| Absolute (= sample size) and relative (= percentages) frequencies of categories | Mean and standard deviation (SD) | Median and inter-quartile range (IQR) or Median and range |
| *Examples* | | |
| 63 (42.0%; n=150) male participants | Mean weight 22.5 kg (SD 6.5) | Median number of cigarettes smoked per day 10 (IQR = [5, 20]) |
| **Graphical display** | | |
| Bar chart | Histogram Stem-and-leaf plot Plot of mean and standard deviation | Histogram Stem-and-leaf plot Box-and-whiskers plot |

## Box 12.2

### MEASURES OF CENTRAL TENDENCY

The arithmetic mean of a sample with n observations $x_1, x_2, x_3, ..., x_n$ is:

$$\bar{x} = \frac{x_1 + x_2 + x_3 + ..... + x_n}{n}$$

The age of 7 participants (n=7) in a study was recorded as: 62, 71, 59, 67, 88, 77, 59.

Calculation of the arithmetic mean ($\bar{x}$) for this small example:

$$\bar{x} = \frac{62 + 71 + 59 + 67 + 88 + 77 + 59}{7} = 69$$

The median ($x_{0.5}$) of a sample with n observations $x_1, x_2, x_3, ..., x_n$ in ascending order is dependent on whether the sample size (n) is odd or even.

If sample size (n) is odd:

$$x_{0.5} = \frac{(n+1)}{2} \text{ th largest observation}$$

Calculation of the median ($x_{0.5}$) for the small example with sample size n=7.
First sort values in ascending order: 59, 59, 62, 67, 71, 77, 88.
Calculate position of median value:

$$x_{0.5} = \frac{(7+1)}{2} = \frac{8}{2} = 4^{\text{th}} \text{ largest observation}$$

hence the median is 67, which is the fourth largest value.
If the sample size (n) is even:

$x_{0.5}$ = average of $\frac{(n)}{2}$ th + ($\frac{(n)}{2}$ + 1) = th largest observation

Calculation of the median ($x_{0.5}$) for a small example with sample size n=6:
Sorted values in ascending order: 59, 62, 67, 71, 77, 88.

Calculate the position of median value:

$x_{0.5}$ = average of $\frac{(6)}{2}$ th + ($\frac{(6)}{2}$ +1) = th largest observation

     = average of 3rd + (3+1) th largest observation

     = average of 3rd + 4th largest observation

hence the median is $\frac{67+71}{2}$ = 69

A measure of central tendency for numerical data is usually accompanied by a measure of dispersion indicating the spread (variability) of the data. If the arithmetic mean is used as the measure of central tendency, the standard deviation (SD) is the dispersion measure of choice. If the median is used, the inter-quartile range (IQR) is an adequate dispersion measure. Providing minimum and maximum values (i.e. the range) is sometimes informative, in particular when the observed values show little variation. Please read the chapter on summary statistics in Burt Gerstman's book (2008) for further detailed information.

The standard deviation is an important measure of variability. The basic idea of the standard deviation is measuring the combined distance between the mean value and each individual observation. In Box 12.2 we show an example for how the mean is calculated from seven individual age values. The mean was 69 years. The standard deviation for this mean value would take into account the distances, which are the differences between each value and the mean: 62–69, 71–69, 59–69, 67–69, 88–69, 77–69 and 59–69. If we added up just these seven differences we would end up with 0, because positive and negative differences would cancel each other out—this is the definition of the mean value! Hence the formula for the standard deviation is a little more complicated, but the basic idea is looking at these differences to the mean value as a measure of the variability of the data.

*Mean or median—when to use which?*

This question can only be answered by checking the distribution of the numerical variable. If the distribution is convex and symmetrical (Figure 12.1a), the mean will be similar to the median and the arithmetic mean and standard deviation are used for descriptive purposes. If the distribution is convex but asymmetrical (Figure 12.1b), or there are too few observations to judge the distribution, then median and inter-quartile range are the descriptive measures of choice. Figure 12.1b below shows negatively and positively skewed data. Non-convex distributions (including bimodal and concave distributions) (Figure 12.1c) are rare and require expert advice.

Figure 12.1a    Convex and symmetrical distribution

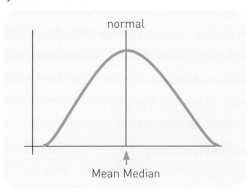

Figure 12.1b    Convex and asymmetrical distribution

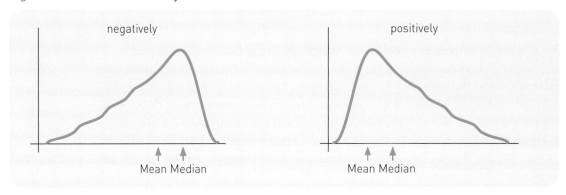

Figure 12.1c    Non-convex distribution

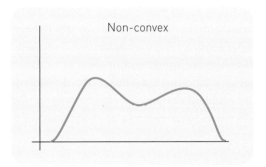

*Please note*

The mean is notoriously sensitive to outliers; the median, in contrast, is a very robust measure. Checking the shape of the distribution under question is a reasonable start and generally provides a good decision base for the choice between mean and median.

Graphical display

Graphical displays are often used in the description of variables since they may show complex data and relationships more clearly than tables alone. As before, the correct graphical display depends on the type(s) of variable(s) involved.

# TIPS AND SKILLS

How to describe quantitative data?

a  Categorical data (e.g. level of education): absolute and relative frequency per category.

b  Numerical data (e.g. age):
Check distribution of numerical data.
If it is convex and symmetrically distributed use mean and standard deviation.
If it is skewed use median and inter-quartile range.

----

*Graphical displays for one variable ('univariate')*

The standard graphical display for a categorical variable is a bar chart (Figure 12.2a). In bar charts the height of the bar represents the absolute (= sample size) or the relative frequency (= percentage) of the category.

The histogram (Figures 12.2b [symmetrical distribution] and 12.2c [skewed distribution]) is the graph of choice for numerical data. In a histogram the bars are not spaced as in a bar chart but joined, indicating that the different categories displayed follow each other directly. In a histogram, the area of the bar indicates the absolute or relative frequency. Please note that in histograms the width of the bars can change and that the impression given by a histogram might vary considerably with the chosen width of the bars. If the widths of all bars are the same as in our examples 12.2b and 12.2c then it is again the height of the bar that conveys the information.

Figure 12.2a–c   Graphic displays for one variable

a

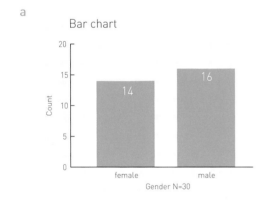

b

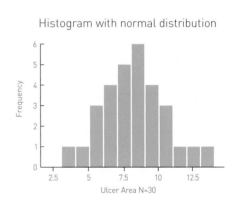

c

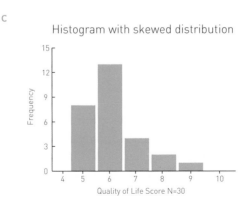

*Graphical display involving two variables ('bivariate')*

If both variables concerned are categorical, for example gender and smoking status, the depiction of choice is a cross-tabulation, which is a table where the categories of one variable define the columns and the categories of the second variable define the rows. If both variables are numerical, for example age and blood pressure, a scatter plot (Figure 12.2d) is used to show their relationship graphically. A scatter plot is a two-dimensional coordinate system with two axes (X-axis and Y-axis) and each participant is marked by a dot where the readings from the X-axis and from the Y-axis intersect.

If one variable is categorical and the second one is numerical there are two options, depending on the appropriate measure of central tendency for the numerical variable. If the numerical variable is convex and symmetrically distributed then mean and standard deviation are used, and a mean and standard deviation plot (Figure 12.2e) can be created depicting the numerical variable in each category of the categorical variable using mean and standard deviation. In case the numerical variable is skewed and hence described by median and inter-quartile range, then a box-and-whiskers plot (Figure 12.2f) can be used where, for each category, the box is defined by the 25%- and the 75%-quantile; the bar in the box is the median, and the whiskers show minimum and maximum value of the distribution.

**Figure 12.2d–f**   Graphic displays involving two variables

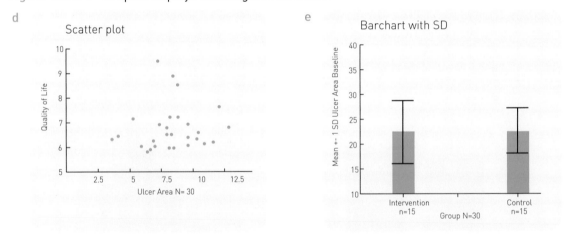

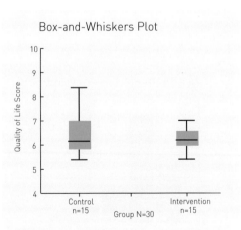

## Box 12.3

### DESCRIPTIVE STATISTICS

Percentage of categorical data and measures of central tendency and dispersion for numerical data are used to describe a data set. Descriptive statistics are used in all quantitative studies, because describing the data is always the first step of statistical analysis.

Example: A study investigated the perceived quality of life of patients who underwent coronary artery bypass graft surgery (Ballan & Lee 2007). Quality of life was measured pre- and post-operatively using the validated SF-36 questionnaire separated into physical and mental health. These two scores range from 0 (= worst) to 100 (= best).

An abridged description of the 62 participants is given in the following table, an example of descriptive statistics display.

| Variable | Descriptive statistics (n=62) |
|---|---|
| Mean age (SD)* [years] | 66.4 (10.2) |
| % Male | 87.1% |
| % Hypertensive | 93.5% |
| Smoking status<br>% Ex-smokers<br>% Current smokers | 42.0%<br>24.2% |
| Median number of cigarettes of current smokers smoked per day (IQR)** | 10 (5, 20) |
| Pre-operative SF-36 results<br>Mean physical functioning score (SD)<br>Mean mental health score (SD) | 26.1 (8.0)<br>53.4 (12.7) |

*SD = standard deviation; **IQR = inter-quartile range

Source: Adapted from Ballan & Lee 2007

## THINKING DEEPLY

### Descriptive statistics

Reading tables like the one given in Box 12.3 is an important skill that any nurse or midwife needs to develop in order to read and understand publications. Please go back to Box 12.3 and look at the numbers given. What do they tell you?

They tell me, for example: The majority (87.1%) of the 62 participants were male and the mean age of participants was 66 years (SD10.2). This implies that the age was convex and symmetrically distributed. The median number of cigarettes smoked was 10. This implies that the distribution of numbers of cigarettes was skewed. It also implies that 50% of current smokers smoked less or equal to 10 cigarettes per day. The inter-quartile range was from 5 to 20 cigarettes, implying that 25% of current smokers smoked less or equal to 5 cigarettes per day while 75% smoked less or equal to 20 cigarettes per day.

## Inferential statistics

Quantitative researchers want to generalise the findings from the data of their participants or sample to a wider population. The ability of statistics to use information from a sample and transfer the results to a wider target population is called inferential statistics. It is one of the main reasons for using statistics in the health sciences. Inferential statistics offers two main tools: (1) hypothesis testing and (2) the confidence interval, which are both grounded in the same theory.

### Confidence interval

**Confidence interval:**
A statement about the target population based on values derived from a sample. It tells us where the true value from the target population is likely to be.

The **confidence interval** is a statement about the wider population, taking information exclusively from a sample. The confidence interval is given with some measure of certainty (usually 95%). If a 95%-confidence interval is given, we are 95% sure that the confidence interval includes the true target population value. If a 99%-confidence interval is given, we are 99% sure that the interval includes the true value from the target population. Hence when calculating a confidence interval we allow some

---

## Box 12.4

### CONFIDENCE INTERVAL

A 95%-confidence interval tells us that the true but unknown population parameter of interest (e.g. the mean value) lies within the interval with a probability of 95%.

Example: A study investigated the perceived quality of life of patients who underwent coronary artery bypass graft surgery (Ballan & Lee 2007). Quality of life was measured pre- and post-operatively using the validated SF-36 questionnaire separated into physical and mental health. These two scores range from 0 (= worst) to 100 (= best) and were summarised using mean values and standard deviations.

| SF-36 | Pre-operation | Post-operation | Difference |
|---|---|---|---|
| Mean physical functioning score (SD) | 26.1 (8.0) | 33.5 (10.2) | 7.4 |
| Mean mental health score (SD) | 53.4 (12.7) | 53.7 (10.1) | 0.3 |

One can calculate 95%-confidence intervals for the post- to pre- differences in the physical and mental health scores.

Difference in physical functioning score: 95%-confidence interval = (2.8, 12.0)
Difference in mental functioning score: 95%-confidence interval = (-0.35, 0.95)

The 95%-confidence interval for the post- to pre- difference in the physical functioning score implies that we can be 95% confident that the true difference in the target population is between 2.8 and 12.0. This interval does not include 0, and the difference of 7.4 between pre- and post- will be called 'statistically significant' (see below for what this means).

The 95%-confidence interval for the post- to pre- difference in the mental health score implies that we can be 95% confident that the true difference in the target population is between −0.35 and 0.95. This interval does include 0, and the difference of 0.3 between pre- and post- is not statistically significant.

Source: Adapted from Ballan & Lee 2007

pre-specified uncertainty most often chosen to be 0.05 (or 5%)—a completely arbitrary but internationally accepted choice.

*Please note*

1  Confidence intervals can be calculated for many different parameters, including mean values, proportions, medians, odds-ratios, relative risks and many others.
2  Generally, all confidence intervals include the sample estimate (e.g. the sample mean, sample proportion). However, confidence intervals do not refer to the sample but to the population.
3  The larger the sample size the narrower the confidence interval. Hence an increase in sample size will make a confidence interval more precise and this is what we want: a precise statement!

## Statistical hypothesis testing for difference

Many health science researchers conduct research to find out whether one type of care is better than another type of care, ultimately comparing groups of people for difference. A comparative research question, such as: 'Is there a difference in the quality of life in patients participating in the Lindsay Leg Club® compared to normal community nursing care?' can be answered statistically by judging how likely it is that an observed difference between the groups is due to chance alone.

This judgment can be based on either of two statistical tools:

1  Calculating the 95%-confidence interval for the difference of the proportions between the groups. If the 95%-confidence interval does not include zero, the groups are called 'statistically significantly different'. Please see examples in Box 12.4 of the 95%-confidence intervals for the differences in physical and mental functioning scores.
2  Conducting a statistical test which directly gives the probability that the difference arose by chance alone.

Often a statistical test is used to assess whether an observed difference is due to chance. A large number of different statistical tests are available and depending on the types of variables involved and the research hypothesis, one particular test is usually most appropriate (Figure 12.3).

The result of a statistical test is called the p-value. The p-value gives the probability that the observed difference between groups (or an even larger difference) is due to chance alone. By convention, a p-value below 0.05 is considered statistically significant. Again, allowing 5% uncertainty is completely arbitrary, though internationally accepted. For example, p = 0.026 implies that there is a 26 in 1000 probability (or 2.6%) that the observed difference (or an even greater difference) is due to chance alone, assuming that in reality there is no difference. A p = 0.026 would be interpreted as a 'statistically significant' result.

*Please note*

1  In the scientific literature the word 'significant' should be used in a statistical context only, that is, only when a statistical test was conducted that resulted in a p-value of less than 0.05.
2  Statistical significance does not automatically imply medical relevance. Small differences can be statistically significant if only the sample size is large enough, but may not be medically relevant. For example, in the Lindsay Leg Club® intervention

**Statistical hypothesis test:** Part of inferential statistics and a decision-making tool used to confirm or reject a research hypothesis. A statistical test judges how likely it is that an observed difference between groups, or an association between characteristics, is likely to be due to random error (chance) alone. A statistical test makes inferences from findings of the sample to the wider population. The appropriate statistical test for a given research hypothesis is dependent on the type of the variables involved.

**Alpha error (Type I error):** One of the two types of potential errors when conducting a statistical hypothesis test. An alpha error can only occur when the statistical test result is 'significant' (i.e. p<0.05). In this case, there is still a small chance (below 5%) that the observed difference (or the observed amount of association) is attributable to chance alone and does factually not exist in the wider population.

**Beta error (Type II error):** is one of the two types of potential errors when conducting a statistical hypothesis test. A beta error can only be potentially committed when the statistical test result is 'not significant' (i.e. p⩾0.05). In this case, there is still a chance that the observed difference (or the observed amount of association) actually exists in the wider population but the test failed to detect it. The beta error is controlled by conducting an appropriate sample size calculation during the design phase of the study.

trial, quality of life was measured using Spitzer's quality of life index (1981) for chronically ill patients. This scale has a range from 0 = poor quality of life to 10 = excellent quality of life. If we consider a difference of 1 unit or larger for this index as clinically relevant but the study reveals only a difference of 0.75, then no statistical test should be performed. Even if this statistical test was statistically significant (because of a large sample size), it would not relate to a result that was clinically relevant.

## Errors in statistical testing

When a statistical test is conducted two types of error can occur (Table 12.3): **alpha error** (also called Type I error) and **beta error** (also called Type II error). Alpha error implies that a statistical test finds a significant difference between groups, when in reality there is none. Beta error implies that a statistical test does not detect an existing difference between groups when in reality there is one.

**Table 12.3** Errors in statistical hypothesis testing

| | | Reality | |
|---|---|---|---|
| | | No difference | Difference |
| Statistical test | No difference | 1-Alpha | Beta error (Type II error; false negative) |
| | Difference | Alpha error (Type I error; false positive) | 1-Beta 'Power' of test |

Alpha error is directly linked to the p-value. We usually set alpha to 0.05 and then only p-values below 0.05 will be called statistically significant. Hence alpha can maximally be 0.05.

Beta error is only controlled if a sample size calculation was conducted which, for a given research hypothesis, will ensure that there is adequate power to detect a pre-specified clinically relevant difference. The power of a study is the probability that the study will detect an expected difference if it truly exists in the wider population. In general, studies should be designed large enough to have a power in excess of 80%.

*Please note*

1   When planning a study we set the alpha error (usually to 0.05) and the beta error (usually to 0.2 or 0.1). During the statistical analysis of the data of the study we calculate the p-value. This p-value is then compared with alpha to assess whether a statistically significant difference was observed.

2   Confident statistical hypothesis testing can only be performed if an appropriate research hypothesis is specified and a sample size calculation is conducted during the design phase of the study. The sample size calculation will allow for controlling the beta error.

Box 12.5

### THE RESULT OF A STATISTICAL TEST
A p-value is the result of a statistical test. The p-value gives the probability that an observed difference or an even more extreme difference happened by chance alone (given that in reality there is no difference).

Example 1: The Lindsay Leg Club® intervention study investigated whether participants receiving care under the Leg Club model would show improved quality of life in comparison with participants receiving individual home care. In this study, quality of life was measured with Spitzer's quality of life index (1981) for the chronically ill. This scale has a range from 0 = poor quality of life to 10 = excellent quality of life.

Study results for quality of life (mean and SD)

|  | Before | After | Difference |
| --- | --- | --- | --- |
| Lindsay Leg Club® intervention | 7.61 (1.65) | 8.96 (1.43) | 1.35 |
| Control group | 7.86 (2.27) | 8.11 (2.10) | 0.25 |

The p-value for comparing the differences between the two groups was 0.014. This p-value implies that the observed difference (1.35-0.25 = 1.15; or a more extreme difference) between the intervention and control group happened by chance alone with a likelihood of 0.014 (or 1.4%) if in reality there is no difference between the two groups. Hence it is unlikely that the result happened by chance alone. This result is 'statistically significant'.

Source: Adapted from Edwards et al. 2009

Example 2: A study investigated the perceived quality of life of patients who underwent coronary artery bypass graft surgery. Quality of life was measured pre- and post-operatively using the validated SF-36 questionnaire separated into physical and mental health. These two scores range from 0 (= worst) to 100 (= best) and were summarised using mean values and standard deviations.

SF-36 pre- and post-operatively

| SF-36 | Pre-operation | Post-operation | Difference |
| --- | --- | --- | --- |
| Mean physical functioning score (SD) | 26.1 (8.0) | 33.5 (10.2) | 7.4 |
| Mean mental health score (SD) | 53.4 (12.7) | 53.7 (10.1) | 0.3 |

The p-value for the pre- to post- change of the physical functioning score was less than 0.001; the p-value for the mental health score was 0.902.

The p-value for the physical functioning score implies that the probability that the observed difference between pre- and post-surgery (7.4) occurred by chance alone was less than 0.001 (or less than 0.1%), assuming that in reality there was no difference. Hence it is very unlikely that the observed difference in physical functioning occurred by chance alone. This result is 'statistically significant'.

On the other hand, the p-value for the mental health score implies that the probability that the observed difference between pre- and post-surgery (0.3) occurred by chance alone was 0.902 (or 90.2%), assuming that in reality there was no difference. Hence it is very likely that the observed difference in the mental health score occurred by chance alone. This result is 'not statistically significant'.

Source: Adapted from Ballan & Lee 2007

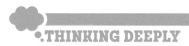

## THINKING DEEPLY

### P-values

The p-value is the result of a statistical test. If a p-value is smaller then 0.05 then we say that the result is called statistically significant. This implies that we have statistically detected a difference between the groups we compared.

If a p-value is larger then 0.05 then this does not mean that there is no difference between the groups we compared. The observed difference was just too small to be detected statistically with the given sample size. If the observed difference was clinically relevant then our study did not have adequate power to detect the difference.

### Selecting an appropriate bivariate test procedure

The choice of the correct statistical test procedure for a specific bivariate (two variables) test situation is dependent on the types of the two variables involved. Once identified, this information leads to the right group of statistical tests as detailed in Figure 12.3.

1   If both variables are numerical (e.g. age and quality of life score) then the correct statistical test procedures can be found in the correlation/regression group.
2   If both variables are categorical (e.g. type of medication and post-operative vomiting) then the correct statistical test belongs to the chi-square group.
3   If one variable is numerical and the other variable is categorical (e.g. gender and quality of life) then the correct statistical test procedure is either a parametric t-test/ Analysis of Variance or a non-parametric Wilcoxon type test.

**Figure 12.3   Classification of bivariate statistical tests**

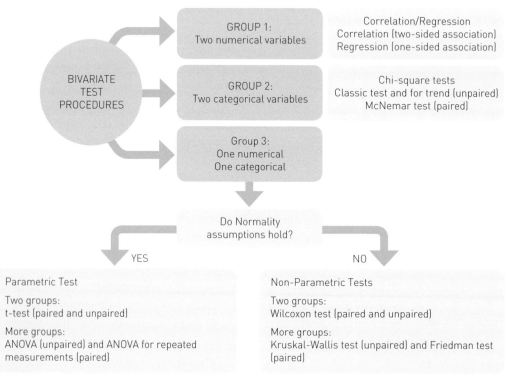

Based on the types of the two variables involved, Figure 12.3 points to the right group of tests for a given study situation. To reach at one particular test, however, additional decisions have to be made as detailed in Figure 12.3 and outlined below.

**Table 12.4**   Examples of research hypothesis, types of data and bivariate statistical tests

|  | Variable 1 | Variable 2 | Test used |
|---|---|---|---|
| **Hypothesis: The mean quality of life improvement is higher in the Lindsay Leg Club® intervention group compared to the control group.** | | | |
| Variable | Intervention or control | Quality of life score (mean value) | |
| Type of variable | Nominal | Numerical | t-test comparing mean values |
| **Hypothesis: In the Lindsay Leg Club® intervention trial the improvements in quality of life are associated with the changes in activities of daily living.** | | | |
| Variable | Quality of life score | Activity of daily living score | |
| Type of variable | Numerical | Numerical | Correlation (two-sided association) |
| **Hypothesis: In the Lindsay Leg Club® intervention trial the gender distribution is similar between intervention and control group.** | | | |
| Variable | Intervention or control | Gender | |
| Type of variable | Nominal | Nominal | Chi-square test |
| **Hypothesis: The median pain severity at baseline is higher in the Lindsay Leg Club® intervention group compared to the control group.** | | | |
| Variable | Intervention or control | Pain severity at baseline (median value) | |
| Type of variable | Nominal | Numerical | Wilcoxon test comparing median values |

Source: Adapted from Edwards et al. 2009

In the following, further terminology is introduced which is additionally required for deciding which statistical test is adequate.

### Paired versus unpaired test

If the research hypothesis under consideration involves the comparison of two (or more) groups who are independent from each other (i.e. different people; e.g. comparing patients in the Lindsay Leg Club® group with patients in the control group), then the unpaired version of the statistical test procedure is used. If the research hypothesis involves comparing the same people who were measured twice or more often (e.g. quality of life is assessed in patients in the Lindsay Leg Club® group at baseline and after six months), then the paired version of the statistical test is correct. This distinction is relevant in statistical test groups 2 and 3 only (Figure 12.3).

## Parametric versus non-parametric test

In test groups 1 and 3 (Figure 12.3) a decision is made as to whether a parametric or non-parametric statistical test is required. The answer to this question is linked to the distribution of the numerical variable(s) involved. If the numerical variable is approximately normally distributed (see below) in all categories of the categorical variable (group 3), or both numerical variables are approximately normally distributed (group 1), then a parametric test is used. Otherwise a non-parametric test will be conducted.

As a rule of thumb, a numerical variable is approximately normally distributed if (1) the distribution is convex and symmetrical; (2) mean and median differ by less than 10%; and (3) the standard deviation is less than a third of the mean value (this last criterion is only appropriate for distributions that are not centrally located around zero). One can also test for normality formally by looking at 'normal plots' or using the Kolmogorov-Smirnov test (Altman 1991; Zar 2010).

## Regression and correlation: One-sided versus two-sided association

Statistical test group 1 (Figure 12.3) differs from the two other groups as regression and correlation procedures are not deciding on a difference, but rather investigating whether an association exists between the two numerical variables involved. This association can be either one-sided or two-sided. When the association between the two variables is one-sided, that is, one variable may influence the other but the reverse is not possible, then we use a regression approach where the independent variable is depicted on the x-axis. A classical regression example is the association between age and blood pressure. Age influences blood pressure (as we get older, blood pressure usually increases), but blood pressure cannot influence age. Age is the independent variable and is depicted on the x-axis.

When the association is two-sided, that is, both variables can influence each other, then a correlation approach is used and the allocation of the variables to the axes of the scatter plot is arbitrary. An example of a two-sided association could be investigating the association between level of physical activity and alcohol consumption as assessed in a survey of young adults. Either characteristic could influence the other; there is no clear independent variable. Hence, this is an example of a correlation problem.

Following the graphical display conventions introduced above, two numerical variables are usually depicted in a scatter plot. Before embarking on regression or correlation analysis we should always look at the scatter plot, as this graph is informative about the nature of the association under study. Standard procedures of regression and correlation statistics assume a linear relationship—that is, as one variable increases, the other increases as well (positive linear relationship: Figure 12.4a); or as one variable increases, the other variable decreases (negative linear relationship: Figure 12.4b). A linear relationship implies that a straight line will be sufficient to summarise the relationship well (see lines in Figures 12.4a and 12.4b).

If the dots of the scatter plot form an indistinct cloud (Figure 12.4c), a negligible association between the two variables exists. This figure shows that whatever value one variable has, the other variable can take any value of its range. Relationships do not need to be all linear, but can be quadratic (Figure 12.4.d), exponential (Figure 12.4.e) or more intricate. In these cases a linear regression or correlation analysis is inappropriate and more complex approaches are necessary.

Figure 12.4  Scatter plots of association

a
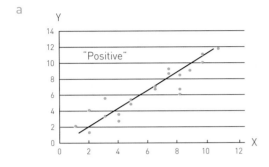

b
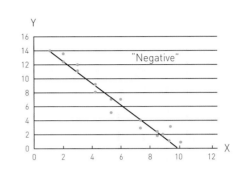

c
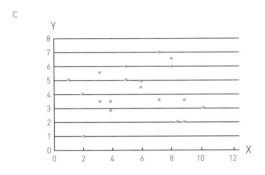

d
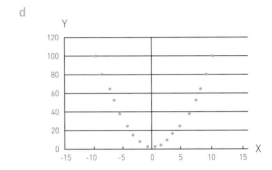

e
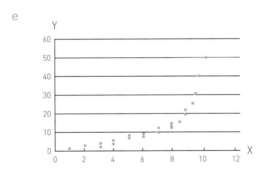

The strength of linear regression or correlation is assessed by the so-called Pearson's correlation coefficient (parametric) or Spearman's rank correlation coefficient (non-parametric). Please always remember when using these statistics to refer back to the scatter plot, as these statistics can be strongly influenced by outliers.

## Survival analysis

One additional bivariate test, the logrank test, is worth mentioning when introducing the most common bivariate test procedures. When a specified event (e.g. death) is observed in a cohort of people who are followed up for a period of time, special statistical procedures (survival analysis) become necessary. The individual survival time (i.e. follow-up time to event) is often unknown for some people in the cohort, because not everybody will have the event during the study period. The cases who do not have the event during the follow-up period or who withdraw from the study are called censored cases. These cases cannot be deleted from the data set because this would lead to an underestimation of the survival probability—as these people did survive for some time. In this situation the logrank test is used to compare survival probabilities between groups. For further details on survival analysis please refer to Altman (1991).

*Please note*

Refer to the chapter 'Choosing the statistical method' in Bland's (2000) book for further details. A description of how to calculate a bivariate statistical test by hand is provided in all standard statistical textbooks (see e.g. Zar 2010 or Bland 2000).

## Multivariable statistical analysis

Studying health phenomena in human populations is usually more complicated than just relating two characteristics, such as age and blood pressure. Blood pressure might be influenced by other characteristics, for example gender and level of fitness of a person. That is, bivariate statistical analysis is often insufficient to adequately address the research question under study. The main advantage of multivariable techniques in the health sciences is that they enable the researcher to assess more than one single study factor at a time and therefore allow adjusting for the influence of factors other than the study factor. These 'other factors' are called confounders or **confounding variables** and they are a common problem in quantitative designs. Confounding occurs when extraneous variables (confounders) that are correlated with both the study factor and the outcome distort the bivariate association under study.

Researchers try to minimise confounding during the design phase of a study by using randomisation. Randomisation allocates participants of a study into intervention and control groups by chance alone. We randomise participants in order to compare groups that are similar with respect to other influencing characteristics (confounders). A randomised controlled trial such as the Lindsay Leg Club® intervention study should have little issue with confounding, since, for example, age and gender distributions should be similar for the two groups that are being compared. Therefore, bivariate analysis is completely sufficient for this trial and for many randomised controlled trails. **Multivariable procedures** usually become necessary in studies in which one cannot randomise or in which randomisation failed.

For example, if one were to investigate the relationship between the number of sexual partners somebody has had during the last year (= study factor) and the likelihood of having a positive test for Chlamydia trachomatis (= outcome), age would need to be considered as a potential confounder. The reasons are that (1) age is related to the number of sexual partners a person has had during the previous year—a younger person is more likely to have changed sexual partners while an older person is more likely to be in a stable relationship. (2) Age is also related to the likelihood of Chlamydia—younger people are more likely to be Chlamydia-positive than older people. Therefore, one could argue that part of the association found between number of sexual partners and Chlamydia is due to age. Age is a potential confounder and one needs to adjust for the effect of age statistically in order to make a valid statement about the association between the number of sexual partners and the occurrence of Chlamydia trachomatis. A multivariable model is required.

### Selecting an appropriate multivariable method

The selection of a suitable multivariable method is dependent on a number of considerations which include the research hypothesis, the type of the target variable (outcome) and to a lesser degree the types of independent variables, and the statistical

**Confounding variable:** An independent variable that varies systematically with the hypothetical causal variable under study. When uncontrolled, the effects of a confounding variable cannot be distinguished from those of the study variable.

**Multivariable procedures:** Used to statistically investigate the relationship between study factor(s) and outcome by simultaneously allowing adjustment for confounding. Multivariable models assess the effects of several variables together on an outcome (= dependent variable). The choice of an appropriate multivariable model (e.g. logistic regression, multiple linear regression, Cox proportional hazard analysis) is foremost dependent on the type of the outcome variable.

assumptions that need to be fulfilled. Table 12.5 provides an overview of the multivariable models used most frequently in the health sciences.

**Table 12.5**  Overview of multivariable methods most frequently used in the health sciences

| Target variable | Multivariate model and use | Main assumptions |
|---|---|---|
| Numerical continuous | Multiple linear regression analysis Assesses strength and direction of relationship | Normality, linearity, homoscedasticity, no outliers |
| Numerical— continuous | Analysis of variance Assesses whether relationship exists | Normality, homoscedasticity, equal sample sizes, random sampling |
| Categorical—binary | Logistic regression Assesses strength and direction of relationship | Linearity, homogeneity of variances, homoscedasticity of residuals, no outliers |
| Survival ('moving binary') | Cox proportional hazard analysis Assesses strength and direction of relationship with mortality | Proportional hazards and linearity |

## Box 12.6

### MULTIVARIABLE METHODS

A multivariable model is used to investigate the relationship between study factor(s) and outcome by simultaneously allowing adjustment for confounding. Multivariable methods can assess the effects of several study factors together. Multivariable methods become necessary for randomised controlled trials when randomisation fails.

Example 1: A study investigates the association between number of sexual partners and prevalence of Chlamydia trachomatis. This research question implies an observational study design because ethically humans cannot be randomised into groups with different numbers of sexual partners. Therefore, a number of confounders might exist which potentially have an effect on the association under investigation and a multivariable analysis is necessary. The confounders might be age, gender, sexual preference, etc.

The outcome is Chlamydia trachomatis (yes/no) and is categorical, binary. Therefore, the multivariable method of choice would be a logistic regression. The logistic regression analysis will assess the effect of the number of sexual partners adjusted for confounding variables.

Example 2: A study on pain management in patients with advanced cancer comparing morning versus evening once only sustained-released morphine sulfate. A visual analogue scale was used to measure pain levels in values ranging

*(Continued)*

PETRA BUETTNER, REINHOLD MULLER AND MONIKA BUHRER-SKINNER

*(Continued)*

from 0 = no pain to 100 = maximal pain. The study randomised patients into the two groups (morning versus evening), but let's assume that this randomisation did not work out for gender. The morning group has many more female participants than the evening group. We also know from other studies that men perceive pain levels differently from women. Hence gender is a potential confounder.

The outcome level of pain is measured as a numerical variable. Therefore, the multivariable method of choice would be a multiple linear regression analysis. Assumptions for linear regression analysis need to be checked. The multiple linear regression analysis will assess the effect of the intervention on level of pain adjusted for gender.

Source: Example 2 adapted from Currow et al. 2007

For technical details on the above introduced multivariable methods, please refer to Feinstein (1996), Kleinbaum et al. (1988), or Kleinbaum and Klein (2002).

## TIPS AND SKILLS

### CHOOSING THE CORRECT STATISTICAL PROCEDURE…

is mostly dependent on the types of variables involved. This is true for descriptive statistics as well as for bivariate and multivariable techniques. It is fundamental for all who want to apply statistics to be able to differentiate between categorical and numerical data. As soon as you know the type of your outcome measure you can at least decide what statistical technique you will need to apply. You may still require expert advice to conduct the actual analysis but you have understood one of the main decision-making processes behind it all.

Implications for evidence-based practice

Nurse and midwife researchers require enough knowledge of statistical procedures to be able to design a study appropriately (sample size), understand and use appropriate statistical procedures, and finally report comprehensively on the findings of their analysis. Similarly, nurses reading published research need first to be able to judge whether statistical methods used were appropriate and second to understand the results of a study in order to interpret nursing or midwifery research results.

## Use of computer programs for data analysis

Nowadays nobody will conduct serious statistical analysis by hand. The rise of faster and faster personal computers and specialised statistical software allows easy access to complicated statistical methodology for everybody. A note of caution should be introduced here: the ready access to statistical software is no substitute for a comprehensive understanding of the implemented statistical tools. Statistical software is a fantastic tool, but only if users have adequate knowledge of statistical reasoning and its underlying assumptions.

There are a multitude of statistical software packages available. Standard statistical software packages which are used by researchers, academic institutions and businesses include, for example, STATA, SPSS, SAS, BMDP, NCSS and S-PLUS. These professional software packages cater for a wide range of statistical problems and have excellent graphic capabilities. The packages are licensed and rather expensive; hence choice might be limited to the software to which your employer or your university has subscribed. There are also a number of freely available statistical packages. For example, Epi Info was developed by the Centers for Disease Control and Prevention (CDC, Atlanta) and is a free-source software targeted towards epidemiologists and public health professionals. You can download Epi Info version 7 from the website <wwwn .cdc.gov/epiinfo/7>. The site links directly to a number of introductory videos which will help you with getting started with EPI-info. Some programs, for example SPSS, offer student and graduate versions that are much more affordable but that are also limited in their statistical capabilities. Most software programs can be checked out for free on the internet for a limited time. There is also a large number of statistics websites on offer (see Useful websites for a start) as well as supporting YouTube videos. We will use Quickcalcs from Graphpad in the second appendix exercise <http://graphpad.com/ quickcalcs>.

At the beginner's level differences between the professional statistical software packages are rather more formal than content-based. Programs such as STATA, SPSS, S-PLUS, BMDP, NCSS or SAS all cover the basic bivariate and multivariable statistical procedures, and differences come only with the perceived user-friendliness of the program. But this is a personal matter, so you need to find the program that suits you best yourself. All statistical software packages come with handbooks, extensive help functions, and there are YouTube videos for many topics. Please read up or ask a specialist, when in doubt.

# SUMMARY

- Statistics is a tool that allows us to analyse data collected during quantitative research projects. It enables us to confirm or reject quantitative research hypotheses.
- Researchers need to understand the type of data they collect that are determined by their research questions.
- Most data analyses require more complex approaches than bivariate statistics and some multivariable methods have been introduced.
- Researchers need to interpret the results of the data analyses. Knowledge and understanding of the research issues will assist the researchers to know the meaning of the results.

---

### PRACTICE EXERCISE 12.1

You are part of a research team which is investigating whether a difference exists in perceived pain during burns dressing for patients receiving intramuscular injection of Pethidine versus inhaling Entonox.

What characteristics do you need to develop a falsifiable research hypothesis?

Try to formulate a research hypothesis for this scenario.

Source: Adapted from Ruegg et al. 2009

---

### PRACTICE EXERCISE 12.2

You are part of a research team which is investigating whether a difference exists in perceived pain during burns dressing for patients receiving intramuscular injection of Pethidine versus inhaling Entonox.

Data is collected on the following characteristics: age, gender, ethnicity, body mass index, surface area of burns, pain score (measured using a visual analogue scale ranging from 0 = no pain to 100 = worst pain), and perceived pain tolerance (scale: low tolerance, moderate tolerance, high tolerance).

a  Classify these variables into categorical (nominal/ordinal) and numerical (discrete/continuous).

- A total of 48 patients participated in the study: 32 participants were male (Graphic 1) and 41 were Caucasian (Graphic 2). Low pain tolerance was recorded for 2 patients, 11 patients showed moderate and 35 showed high pain tolerance (Graphic 3).
- Descriptive statistics for body mass index are: mean 29.1, SD 2.6, median 29.4, IQR [27, 31]; range 23.9. to 34.9 (Graphic 4).
- Descriptive statistics for age in years are: mean 57.0, SD 15.8, median 58.8, IQR [47.7, 65.4]; range 18 to 96 (Graphic 5).
- Descriptive statistics for surface area of burns in cm2 are: mean 8.0, SD 15.3, median 3, IQR [2, 5]; range 2 to 96 (Graphic 6).
- Descriptive statistics for pain score for patients using Entonox are: mean 36.5, SD 15.1, median 37.0, IQR = [26, 51], range 7 to 57 (Graphic 7).

The data are graphically displayed below.

b  Choose the correct descriptive statistics based on the information given for the variables: gender, ethnicity, pain tolerance, BMI, age, wound surface area and pain score.

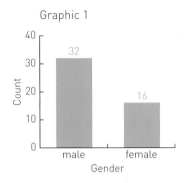

Graphic 1

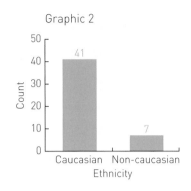

Graphic 2

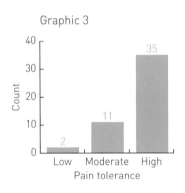

Graphic 3

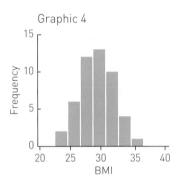

Graphic 4

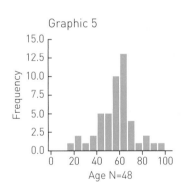

Graphic 5

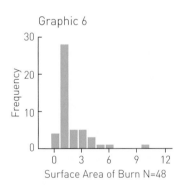

Graphic 6

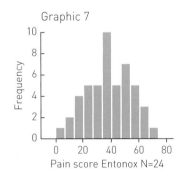

Graphic 7

Source: Adapted from Ruegg et al. 2009

PRACTICE EXERCISE 12.3

### Bivariate statistical tests

You are part of a research team that is investigating whether a difference exists in perceived pain during burns dressing for patients receiving intramuscular injection of Pethidine versus inhaling Entonox.

Data is collected on the following characteristics: age, gender, ethnicity, body mass index, surface area of burns, pain score (measured using a visual analogue scale ranging from 0 = no pain to 100 = worst pain), and perceived pain tolerance (scale: low tolerance, moderate tolerance, high tolerance).

a  Which group of bivariate statistical tests would be appropriate for investigating relationships between the following variables (refer to Figure 12.3)?

- pain score and type of pain relief
- pain score and body mass index
- gender and perceived pain tolerance
- age and gender
- gender and type of pain relief
- ethnicity and pain score
- age and pain score.

Further analysis of the data showed the following: a total of 48 patients participated in the study: 32 participants were male and 41 were Caucasian. Low pain tolerance was recorded for 2 patients, 11 patients showed moderate and 35 showed high pain tolerance (see Graphics 1 to 3 in Practice exercise 12.2).

Descriptive statistics for body mass index are: mean 29.1, SD 2.6, median 29.4, Interquartile range (IQR) [27, 31]; range 23.9. to 34.9 (see Graphic 4 in Practice exercise 12.2).

Descriptive statistics for age are: mean 57.0, SD 15.8, median 58.8, IQR [47.7, 65.4]; range 18 to 96 (see Graphic 5 in Practice exercise 12.2). In the category of male gender the descriptive statistics for age are: mean 55.3, SD 15.9, median 57.3, IQR [45.4, 65.4], range 18 to 96 (Graphic 1). In the category of female gender the values are: mean 60.6, SD 15.6, median 59.4, IQR [53.4, 68.8], range 36 to 90 (Graphic 2).

Descriptive statistics for surface area of burns are: mean 8.0, SD 15.3, median 3, IQR [2, 5]; range 2 to 96 (see Graphic 6 in Practice exercise 12.2).

Descriptive statistics for the total pain score are: mean 41, SD 14.6, median 42.2, IQR [31.3,51.2], and range 7 to 71 (n=48 Graphic 3) and for the pain score using Entonox are: mean 36.5, SD 15.1, median 37.0, IQR = [26, 51], range 7 to 57 (see Graphic 7 in Practice exercise 12.2).

Descriptive statistics for pain score using Pethidine are: mean 45.5, SD 12.8, median 44.8, IQR [39.4, 51.7], and range 17 to 71 (Graphic 4).

Descriptive statistics for pain score in the category of non-Caucasian ethnicity are: mean 45.6, SD 18.1, median 51.1, IQR [30.3, 56.9], range 16 to 71 (Graphic 5).

b  Based on the information you have, which particular bivariate statistical test would be appropriate for investigating relationships between the above mentioned variables?

Source: Adapted from Ruegg et al. 2009

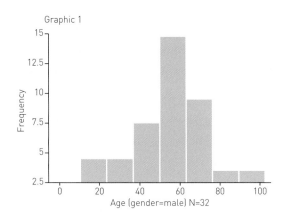

Graphic 1

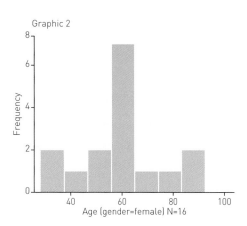

Graphic 2

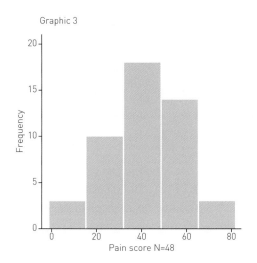

Graphic 3

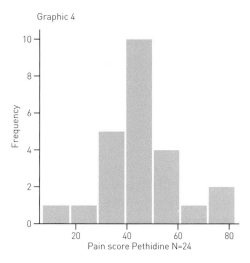

Graphic 4

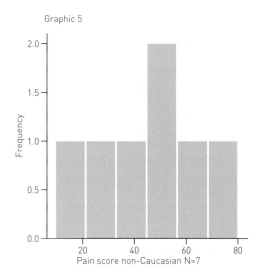

Graphic 5

PRACTICE EXERCISE 12.4

You are part of a research team which is investigating whether a difference exists in perceived pain during burns dressing for patients receiving intramuscular injection of Pethidine versus inhaling Entonox. The research team has now analysed some of the data on pain calculating 95% confidence intervals for the pain score.

a   The 95% confidence interval for the pain score of patients who inhaled Entonox is [30.1, 42.9]. The 95% confidence interval for the pain score of patients who received intramuscular injection of Pethidine is [40.1, 50.9]. Explain these two confidence intervals.

b   Further, the 95% confidence interval for the difference in the pain scores between Entonox and Pethidine groups is [0.86, 17.1]. Interpret this confidence interval.

Source: Adapted from Ruegg et al. 2009

PRACTICE EXERCISE 12.5

You are part of a research team which is investigating whether a difference exists in perceived pain during burns dressing for patients receiving intramuscular injection of Pethidine versus inhaling Entonox.

a   The research team started their analysis by comparing the patients in the two treatment groups at baseline to see whether the groups were initially comparable. They used bivariate statistical tests comparing the two treatment groups with respect to age, gender and pain tolerance among other characteristics. What statistical tests would they have used?

b   The results of these three statistical tests were p = 0.125 for age, p = 0.559 for gender and p = 0.418 for pain tolerance. Interpret these three p-values.

c   Further the authors compared the perceived level of pain between the two treatment groups and the p-value was 0.031. What statistical test was used? Please interpret the p-value.

Source: Adapted from Ruegg et al. 2009

Answers to practice exercises

12.1

You would consider defining the following characteristics:

*Study factor:* Type of pain relief (Pethidine or Entonox);

*Outcome:* Perceived pain (measure pain using a validated instrument, e.g. Visual Analogue Scale);

*Quantitative statement about the expected result:* The expected difference can be either expressed as a total difference between average values (either mean or median) of the pain score, e.g. the mean pain scores in the participants who use Pethidine versus those who use Entonox or as a relative difference between the two study groups, e.g. the pain score in the one group will be x% different (possibly higher or lower) from the pain score in the other group. Always remember that the difference that you are trying to detect should be clinically relevant.

   In addition a measure of the variability (e.g. standard deviation) of the pain score will be needed. Additionally you would need to clearly define inclusion and exclusion criteria of participants.

*Possible research hypothesis:* The mean pain score of patients who receive Pethidine during burns dressing is 5 units (standard deviation 3 units) lower than the mean pain score of patients who received Entonox.

12.2a

| Characteristic | Type of variable |
|---|---|
| Age | Numerical<br>Discrete if measured as age at last birthday<br>Continuous if measured as time since birth |
| Gender | Categorical nominal |
| Ethnicity | Categorical nominal |
| Body Mass Index (BMI) | Numerical continuous |
| Surface area of burns | Numerical continuous |
| Pain score | Numerical continuous between 0 and 100 |
| Perceived pain tolerance | Categorical ordinal |

12.2b

| Characteristic | Values | Rationale |
|---|---|---|
| Gender male n=32 | 66% | Categorical variable with two categories, the second category (female n=16, 33%) is implied |
| Ethnicity Caucasian n=41 | 85.4% | Categorical variable with two categories, the other category (non-Caucasian n=7, 14.6%) is implied |
| Pain tolerance<br>Low n=2<br>Moderate n=11<br>High n=35 | 42%<br>22.9%<br>72.9% | Categorical variable with three categories, data is given for all categories |
| Mean BMI (SD)* [kg/m$^2$] | 29.1 (2.6) | Numerical variable, histogram shows a symmetrical distribution (Graphic 4) |
| Mean age (SD) [years] | 57 (15.8) | Numerical variable, histogram shows a symmetrical distribution (Graphic 5) |
| Median surface area of burns (IQR)**[cm$^2$] | 3 (2, 5) | Numerical variable, histogram shows asymmetrical distribution (Graphic 6) |
| Mean pain score using Entonox (SD) | 36.5 (15.1) | Numerical variable, histogram shows a symmetrical distribution (Graphic 7) |

*SD = standard deviation; **IQR = inter-quartile range

12.3a

| Variable | Type of variable |
|---|---|
| Age | Numerical |
| Gender | Categorical/2 categories |
| Ethnicity | Categorical/2 categories |
| Body mass index (BMI) | Numerical |
| Surface area of burns | Numerical |
| Pain score | Numerical |
| Perceived pain tolerance | Categorical ordinal/3 categories |
| Type of pain relief | Categorical/2 categories |

| Variable | Group of bivariate statistical test | |
|---|---|---|
| Pain score and type of pain relief | Numerical/categorical | Group 3 |
| Pain score and BMI | Numerical/numerical | Group 1 |
| Gender and perceived pain tolerance | Categorical/categorical | Group 2 |
| Age and gender | Numerical/categorical | Group 3 |
| Gender and type of pain relief | Categorical/categorical | Group 2 |
| Ethnicity and pain score | Categorical/numerical | Group 3 |
| Age and pain score | Numerical/numerical | Group 1 |

12.3b

| Variables | Statistical test | Rationale |
|---|---|---|
| Pain score and type of pain relief | Unpaired t-test | Symmetrical distribution of pain score in both categories |
| Pain score and BMI | Regression | One-sided association: BMI could influence pain score but not the other way around; both variables are symmetrically distributed |
| Gender and perceived pain tolerance | Unpaired chi-square test or Fisher's exact test (small sample size) | Pain tolerance is an ordinal categorical variable, but the sample size in the example is small |
| Age and gender | Unpaired t-test | Symmetrical distribution of age in both categories |

*(Continued)*

*(Continued)*

| Variables | Statistical test | Rationale |
| --- | --- | --- |
| Gender and type of pain relief | Unpaired chi-square test or Fisher's exact test (small sample size) | Both categorical variables have two categories; small sample size |
| Ethnicity and pain score | Unpaired Wilcoxon test | Asymmetrical distribution of pain score in one of the categories; small sample size |
| Age and pain score | Regression | One-sided association: age might influence pain score but not the other way around; both variables are symmetrically distributed |

## 12.4

a   The 95% confidence interval for the pain score of patients who inhaled Entonox is [30.1, 42.9]. This implies that we can be 95% confident that the true pain score in the wider target population of patients who inhale Entonox while receiving burns dressing is between 30.1 and 42.9.

   The 95% confidence interval for the pain score of patients who received intramuscular injection of Pethidine is [40.1, 50.9]. This implies that we can be 95% confident that the true pain score in the wider target population of patients who get an injection of Pethidine while receiving burns dressing is between 40.1 and 50.9.

b   The 95% confidence interval for the difference in the pain scores between Entonox and Pethidine groups is [0.86, 17.1]. This implies that we can be 95% confident that the true difference in the pain scores between patients receiving Entonox and patients receiving Pethidine is between 0.86 and 17.1. Note that this confidence interval does not include '0' (= no difference in pain scores). Based on this 95% confidence interval we could therefore conclude that there is a statistically significant difference in the pain scores between the two treatment groups and that this difference might be as small as 0.86 scores or as large as 17.1.

## 12.5

a   Statistical tests used for comparing two treatment groups (= categorical variable) with age (= numerical variable, distributed symmetrical and konvex; see Practice exercise 12.2, Graphic 5): unpaired t-test; with gender (= categorical variable): Chi-square test; with pain tolerance (= categorical variable): Chi-square test.

b   p-values are results of statistical tests. For the comparison between the two treatment groups and age the p-value was 0.125. This result tells us that there is a 12.5% chance that the observed difference in age between the two treatment groups was due to chance alone (assuming that in reality there

is no difference). Thus the probability that the differences occurred by chance (= 0.125) is larger than the usual cut-off of 0.05 and the result of this statistical test would be called 'not significant'.

The results of the other two tests for gender (p = 0.559) and for pain tolerance (p = 0.418) were also not statistically significant. These results are in favour of the study design as it supports the notion that the two treatment groups were similar at baseline and hence comparable.

c   The statistical test used for comparing two treatment groups (= categorical variable) with pain score (= numerical variable, distributed symmetrical and konvex; see Practice exercise 12.2, Graphic 7, and Practice exercise 12.3, Graphic 4): unpaired t-test.

For the comparison between the two treatment groups and perceived level of pain the p-value was 0.031. This result tells us that there is a 3.1% chance that the observed difference in pain between the two treatment groups was due to chance alone (assuming that in reality there is no difference). Thus the probability that the differences occurred by chance (= 0.031) is smaller than the usual cut-off of 0.05 and the result of this statistical test would be called 'significant'. Note that this result agrees with the result of the 95% confidence interval for the difference in pain (Practice exercise 12.4b).

Remember that this comparison was the reason for the study and that this p-value would be the main result of the study. The research team would conclude that patients receiving intramuscular injection of Pethidine had a significantly higher level of perceived pain (mean 45.5; SD 12.8) when compared with inhaling Entonox (mean 36.5; SD 15.1; p=0.031).

# APPENDIX 12.1
## READ AND UNDERSTAND STATISTICS IN A PUBLISHED ARTICLE

Download this published and freely available article:

D. Blackberry, J. S. Furler, J. D. Best, P. Chondros, M. Vale, C. Walker, T. Dunning, L. Segal, J. Dunbar, R. Audehm, D. Liew & D. Young (2013). Effectiveness of general practice based, practice nurse led telephone coaching on glycaemic control of type 2 diabetes: The Patient Engagement And Coaching for Health (PEACH) pragmatic cluster randomised controlled trial. *British Medical Journal* 2013 Sep 18;347:f5272. <www.bmj.com/content/347/bmj.f5272?view=long&pmid=24048296>.

This article reports about the findings of an Australian study published in 2013; a randomised controlled trial of a nurse-led intervention for glycaemic control of type 2 diabetes.

Read the Abstract of this article. You will now understand the Results part fully and in particular all the numbers in the main Results sentence: 'At 18 months' follow-up the effect on glycaemic control did not differ significantly (mean difference 0.02, 95% confidence interval -0.20 to 0.24, P=0.84) between the intervention and control groups, adjusted for HbA1c measured at baseline and the clustering.'

Read the Results section including the three tables of the article. Text and tables of this article provide an excellent example of how to describe, compare and present quantitative data.

# APPENDIX 12.2
## ANALYSE A SMALL DATA SET USING GRAPHPAD'S QUICKCALCS ONLINE

The following table presents a small practice example data set with 20 participants with a free online software package. The data set includes 4 variables: age, gender, ethnicity and systolic blood pressure.

| Identification number | Age [years] | Gender | Ethnicity | Systolic blood pressure [mm Hg] |
|---|---|---|---|---|
| 1 | 49.00 | female | Caucasian | 95.00 |
| 2 | 60.00 | female | Caucasian | 138.00 |
| 3 | 48.00 | male | Caucasian | 120.00 |
| 4 | 85.00 | male | non-Caucasian | 145.00 |
| 5 | 65.00 | male | non-Caucasian | 127.00 |
| 6 | 60.00 | male | non-Caucasian | 155.00 |
| 7 | 65.00 | male | non-Caucasian | 162.00 |
| 8 | 72.00 | female | non-Caucasian | 140.00 |
| 9 | 62.00 | female | Caucasian | 132.00 |
| 10 | 75.00 | male | non-Caucasian | 165.00 |
| 11 | 57.00 | male | Caucasian | 90.00 |
| 12 | 57.00 | female | non-Caucasian | 145.00 |
| 13 | 61.00 | male | Caucasian | 136.00 |

| Identification number | Age [years] | Gender | Ethnicity | Systolic blood pressure [mm Hg] |
|---|---|---|---|---|
| 14 | 58.00 | male | non-Caucasian | 147.00 |
| 15 | 45.00 | female | non-Caucasian | 115.00 |
| 16 | 53.00 | male | Caucasian | 152.00 |
| 17 | 63.00 | female | Caucasian | 145.00 |
| 18 | 61.00 | female | non-Caucasian | 159.00 |
| 19 | 59.00 | female | Caucasian | 120.00 |
| 20 | 55.00 | female | Caucasian | 125.00 |

We want to investigate the following three research questions:

a) Is there an association between gender and ethnicity?

b) Is there an association between ethnicity and blood pressure?

c) Is there an association between age and blood pressure?

Step 1

In order to decide which statistical test to use we need to decide which types of variables we have. This will give us some first indication about the statistical tests to use.

a) Gender and ethnicity: both categorical; Unpaired Chi-square test or better Fisher's exact test (because the sample size is small!)

b) Ethnicity and blood pressure: one categorical and one numerical; Unpaired t-test (we assume normal distribution of blood pressure in this exercise)

c) Age and blood pressure: both numerical; linear regression (we assume normal distributions for age and blood pressure in this exercise)

Step 2

We will use GraphPad QuickCalcs online. When you enter <http://graphpad.com/quickcalcs> then the following screen will appear:

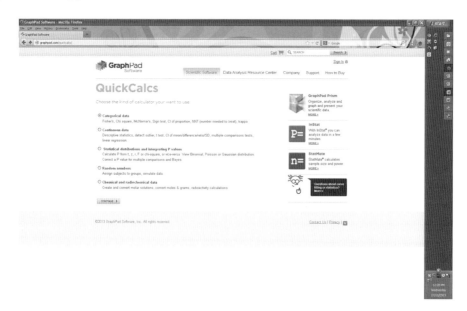

In order to answer research question (a) we need to calculate an unpaired Chi-square test or, better, Fisher's exact test because of the small sample size. By default the QuickCalcs site has ticked the correct calculator already ('Categorical data') and we just need to click 'Continue'. On the following site we need to choose 'Fisher's and chi-square. Analyse a 2×2 contingency table' and the following site comes up which allows us to enter our data directly:

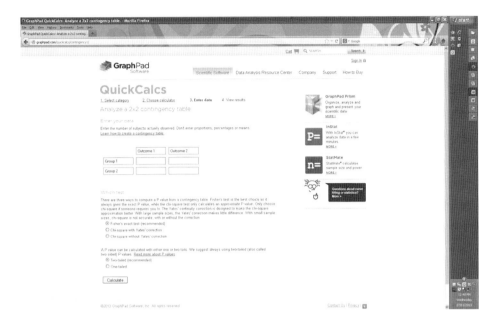

The data set included a total of 10 women, 6 of them Caucasian, while of the 10 men 4 were of Caucasian descent. See output window below. The p-value for Fisher's exact test is 0.6563. Interpret the result.

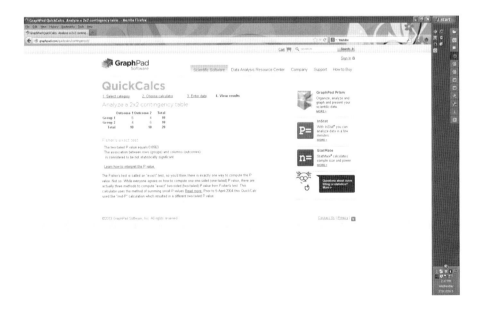

In order to answer research question (b) we need to go back to <http://graphpad.com/quickcalcs/> and now click 'Continuous data' and 'Continue'. Within the exercise we assume that blood pressure is approximately normally distributed and so we can click '*t* test to compare two means' and 'Continue'. The following site comes up:

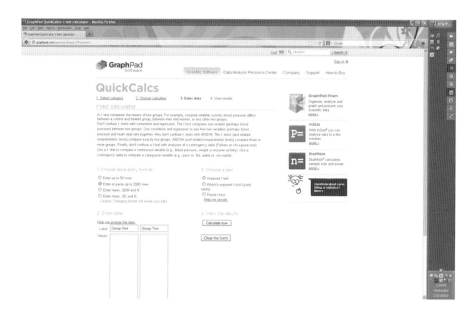

Now you need to enter blood pressure of Caucasian participants as 'Group One' and blood pressure of non-Caucasian participants as 'Group Two' in the available table and click on 'Calculate now' to get the result.

In order to answer research question (c) we need to go back to <http://graphpad.com/quickcalcs> and click again 'Continuous data' and 'Continue'. This time you need to choose the 'Linear regression' calculator to be able to answer the question.

## FURTHER READING

Altman, D. G. (1991). *Practical Statistics for Medical Research*. Cornwall, UK: Chapman & Hall, T. J. Press.

Gerstman, B. B. (2008). *Basic Biostatistics: Statistics for Public Health Practice*. Sudbury, MA: Jones & Bartlett.

Kleinbaum, D. G. & Klein, M. (2002). *Logistic Regression: A Self-Learning Text*, 2nd edn. New York: Springer Verlag.

Kleinbaum, D. G., Kupper, L. L. & Morgenstern, H. (1982). *Epidemiologic Research: Principles and Quantitative Methods*. New York: Van Nostrand Reinhold.

## USEFUL WEBSITES

Statistical calculation pages allow you to calculate numerous statistical processes. The pages offer a good explanation to the various statistics being calculated. <http://statpages.org>

GraphPad allows you to calculate bivariate statistical tests online. GraphPad is easy to use. Try it! <http://graphpad.com/quickcalcs>

## REFERENCES

Altman, D. G. (1991). *Practical Statistics for Medical Research*. Cornwall, UK: Chapman & Hall, T. J. Press.

Ballan, A. & Lee, G. (2007). A comparative study of patient perceived quality of life pre and post coronary artery bypass graft surgery. *Australian Journal of Advanced Nursing* 24(4), 24.

Blackberry, I. D., Furler, J. S., Best, J. D., Chondros, P., Vale, M., Walker, C., Dunning, T., Segal, L., Dunbar, J., Audehm, R., Liew, D. & Young, D. (2013). Effectiveness of general practice based, practice nurse led telephone coaching on glycaemic control of type 2 diabetes: The Patient Engagement And Coaching for Health (PEACH) pragmatic cluster randomised controlled trial. *British Medical Journal* 347:f5272.

Bland, M. (2000). *An Introduction to Medical Statistics*, 3rd edn. Melbourne: Oxford University Press.

Currow, D. C., Plummer, J. L., Cooney, N. J., Gorman, D. & Glare, P. A. (2007). A randomized, double-blind, multi-site, crossover, placebo-controlled equivalence study of morning versus evening once-daily sustained-release morphine sulfate in people with pain from advanced cancer. *Journal of Pain and Symptom Management* 34(1), 17–23.

Edwards, H., Courtney, M., Finlayson, K., Shuter, P. & Lindsay, E. (2009). A randomised controlled trial of a community nursing intervention: Improved quality of life and healing for clients with leg ulcers. *Journal of Clinical Nursing* 18, 1541–9.

Feinstein, A. (1996). *Multivariable Analysis: An Introduction*. New Haven, CN: Yale University Press.

Gerstman, B. B. (2008). *Basic Biostatistics: Statistics for Public Health Practice*. Sudbury, MA: Jones & Bartlett.

Hegney, D. G., Craigie, M., Hemsworth, D., Osseiran-Moisson, R., Aoun, S., Francis, K. & Drury, V. (2013). Compassion satisfaction, compassion fatigue, anxiety, depression and stress in registered nurses in Australia: Study 1 results. *Journal of Nursing Management* 1 November.

Kleinbaum, D. G. & Klein, M. (2002). *Logistic Regression: A Self-Learning Text*, 2nd edn. New York: Springer Verlag.

Kleinbaum, D. G., Kupper, L. L. & Muller, K. E. (1988). *Applied Regression Analysis and Other Multivariable Methods*, 2nd edn. North Scituate, MA: Duxbury Press, Wadsworth Publishing Company.

Ruegg, T. A., Curran, C. R. & Lamb, T. (2009). Use of buffered lidocaine in bone marrow biopsies: A randomized, controlled trial. *Oncology Nursing Forum* 36(1), 52.

Spitzer, W., Dobson, A. & Hall, J. (1981). Measuring the quality of life of cancer patients: A concise QL-Index for use by physicians. *Journal of Chronic Diseases* 34, 585–97.

Zar, J. H. (2010). *Biostatistical Analysis*, 5th edn. Upper Saddle River, NJ: Pearson/Prentice Hall.

CHAPTER 13

# MIXED METHODS RESEARCH

Janice Lewis

## KEY TERMS

mixed methods
 research
incompatibility
 thesis
pragmatism
notation system
emphasis dimension
time dimension
concurrent mixed
 methods design
sequential mixed
 methods design

## CHAPTER LEARNING OBJECTIVES

By the end of this chapter you will be able to:

- understand the purpose of mixed methods research
- identify the differences between quantitative and qualitative research
- describe the different approaches to mixed methods research
- discuss sampling techniques in mixed methods research
- discuss issues of validity in mixed methods research
- identify the opportunities for mixed methods research in evidence-based nursing and midwifery.

# Introduction

In previous chapters we have described aspects of quantitative and qualitative research designs, approaches to data collection and the analysis of data. Recent times, however, have seen the evolution throughout the social and behavioural sciences, as well as in nursing and midwifery, of an approach to research that Tashakkori and Teddlie (2003) have described as the third methodological movement. This approach, mixed methods research, is the subject of this chapter.

**Mixed methods research** is a term that has come to describe a class of research where the researcher mixes or combines qualitative and quantitative research methods in the same project. The other movements described in other chapters of this book are quantitatively oriented research and qualitatively oriented research. Mixed methods research represents a change in that the researchers are primarily interested in both narrative and numerical data and their analysis.

The use of mixed methods has a long history, with examples of research using this approach being identified throughout most of the 20th century and into the 21st. Mixed methods research as an identifiably different methodology, however, is fairly recent, emerging mostly since the late 1980s (Plano Clark & Cresswell 2008). Tashakkori and Teddlie (2003) recognise this recent development in methodology but suggest that the field of mixed methods research has now progressed beyond infancy into adolescence. Adolescence is a good description of the current position. Mixed methods as a research methodology is experiencing rapid growth, as evidenced by the expanding body of literature and, advancing the field, the launch of several journals (e.g. the *Journal of Mixed Methods Research* and the *International Journal of Multiple Research Approaches*) and the proliferation of journal articles across all disciplines reporting on research using mixed methods approaches. On the other hand, as with most adolescents, mixed methods research is still undergoing some difficulties with identity and differences of opinion.

> **Mixed methods research:** Research that systematically combines the collection and analysis of both qualitative and quantitative data in the same study.

# Why conduct mixed methods research?

Following a review of the growing body of research using mixed methods, Greene and associates (1989) identified five purposes for conducting mixed methods research. These justifications have been quite influential and remain relevant today. These purposes are:

- Seeking convergence and corroboration of results from different methods that are studying the same phenomena. For example, in case studies several sources of data are used to describe a single case. This approach is frequently referred to as *triangulation*.
- Seeking to elaborate, augment or add clarification to results from one method with the results of another method. For example, interviews may be conducted to explain contradictory findings in the analysis of questionnaire data.
- Using the results from one method to inform or develop another method. For example, interviews or focus groups may be conducted before a questionnaire is developed. Or direct observation may be used to access small populations and questionnaires may be used to access larger populations, both in the same research project.
- Using one method to discover new perceptions in an area of research enquiry leads to new perspectives and possible reframing of the research question. For example, interviews may be conducted with people who are known to have differing opinions, so that the researcher can acquire an in-depth understanding of the issues before framing the research question and developing the research design.

There are other justifications for combining qualitative and quantitative research than these. Bryman (2006), for example, suggested 16 reasons for mixing research methods in the one study. Nevertheless, all the justifications offered reflect the underpinning notion that mixing methods offers a richer explanation than the sole use of quantitative or qualitative methods, drawing on the strengths of each approach and overcoming its weaknesses.

## Differences between quantitative and qualitative research methods

The possibilities of mixed methods are more clearly understood by considering the differences between quantitative and qualitative research methods. The strengths and weaknesses of the respective methods are worthy of reflection. The following tables have been adapted from Burke Johnson and Onwuegbuzie (2004).

Traditional quantitative and qualitative approaches to research have their strengths and weaknesses (Tables 13.1 and 13.2). One approach is not necessarily appropriate for addressing all research questions. Most mixed methods researchers (e.g. Plano Clark & Cresswell 2008; Tashakkori & Teddlie 2003) take the position that the research questions should drive the choice of method. That is, the method used should be the one that is thought to answer the question best. Not all researchers, however, agree with this position and argue that one approach is preferable and that mixing methods is not appropriate. This debate, although not as intense as it has been in the past, is not yet fully resolved and despite the rapidly growing support for mixed methods research, there is a lack of universal acceptance.

**Table 13.1**   Quantitative research: Strengths and weaknesses

| Strengths | Weaknesses |
|---|---|
| • testing and validating already constructed theories<br>• hypotheses are constructed before the data are collected<br>• may be replicated in different settings<br>• may generalise findings to larger populations<br>• the researcher can construct situations that reduce confounding influences<br>• the researcher can generate theory deductively<br>• data collection may be relatively quick<br>• produces numerical data<br>• accommodates variation in researcher abilities<br>• is useful for studying large numbers of people | • the categories or themes explaining the data generated by the researcher may not reflect the understanding of the subjects<br>• underpinning theories may not be useful or reflect the subjects' understanding<br>• hypothesis testing rather than hypothesis generation<br>• knowledge produced may only be specific to local situations, context or individuals |

**Table 13.2**   Qualitative research: Strengths and weaknesses

| Strengths | Weaknesses |
|---|---|
| • the data are based on the participants' categories of meaning<br>• useful for studying a limited number of cases in depth | • knowledge produced may not be generalisable to other populations or other settings |

| Strengths | Weaknesses |
|---|---|
| • useful for describing complex phenomena<br>• useful for research in areas about which there is limited prior research<br>• study dynamic situations, exploring patterns of change<br>• can identify contextual and setting factors that influence findings<br>• can accommodate changes that occur during the study<br>• can determine the course of the particular event<br>• can generate theory inductively | • it is more difficult to test hypotheses and theories<br>• data collection and analysis may be time-consuming<br>• data collection and analysis is influenced by the researcher's abilities<br>• results are more easily influenced by the researcher's personal biases |

## TIPS AND SKILLS

To understand mixed methods research it is necessary to have a good grasp of both qualitative and quantitative methods. Quantitative and qualitative research methods are explained in Parts 2 and 3 of this book.

- - - - - - - - - - - - - - - - - - - - - - - - - - - - - - - - - - - - - - - - - - - - - - - - -

# Views of mixed methods research

## Incompatibility thesis

Much of the early debate about mixed methods research was based in what Bryman (2007, 2008) described as the *paradigm* argument. Schwandt (2001) defined a paradigm as a worldview or general perspective. In the research context, the word has come to mean the commitments, beliefs and values, methods and outlooks shared across a research discipline. Quantitative and qualitative research may be understood as belonging to particular and identifiably different paradigms. Quantitative research resides in the positivist paradigm, which takes the view that research must be value-free, with the researcher being independent of what is being researched. Objectivity is then the researcher's aim. Knowledge is arrived at by gathering facts that provide the basis for proving or disproving hypotheses. The aim of the research is to identify a single truth. Qualitative research, on the other hand, is considered to be in the constructivist paradigm, which views the researcher as inseparable from what is being researched. Research is bound by the values of the researcher and the notion of objectivity is rejected. Also rejected is the notion of a single reality. For those whose beliefs lie in the constructivist paradigm reality is multiple and is constructed by the observers.

Applying these worldviews to mixed methods research raised some apparently insurmountable issues. For example, many saw it as impossible to be objective and subjective in the same piece of research. This has led to the view held by some that qualitative and quantitative research paradigms, including their associative methods, cannot and should not be mixed. This is the position that Howe (1988) labelled the **incompatibility thesis** where accommodation between paradigms is viewed as not being feasible because the two worldviews or paradigms are in opposition. Nevertheless, not all take that position; some argue that examining the same question from different

**Incompatibility thesis:** The assumption that accommodation between paradigms is not feasible.

perspectives adds depth and understanding, that having different views adds value to the research rather than detracting from it.

## Pragmatism and mixed methods

**Pragmatism:** A worldview which accepts multiple realities that reflect both biased and unbiased perspectives and supports practicality when addressing the research question. It has been proposed as a paradigm that best fits mixed methods research.

For some researchers, the conflict between paradigms remains unresolved. Others (e.g. Creswell & Plano Clark 2007; Burke Johnson & Onwuegbuzie 2004; Morgan 2007) have taken a different position, arguing that research should not be limited to the positivist or constructivist paradigms. They point out that there are other worldviews and one of them contends that **pragmatism** best fits mixed methods research.

Pragmatism is a philosophical movement that began in the USA in the late 19th century. It aimed to find the middle ground between dogmatism and scepticism (Creswell 2003). Its focus was on rejecting traditional dualisms such as facts versus values or subjectivism versus objectivism, and finding workable solutions. Truth, meaning and knowledge were viewed as tentative in that they can and do change over time. Because of this, the emphasis is on practical theory and what works. By taking a pragmatic position researchers can reject the forced choice between methods based on paradigmatic position and in doing so also reject the incompatibility thesis. Thus for mixed methods researchers, the research question is more important than the paradigm that underlies the method. The research method that is used should be one that best answers the research question.

### °.THINKING DEEPLY

In any research, the researchers start with some assumptions about what they will learn and how they will learn it. These assumptions are based in the researchers' beliefs about what they consider to be valid knowledge, what constitutes evidence and what data are needed to contribute to this knowledge.

In this chapter we argue that pragmatism is a philosophical position that can inform mixed methods research. It provides a theoretical perspective which lies behind the methodology. In previous chapters in this book you have learnt about quantitative and qualitative methods and methodologies. What theoretical perspectives underpin these methodologies? How do they differ? How do these theoretical perspectives impact on the research design, data collection and data analysis?

## Status of quantitative and qualitative elements

Another issue that emerged in the development of mixed methods research was debate about the way in which the methods would be used in the same study and whether or not one element of the research was more important than others. Morse (1991, 2003) took the position that mixed methods are possible but that paradigmatic positions must be kept clearly separate. She advanced the thinking on mixed methods research by suggesting that mixed methods studies could be designed in different ways. Quantitative and qualitative methods could be used at the same time or they could be used sequentially, with one method being used to plan the next. Morse also suggested that in a mixed methods study the quantitative and qualitative phases can have equal importance. When mixing methods the role of each method should be clearly stated. In order to clarify the role of each method in this study, Morse developed a **notation system**. The elements of the system are summarised thus:

- use of the abbreviations QUAN for quantitative and QUAL for qualitative
- use of **+** to indicate that data are collected simultaneously
- use of → to indicate that data are collected sequentially
- use of UPPER CASE to denote that more priority is given to that orientation and use of lower case to denote a lesser role, thus indicating the relative weights of QUAL and QUAN.

**Notation system:**
A systematic way of describing how a mixed methods study is conducted.

## THINKING DEEPLY

The research question is crucial for all research. It guides the design of your research, the data you collect and analysis of that data. Bryman (2008) points out that the lack of a good research question often leads to unfocused and confusing research. The research question must be stated in a way that is researchable, that is, expressed in sufficiently specific terms that the question can be answered. It is most important to remember that it is the research question that drives the methodology and not the other way around.

In previous chapters you have considered both quantitative and qualitative research and the types of questions that these research methods can answer. For this reason quantitative questions often relate to the relationship between a dependent and independent variable. Qualitative research questions frequently relate to human experience and behaviour in defined circumstances.

What do you think a mixed methods research question will look like? What features of the research question would make the researcher think that they need to use a mixed methods approach in order to answer the question?

The status of the quantitative and qualitative elements in mixed methods research continues to be a matter of debate. Decisions relating to priority (Morse 2003), weighting (Creswell & Plano Clark 2007) or dominance (Leech & Onwuegbuzie 2009) of the elements or phases of a mixed methods study are considered by many to be core considerations in mixed methods study designs.

## Mixed methods as a continuum

Not all agree with Morse's position on the dichotomy between quantitative and qualitative research methods. Newman and colleagues (2003) argue that considering the comparative worth of the two approaches is pointless and suggest that quantitative and qualitative methods should be viewed as a continuum rather than a dichotomy (Figure 13.1). From this perspective, the weighting or dominance of the element is not as important as the sequence and how the elements interface.

In Figure 13.1 mixed methods research is represented by Zones B, C and D. It is in Zone C that totally integrated mixed methods research occurs. This approach supports the notion of partially mixed methods and fully mixed methods proposed by some theorists such as Leech and Onwuegbuzie (2009). Nonetheless, the continuum approach suggests that the researcher can take a position at any point along the continuum. The choice of position will be driven by the optimal way in which to answer the research question.

Figure 13.1    The QUAL-MM-QUAN Continuum

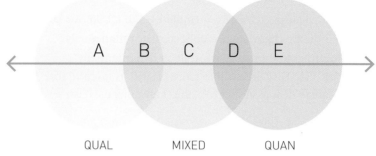

QUAL              MIXED              QUAN

Source: Adapted from Teddlie & Tashakkori 2009

Debates about methodological elements of mixed methods are still ongoing. Much of the debate relates to the best way to design a mixed methods study.

## Mixed methods design

**Emphasis dimension:** This considers the status of the qualitative and quantitative elements in a mixed methods study.

The ways in which researchers have combined quantitative and qualitative methods in any one study vary greatly. Bryman (2006) investigated 232 published articles using mixed methods and identified 18 different ways of mixing methods. In order to provide some consistency, several authors have proposed typologies of mixed methods designs. Creswell and Plano Clark (2007) proposed four basic designs with a number of variants. Teddlie and Tashakkori (2009) suggested nine designs, while Leech and Onwuegbuzie (2009) proposed eight. The lack of clarity in mixed methods research designs is no doubt confusing and reflects the evolutionary stage of the methodology. The research designs proposed by these authors address in various ways two underpinning design issues: the **emphasis dimension** and the **time dimension**. Decisions relating to these issues must be, as Maxwell and Loomis (2003) point out, clearly driven by the purpose of the study and the research question, by the questions that guide the study.

**Time dimension:** This relates to when the phases of a mixed methods study are carried out.

### Emphasis dimension

This emerges from the notion that in the design of the study the status of the quantitative and qualitative elements should be identified. It now appears to be generally accepted that the quantitative or qualitative elements of a mixed methods study can have equal status or that one can be dominant.

### Time dimension

The time dimension relates to when the elements or phases of the mixed methods study are carried out. In a concurrent study, the quantitative and qualitative elements of the study are carried out at the same time. The interpretation of the findings of the research follows the integration of the findings from both elements. In the sequential mixed methods study one phase is carried out before the next and the first phase will inform or shape the second phase.

It is the various combinations of these two dimensions, time and emphasis, that generate the multiple research designs.

**Concurrent mixed methods design:** A design where the quantitative and qualitative data collection and data analysis are carried out within the same timeframe.

### Concurrent mixed methods study design

Figure 13.2 illustrates a **concurrent mixed methods design**. In this study the quantitative and qualitative data collection and data analysis are carried out in the same timeframe. Although there are two elements to the concurrent approach, it is a one-phase study. The interpretation of the research appears when the results of the elements are combined. In the study design illustrated in Figure 13.2 the quantitative and qualitative elements are considered to have equal status (both are represented in upper case). Alternatively, one particular element could have been dominant (with one represented in upper case and one in lower case) if that was what the research question required. For this reason there are a number of possible variations on the concurrent design, depending on the emphasis of the methods. The purpose of this particular research design is to add to the explanation offered to one source of data by another source of data. It is based on the assumption that one method can add to the explanation offered by the other. This is often referred to as triangulation.

Figure 13.2   A concurrent mixed methods study design

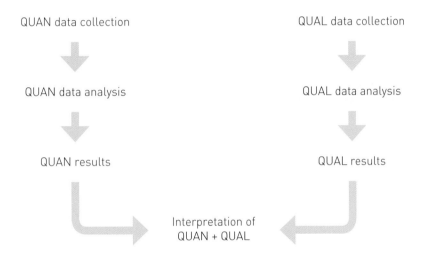

Concurrent mixed methods studies in nursing

The following examples of nursing research studies used concurrent mixed methods designs:

- Ream and others (2006) conducted an exploratory study to enable a detailed understanding of the phenomenon of fatigue in adolescents living with cancer. The researchers used a concurrent mixed methods design. The quantitative phase of the study was a life diary that used numerical rating across a number of items derived from previously developed scales. The qualitative phase of the study consisted of written responses to unstructured open-ended questions and semi-structured in-depth interviews. The qualitative element was dominant in the study.
- Lehana and McNeil (2008) conducted a concurrent mixed methods study to determine how different parent groups (English-speaking and Spanish-speaking) understand medical care provided to their children and the procedural and research consent forms required by that care. The quantitative element of the research was a 36-item questionnaire requiring numerical responses, which measured comprehension or ability to read and understand health information. The questionnaire also collected demographic data. The qualitative element of the study

was focus groups and individual interviews. The strength of the research was that the qualitative analysis enriched the quantitative results, hence strengthening the research. In the article reporting this study the status of the phases was not identified.

### Sequential mixed methods study design

**Sequential mixed methods design:**
A design where the quantitative and qualitative data collection and data analysis are carried out in different timeframes and in two distinct phases.

Figure 13.3 describes a generic **sequential mixed methods design**. Characteristic of this design is that there are two distinct phases that are conducted in separate timeframes. The first phase is used to develop and inform the second. Phase 1 can either be quantitative or qualitative, as can Phase 2. Similarly, Phase 1 or Phase 2 can be dominant or have equal status. For this reason there can be a number of variations of a sequential mixed methods study design, depending on decisions about sequence, timeframes and emphasis. The results of a study are normally in the interpretation of the data following the second phase. The dotted line connecting the results of Phase 1 indicates how results from both phases can influence the interpretation of the results of the study.

**Figure 13.3    A sequential mixed methods research design**

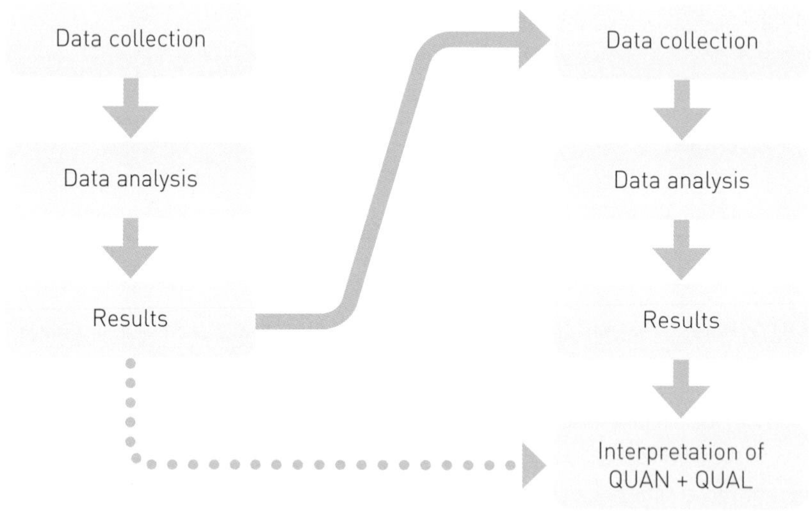

### Sequential mixed methods in nursing

The following nursing research studies used sequential mixed methods designs:

- Davila (2006) used a sequential mixed methods design to develop and evaluate an in-service program aimed at increasing nurses' knowledge and skills in responding to intimate partner violence. Phase 1 used interviews with nurses to identify their learning needs. The analysis of the qualitative data led to the development of an in-service training program designed to meet the expressed needs of nursing staff for enhancing their intervention skills with the intimate partner. Phase 2 of the study was a one-group pre-test/post-test design to evaluate the effectiveness of the program. This phase used quantitative methods.
- In an Australian study, Farrell and Rose (2008) used a sequential mixed methods design to investigate whether personal digital assistants would enhance students' pharmacological and clinical contextual knowledge. In the first phase of the study, a quantitative phase, a quasi-experimental, non-equivalent experimental group design

was used. Some student nurses were allocated to a clinical area with the use of PDAs and some were allocated to areas without the use of PDAs. Before the clinical placement both groups completed a questionnaire requiring numerical responses designed to assess pharmacological knowledge. Later both groups completed the same test on the completion of the clinical placement. The qualitative phase was also conducted on the completion of the clinical placement to explore issues related to the use of PDAs and the influence on students' pharmacological learning. Data were collected using focus group interviews.

## Sampling techniques for mixed methods studies

In both quantitative and qualitative research, data are collected. Sampling techniques appropriate for each approach need to be considered. Qualitative sampling strategies normally employ purposive sampling techniques, whereas quantitative studies use probability sampling. See Table 13.3 for a brief overview of the essential differences between purposive and probability sampling.

**Table 13.3** Purposive and probability sampling

| | Purposive sampling | Probability sampling |
| --- | --- | --- |
| Purpose | To generate a sample that will address research questions | To generate a sample that will address research questions |
| Generalisability | Form of generalisability (transferability) | Form of generalisability (external validity) |
| Selection of cases | Those that can best inform the research | Those that are collectively representative of the population |
| Sample size | Usually less than 30 | Usually more than 50 |
| Time of sample selection | Before and during study | Before study |
| Selection method | Expert judgment | Mathematical formula |
| Data | Narrative data | Numeric data |

### TIPS AND SKILLS

Both quantitative and qualitative sampling techniques must be considered. See Chapter 5, Sampling in Qualitative Research and Chapter 9, Sampling in Quantitative Research.

The researcher using mixed methods would follow the assumptions of the technique being used. Mixed methods research, however, presents some issues to be resolved. As mixed methods research has at least two components/elements/phases, how to draw the research sample for each of these components remains unspecified.

Teddlie and Yu (2007) reviewed the literature for examples of mixed methods sampling techniques. They found that generally in concurrent mixed methods studies the sampling procedures occurred independently. Most of the reported literature appears to use only one research sample. In this approach, the quantitative element of the study has a larger sample and the purposive sample for the qualitative element is drawn from the larger probability sample. There are nevertheless examples of studies that used two independent research samples. Sampling decisions were made according to the research question.

With sequential mixed methods studies sampling is determined by the research design and the related emphasis and sequence decisions. It was apparent, however, in most reported research that the results of Phase 1 influenced the sampling for Phase 2. Again the sample for Phase 1 may be drawn upon for Phase 2 or alternatively separate samples could be chosen. Teddlie and Yu (2007), drawing on other authors and their own research, developed guidelines for mixed methods sampling:

- The sampling strategy should stem logically from the research question.
- The assumptions of the probability and purposive sampling techniques should be followed.
- The sampling strategy should generate quantitative and qualitative databases containing enough data to answer the research question and support the reported findings of the research.
- The sampling strategy must be ethical.
- The sampling strategy must be possible and realistic.
- The sampling strategy should be described in enough detail so that other researchers can assess the credibility of the research.

## Analysis of mixed methods data

The analysis of qualitative and quantitative data is discussed elsewhere in this book (Chapters 8 and 12). In mixed methods research analysis offers some unique challenges. The way in which mixed methods studies may be differentiated from other studies is in the integration of the quantitative and qualitative elements. Integration of the datasets is a key feature of a mixed methods study. Without integrating or mixing the elements or phases, the study becomes two separate studies rather than one cohesive whole. This integration, however, is not without problems and the procedures for doing so are still underdeveloped. Following a review of published articles in health services research, Zhang and Creswell (2013) identified three general approaches that have been used to integrate the data. In the first approach researchers analyse the two types of data at the same time, but separately, and integrate results only during interpretation. This was consistent with the findings of Bryman (2006) and also Bazeley (2006) that most studies do not integrate data until the final interpretation of the findings. In another approach to mixing identified by Zhang and Creswell, the researchers connected the two phases in such a way that the second phase was built on the findings of the first. This approach is consistent with a sequential mixed methods study. The third approach is mixing the data types by embedding the analysis of one data type within the other. This is a much more complex approach and could be expected to be used in a concurrent mixed methods study.

The concurrent mixed methods study is more challenging as this is a one-phase study and the results are dependent on combining the elements and require the data sets to be combined in some way. The development of approaches to the integration of mixed methods data sets has been slow. Computer software is available for the numerical coding of qualitative data ('quantitising'), thus making qualitative data accessible for statistical analysis. Converting quantitative data into narrative ('qualitising') remains problematic.

Bazeley (2006) suggests that although a number of factors may have influenced this protracted development, the principal issue relates to the skills required to manage large data sets. In addition, if the integration of the data sets becomes too complex, this may place the satisfactory completion of the research at risk. The difficulty of the integration process is supported indirectly by Teddlie and Tashakkori (2009), who present a complex typology of mixed methods data analysis techniques related to the purpose of the research and the research design. The diversity of approaches and the skill mix needed by the researcher are intimidating, and as Bazeley (2006) points out, it is for this reason that integration is frequently put in the 'too hard basket'.

Despite difficulties, researchers are endeavouring to develop a method for achieving integration in mixed methods. Fetters and associates (2013) found that integration may occur in the structure of the research question, in data collection and data analysis, or at the point of interpretation or some combination of these. The approach of the integration of the data will depend on the research design. There is evidence of wider use of mixed methods and a growing understanding of approaches to integrating quantitative and qualitative methods in the same study. For example, Plano Clark and associates (2013) explored practices for embedding qualitative data within a randomised clinical trial. It is likely that techniques for integrating quantitative and qualitative data sets will be the next step in the development of mixed methods research.

## Issues of validity in mixed methods research

Issues of validity in mixed methods research are challenging because quantitative and qualitative research have different developmental pathways. While such issues in quantitative research have a long history, validity in qualitative research is less clearly understood. The way to address issues of validity in mixed methods is still evolving. Teddlie and Tashakkori (2009) report that at this stage there is no cohesive and comprehensive framework for establishing the validity of mixed methods studies. Onwuegbuzie and Johnson (2006) argue that because of the unique nature of mixed methods research a new nomenclature should be developed; they recommend that validity in mixed methods research should be thought of in terms of legitimation. Regardless of how validity is labelled, it is essential that the researcher establishes the credibility of mixed methods research. Drawing on Teddlie and Tashakkori (2009), the researcher needs to attend to several principles:

- establishing the suitability of the research design by clearly articulating the relationship between the research question and the methods of study
- ensuring that all the elements of the quantitative and qualitative components of the research design are conducted in a manner that demonstrates the established standards of research rigour required by each method
- demonstrating the relationship between the quantitative and qualitative elements of the study and how this relationship contributes to the findings of the study. In a concurrent mixed methods study this relates to how the findings of the concurrent elements are combined, and in a sequential mixed methods study to how the findings of Phase 1 inform Phase 2 and how the two phases inform the findings of the study.

It is worthwhile remembering that

> Mixed methods are inherently neither more nor less valid than specific approaches to research. As with any research, validity stems more from the appropriateness, thoroughness and effectiveness with which those methods are applied and the care given to thoughtful weighing of the evidence than from the application of a particular set of rules or adherence to an established tradition. (Bazeley 2006, p. 150)

## TIPS AND SKILLS

Demonstrating the relationship between the quantitative and qualitative elements of the study is essential to establishing the credibility of the research.

### Implications for evidence-based practice

Evidence from empirical studies using mixed methods research is as important in healthcare services as studies that use a single approach. Mixed methods research is likely to be increasingly used by nurse/midwife researchers to explore health problems so that health services can be improved. Users and readers can use its principles to critique both quantitative and qualitative research to identify the strengths and weaknesses of research publications. These may be challenging tasks but they are achievable, even by those who lack experience, in particular novice researchers or clinicians. Guidelines for synthesising evidence based on mixed methods research are not yet well developed.

## The future of mixed methods research

The rapid growth of mixed methods suggests that the approach is offering something innovative to research. That narrative can be used to add meaning to numbers and numbers can be used to add precision to narrative is being recognised across many disciplines. A mixed methods approach draws on the strengths of both qualitative and quantitative methods and overcomes their weaknesses, and can conceivably be used to answer a broader and more complex range of research questions. In addition, a mixed methods approach can provide strong evidence through the convergence or corroboration of findings and can add insights and understandings that may be missed when only one method is used. In line with current trends, in the future mixed methods research is likely to make a considerable contribution as one of the methods available to study the complex phenomena that are of interest to nurses and midwives.

Mixed methods research still offers many challenges. The diversity of definitions, conceptualisations and nomenclature, in addition to the confusing variety of research designs, reflects the developmental stage of mixed methods as a research methodology. This lack of clarity can be confusing to students and researchers alike. There are also some methodological issues which have yet to be resolved satisfactorily. The biggest emerging challenge relates to the way in which the quantitative and qualitative strands of the study are integrated. Generally understood methods for integration are yet to be forthcoming. This integration is nevertheless central to the concept of mixed methods research.

A mixed methods study is not two separate studies that happen to be addressing the same issue in a different way; it is one study that uses different methods to address a clearly expressed research question. Developing protocols for the integration of these methods is essential if mixed methods research is to continue to develop.

On a more practical level, mixed methods research is often more complex and time-consuming, requiring high-level skills in the researcher. It can be difficult for a single researcher to carry out both phases of the study, especially when a concurrent design is being used. Having skills in both quantitative and qualitative methods could be particularly challenging for a student researcher.

Nevertheless, mixed methods is an exciting area of research and offers possibilities to explain the complexities of nursing practice in new ways. As Tashakkori and Teddlie (2003) say, 'Study what is of interest to you and what is of value to you, study it in different ways that you deem appropriate, utilise the results in a way that brings about positive consequences within your value system' (p. 21).

# SUMMARY

- Mixed methods research studies generally describe a class of research where quantitative and qualitative research methods are combined in the same study.
- There has been rapid growth in the use of mixed methods research. There remains lack of general agreement regarding nomenclature, a standardised reseach design and analysis.
- Quantitative and qualitative research is based on different worldviews or paradigms and some argue that to look at the same issue from different viewpoints is not feasible.
- Proponents of mixed methods research believe the approach offers a way to combine the quantitative approach with its statistical rigour with the qualitative approach, which relies less on statistical rigour but may be considered richer in its description.
- Sampling techniques for mixed methods studies follow protocols for purposive and probablity sampling.

## PRACTICE EXERCISE 13.1

Jirojwong and colleagues (2007) explored identity and self-perception among young Muslim people in Queensland. A major aim of this research project was to explore the identity and self-perception of young Muslim people aged 9–19 years in three Queensland locations. They investigated social, cultural, political and structural environments which influenced the identity and self-perception of young people as described by them. Mixed methods research was used to collect quantitative and qualitative data from 117 youths. They took part in a group discussion and completed a short questionnaire. Social, cultural and political environments that influence the identity of young people were explored.

Based on the given information, was this a concurrent mixed methods design or sequential mixed methods design?

ANSWER: This is a concurrent study. The two data sets were collected at the same time and the collection of one did not influence the collection of the other.

## PRACTICE EXERCISE 13.2

An organisation funding a domiciliary palliative care service wishes to assess the impact of the service. How might a mixed methods study contribute to answering this question?

ANSWER: A number of research designs could be used to answer this question. For example, in a sequential mixed methods study a questionnaire could be developed with the funding body on the aims and objectives of the service, and interviews with the identified stakeholders on their needs from the service. Stakeholders could include general practitioners, pharmacists, carers and the patients. The questionnaire would then be administered to all people accessing the service over a given timeframe.

## PRACTICE EXERCISE 13.3

A colleague had been involved in some research during which a questionnaire was distributed to a probability sample of respondents. The questionnaire asked for a ticked box type of response and this was to be analysed statistically. At the end of the questionnaire was a section headed 'Any additional comments', inviting respondents to make any written comments that they felt they needed to make. There was now quantitative and also some qualitative data.

The colleague claimed that they had done mixed methods research. What would be your response?

ANSWER: It is an imperative of mixed methods research that both quantitative and qualitative elements of the research are conducted in a manner that demonstrates the established standards of research rigour. In this case the sampling for the qualitative element does not meet the requirements of purposive sampling. The respondents are not identified by the research as those best able to inform the research. The questions asked of them are no more particular than 'Any other comments?' It is unlikely that the qualitative element of the research would be integrated with the quantitative data in any meaningful way and most likely reported as a separate result. Having both quantitative and qualitative data does not necessarily make a mixed methods study.

## PRACTICE EXERCISE 13.4

You are planning to answer the question: What are the health beliefs of patients who are hospitalised with myocardial infarction? Which quantitative and qualitative data would best answer this question? What time and emphasis factors need to be considered in the research design?

ANSWER: The quantitative phase of the research could be the administration of a questionnaire designed to identify health beliefs. The qualitative phase of the study could be an interview with the patient to identify whether or not they have beliefs that may or may not be represented in the questionnaire and to seek explanations for this difference. The emphasis factors relate to whether the quantitative or the qualitative phases are going to be considered the dominant part of the research or are going to have equal weight. The time factor relates to whether these phases are going to be conducted sequentially or concurrently. If the phases are to be conducted sequentially the decision needs to be made whether the quantitative is going to be conducted first or second. This will depend on the design of the research. For example, if the questionnaire being used is a standardised questionnaire used in other studies this may be used first and then any interesting findings related to this particular sample identified and followed up with a face-to-face interview. Alternatively, interviews could be conducted and from those interviews a questionnaire developed.

## PRACTICE EXERCISE 13.5

A randomised controlled trial is to be conducted to assess the efficacy of a new treatment for type 2 diabetes. How may a qualitative element contribute to the study and how may data be integrated in the manner expected of a mixed methods study?

ANSWER: Randomised controlled trials normally have large samples. Data collected will be quantitative, such as blood and urine tests (see Chapter 10). A purposeful sample from each research group in the RCT could be interviewed at different points of the treatment (with the drug or placebo). Interviews would relate to side-effects, acceptability and tolerance, and to the personal experience of those taking the drug. These elements frequently contribute to patient compliance with drug regimens. Interviews could be conducted at different times throughout the study. Qualitative findings could offer an explanation for any unexpected variation in the quantitative findings and offer information about compliance issues.

## FURTHER READING

Andrew, S. & Halcombe, E. (eds) (2009). *Mixed Methods of Research for Nursing and Health Sciences.* Oxford: Blackwell.

Brannen, J. (2005). Mixing methods: The entry of qualitative and quantitative approaches into the research process. *International Journal of Social Research Methodology* 8(3), 173–84.

Burke Johnson, R., Onwuegbuzie, A. & Turner, A. (2007). Toward a definition of mixed methods research. *Journal of Mixed Methods Research* 1(2), 112–33.

Freshwater, D. (2007). Reading mixed methods research: Contexts for criticism. *Journal of Mixed Methods Research* 1(2), 134–46.

Giddings, L. (2006). Positivism dressed in drag? *Journal of Research in Nursing* 11(3), 195–203.

Morse, J. (2005). Evolving trends in qualitative research: Advances in mixed-method design. *Qualitative Health Research* 15(5), 583.

Onwuegbuzie, A. & Leech, N. (2005). On becoming a pragmatic researcher: The importance of combining quantitative and qualitative research methodologies. *International Journal of Social Research Methodology* 8(5), 375–87.

Weaver, K. & Olson, J. (2006). Understanding paradigms used for nursing research. *Journal of Advanced Nursing* 53(4), 459–69.

Wilkins, K. & Woodgate, R. (2008). Designing a mixed methods study in paediatric oncology nursing research. *Journal of Paediatric Oncology Nursing* 25(1), 24–33.

## USEFUL WEBSITES

The web is offering an increasingly important resource for students. As with much of the materal on the web, the quality is variable and discrimination is advised. The following are recommended.

The first three sites provide short lectures from individuals recognised in the field of mixed methods research.

*What is Mixed Methods Research?*, John Cresswell

<www.youtube.com/watch?v=1OaNiTlpyX8>

*Conducting Mixed Methods Research* Pt.1 with Alan Bryman

<www.youtube.com/watch?v=L8Usq_TPfko>

*Mixed Methods Research*, Tony Onwuegbuzie

<http://videolectures.net/ssmt09_onwuegbuzie_mmr>

Best practices for mixed methods research in the health sciences

Commissioned by the National Institute of Health Office of Behavioural and Social Sciences Research in the US. It can be downloaded in PDF version or downloaded on e-readers.

<http://obssr.od.nih.gov/scientific_areas/methodology/mixed_methods_research>

An example of a research methods research proposal is available at

<www.sagepub.com/creswellstudy/Sample%20Student%20Proposals/Proposal-MM-Ivankova.pdf>

## REFERENCES

Bazeley, P. (2006). The contribution of computer software to integrating qualitative and quantitative data and analyses. *Research in the Schools* 13(1), 64–74.

Bryman, A. (2006). Integrating quantitative and qualitative research. *Journal of Mixed Methods Research* 1(1), 8–22.

Bryman, A. (2007). Barriers to integrating quantitative and qualitative research. *Journal of Mixed Methods Research* 1(1), 8–22.

Bryman, A. (2008). *Social Research Methods*, 3rd edn. Oxford: Oxford University Press.

Burke Johnson, R. & Onwuegbuzie, A. (2004). Mixed methods research: A research paradigm whose time has come. *Educational Researcher* 33(7), 14–26.

Creswell, J. W. (2003). *Research Design: Qualitative, Quantitative, and Mixed Methods Approaches*, 2nd edn. Thousand Oaks, CA: SAGE.

Creswell, J. W. & Plano Clark, V. (2007). *Designing and Conducting Mixed Methods Research*. Thousand Oaks, CA: SAGE Publications Inc.

Davila, Y. (2006). Increasing nurses' knowledge and skills for enhanced response to intimate partner violence. *Journal of Continuing Education in Nursing* 37(4), 171–7.

Farrell, M. & Rose, L. (2008). Use of mobile hand-held computers in clinical nursing education. *Journal of Nursing Education* 47(1), 13–9.

Fetters, M., Curry, L. & Creswell, J. (2013). Achieving integration in mixed methods designs—Principles and practices. *HSR: Health Services Research* 48 (6), 2134–55.

Greene, J., Caracelli, J. & Graham, W. (1989). Towards a conceptual framework for mixed method evaluation designs. *Educational Evaluation and Policy Analysis* 11(3), 255–74.

Howe, K. (1988). Against the quantitative-qualitative incompatibility thesis, or, dogmas die hard. *Educational Researcher* 17, 10–6.

Jirojwong S., Hay, D., Apellado H. & Ferdous, T. (2007). *The Nurturing Migrants Project: Outcomes and Achievements*. Report submitted to the Multicultural Affairs Queensland. Rockhampton: Central Queensland University.

Leech, N. & Onwuegbuzie, A. (2009). A typology of mixed methods research designs. *Qualitative Quantitative* 43, 265–75.

Lehana, C. & McNeil, J. (2008). Mixed methods exploration of parents' health information understanding. *Clinical Nursing Research* 17(2), 133–44.

Maxwell, J. & Loomis, D. (2003). Mixed methods design: An alternative approach. In A. Tashakkori & C. Teddlie (eds), *Handbook of Mixed Methods in Social and Behavioural Research*. Thousand Oaks, CA: SAGE Publications, pp.241–72.

Morgan, D. (2007). Paradigms lost and the pragmatism regained: Methodological implications of combining qualitative and quantitative methods. *Journal of Mixed Methods Research* 1(1), 48–76.

Morse, J. M. (1991). Approaches to qualitative-quantitative methodological triangulation. *Nursing Research* 40, 120–3.

Morse, J. M. (2003). Principles of mixed methods and multimethod research design. In A. Tashakkori & C. Teddlie (eds), *Handbook of Mixed Methods in Social and Behavioural Research* (pp. 189–208). Thousand Oaks, CA: SAGE Pubications.

Newman, I., Ridenour, C., Newman, C. & DeMarco, G. (2003). A typology of research purposes and its relationship to mixed methods. In A. Tashakkori & C. Teddlie, *Handbook of Mixed Methods in Social and Behavioural Research*. Thousand Oaks, CA: SAGE Pubications.

Onwuegbuzie, A. & Johnson, R. (2006). The validity issue in mixed research. *Research in the Schools* 13(1), 48–63.

Plano Clark, V. & Cresswell, J. (2008). *The Mixed Methods Reader*. Thousand Oaks CA: SAGE Publications.

Plano Clark, V., Schumacher, K., West, C., Edrington, J., Dunn, L., Hartzstark, A., Melisko, M., Rabow, M., Swift, P. & Miaskowski, C. (2013). Practices for embedding an interpretive qualitative approach within a randomised clinical trial. *Journal of Mixed Methods Research* 7(3), 745–68.

Ream, E., Gibson, F., Edwards, J., Seption, B., Mulhall, A. & Richardson, A. (2006). Experience of fatigue in adolescents living with cancer. *Cancer Nursing* 29(4), 317–26.

Schwandt, T. (2001). *Dictionary of Qualitative Enquiry*, 2nd edn. Thousand Oaks, CA: SAGE Publications.

Tashakkori, A. & Teddlie, C. (2003). *Handbook of Mixed Methods in Social and Behavioural Research*. Thousand Oaks, CA: SAGE Publications.

Teddlie, C. & Tashakkori, A. (2009). *Foundations of Mixed Methods Research: Approaches in the Social and Behavioural Sciences*. Thousand Oaks, CA: SAGE Publications.

Teddlie, C. & Yu, F. (2007). Mixed methods sampling: A typology with examples. *Journal of Mixed Methods Research* 1(1), 77–100.

Zhang, W. & Creswell, J. (2013). The use of mixing procedures of mixed methods in health services research. *Medical Care* 51(8), 51–7.

**PART 4**

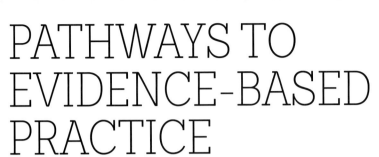

# PATHWAYS TO EVIDENCE-BASED PRACTICE

After the data are analysed, and the results interpreted, it is important that Ann and Bob compare their results to other similar studies through a critical review of the research literature on the topic. Part of a critical review is an evaluation of the researcher's own study, including a self-evaluation by the researcher, and a critique of the rigour of the study—all processes and procedures used as part of the study. Chapter 14 provides important information on how to conduct a critical review of research literature.

A study is not complete until the findings are presented to your peers. The presentation of findings is an obligation that is part of conducting research. There are several ways by which the findings of a study can be communicated to the broader community of scholars and healthcare professionals. Chapter 15 provides a comprehensive description of the steps in synthesising available research on a particular research topic as well as providing a critique of the quality of the research. Chapter 16 explores some ideas about how the research results can be shared with others. The important reason for disseminating results of research studies is to share with colleagues the development of new knowledge and its usefulness in applying the results to current clinical practice. Through the application of research results to clinical practice, current practices can be evaluated and new and improved approaches to practice can be developed supported by the best available evidence. The results of research can play an important role in the development of clinical guidelines and protocols for establishing best practice. As part of choosing the best research evidence to support quality change, a systematic review of available research is needed.

The results of Ann and Bob's studies can now be included in the synthesis of research results. Their results have the potential to contribute to a review of current pain management practices in emergency departments. The findings of these studies also have the potential to generate new research questions leading to new research on pain management. The journey Ann and Bob have embarked on is one important step along the pathway of research, a pathway that will lead to new horizons of understanding and the advancement of nursing and midwifery practice.

# CHAPTER 14

# CRITICAL REVIEW OF RESEARCH

Jane Warland and Phil Maude

## CHAPTER LEARNING OBJECTIVES

After reading this chapter you will be able to:

- understand the definition of critical review
- describe terms associated with critical appraisal
- list strategies for developing critical appraisal skills
- describe the use of common appraisal tools and techniques
- discuss the basic attributes of high-quality primary studies
- analyse how study design and method affect the quality and applicability of clinical-based evidence.

## KEY TERMS

critique
grey literature
peer-reviewed
 journal
impact factor
quantitative
 research methods
qualitative research
 methods
systematic review

# Introduction

It is the responsibility of every registered nurse or midwife (RN/M) to keep up to date with current research (ANMAC 2006a,b), but there are a number of widely known barriers to achieving this (Cheek et al. 2005). Many RN/Ms are unfamiliar with how to tell the difference between well and poorly conducted research. Learning how to critically appraise research literature is therefore a vital skill for all practitioners.

This chapter will guide you through four steps to help you develop your ability to review literature critically:

1    selection and effective reading of the literature
2    critical appraisal and consideration of the level of available evidence
3    collation and description of the literature
4    considering the application of evidence to practice.

A critical review of an article involves analysis and evaluation. Analysis of the article involves objectively reading it and dissecting the information presented in order to identify its purpose, main points, methodology and findings or conclusions. This is done in a systematic way using a reputable critique tool to guide the reviewer/reader (Schneider et al. 2013). The objective of a critical review is not to criticise the article but to **critique** it—to objectively review the research process and verify that the methods the researchers used were sound. Skills in critical appraisal of the literature are essential in the current healthcare environment, which requires RNs and RMs to be proficient in critique and utilisation of healthcare research to inform an evidence base for practice. Note that a critical review is not the same as a systematic review, which is the subject of Chapter 15.

> **Critique:** To critique is to read and examine the strengths and limitations of a published study.

# Selection and effective reading of the literature

A review of the literature classifies and evaluates what scholars and researchers have written on a topic, organised according to a guiding concept such as the research objective(s), hypothesis, thesis or the problem/issue. It is an analysis of the current knowledge concerning a topic.

Your objective is not to list as many articles as possible; rather, it is to demonstrate your intellectual ability to recognise relevant information, and to synthesise and evaluate it according to the guiding concept. You want to know what literature exists and you want to make an informed evaluation or critical appraisal of this literature. To meet both of these needs, you must employ two sets of skills:

> **Grey literature:** Unpublished literature in the form of theses, government reports or conference proceedings.

- *Information-seeking*: the ability to scan the literature efficiently using manual or computerised methods to identify potentially useful articles, books and **grey literature**.
- *Critical appraisal*: the ability to apply principles of analysis to identify unbiased and valid studies. You need to produce more than just a descriptive list of articles and books. You need to show that you understand the study design, sample size and key findings and can critique the methods used. It is usually a bad sign when every paragraph of your review begins with the names of researchers, as this indicates that you are simply accepting what they have said rather than critically appraising what they claim. Instead, organise your review into useful, informative sections that present themes or identify trends.

To begin, you explain the search strategy you used in your literature review so that your approach to finding the literature and deciding what was included and excluded is clear. A list of databases such as MEDLINE, PsycLit, CINAHL or SCOPUS is also needed.

## Box 14.1

### EXAMPLE OF A LITERATURE SEARCH STRATEGY ON AGGRESSIVE PATIENTS

The literature reviewed was drawn from a search conducted using the Cumulative Index to Nursing and Allied Health Literature (CINAHL), MEDLINE and PsycINFO electronic databases. The search was limited to primary research articles published between 2010 and 2015, in English and involving different settings in nursing such as psychiatry, emergency nursing and general wards. The search terms used were: 'violence' or 'violent' or 'aggression' or 'aggressive' and 'nurses'. Of the 77 articles that were found, 17 were chosen for inclusion in this review because they were research papers that included data from Australia. Articles concerning horizontal violence and nursing were excluded.

When you are planning to review the literature there are a number of questions you could ask yourself, for example:

1  Do I have a specific thesis, problem or research question that my literature review helps to define?
2  What type of literature review am I conducting? Am I looking at issues of theory? methodology? policy? quantitative research (such as studies of new or controversial procedures)? qualitative research (such as studies determining criteria for allocating healthcare resources)?
3  What is the scope of my literature review? What types of publications am I using, for example journals, books, government documents, popular media? What discipline am I working in? Is it nursing, midwifery, psychology, sociology, medicine or a combination of two or more areas?
4  How good are my information-seeking skills? Has my search been wide enough to ensure that I have found all the relevant material? Has it been narrow enough to exclude irrelevant material? Is the number of sources I have used appropriate and reflective of the scope of the available literature?
5  Is there a specific relationship between the literature I have chosen to review and the problem I have formulated?
6  How have I made decisions to include some works and exclude others?
7  Have I critically analysed the literature I use? Do I just list and summarise authors and articles, or do I assess them? Do I discuss the strengths and weaknesses of the cited material?
8  Have I cited and discussed studies contrary to my perspective?
9  Will the reader find my literature review relevant, appropriate and useful?

As you continue with your review, ask these questions about the specific book or article you are reviewing:

1  Has the author formulated a problem/issue? Is this a research paper or a review paper?
2  Is the problem/issue ambiguous or clearly articulated? Is its significance (scope, severity, relevance) discussed?

*(Continued)*

*(Continued)*

3　What are the strengths and limitations of the way the author has formulated the problem or issue?

4　Could the problem have been approached more effectively from another perspective?

5　What is the author's research orientation such as interpretation, critical science or a combination?

6　What is the author's theoretical framework, for example developmental, feminist or psychoanalytic?

7　What is the relationship between the theoretical and research perspectives?

8　Has the author evaluated the literature relevant to the problem/issue? Does the author include literature taking positions they do not agree with?

9　In a research study, how good are the three basic components of the study design: population, intervention, outcome? How accurate and valid are the measurements? Is the analysis of the data accurate and relevant to the research question? Are the conclusions validly based on the data and analysis?

10　In popular literature, does the author use appeals to emotion, one-sided examples, rhetorically charged language and tone? Is the author objective, or are they merely 'proving' what they already believe?

11　How does the author structure their argument? Can you 'deconstruct' the flow of the argument to analyse if or where it breaks down?

12　Is this a book or article that contributes to our understanding of the problem under study, and in what ways is it useful for practice? What are its strengths and limitations?

13　How does this book or article fit into the thesis or question I am developing?

## THINKING DEEPLY

When you critically review research reports, various questions in Box 14.1 help identify the strengths and weaknesses of each report. However, the applicability of research results in any given situation will vary. As users of research, you also need to know the context and environment of your workplace.

## Making sense of the literature—first pass

When you first come to an area of research, you are filling in the background in a general way, getting a feel for the whole area, an idea of its scope, starting to appreciate the controversies, to see the high points, and to become more familiar with the main authors. This is your starting point.

## Is there too much literature to handle?

At this stage there may seem to be masses of literature relevant to your research. Or you may worry that there seems to be hardly anything. As you read, think about and discuss articles and isolate the issues you are more interested in. In this way, you focus your topic more and more. The more you can close in on what your research question or topic of enquiry actually is, the more you will be able to have a basis for selecting the relevant areas of the literature. This is the only way to bring it down to a manageable size and to ensure you have looked at all the literature across disciplines.

## Is very little literature available?

If initially you cannot seem to find much at all on your research area, and you are sure that you have used all avenues for searching that the library can present you with, there are a few possibilities:

- You could be right at the cutting edge of something new and it is not surprising there is little around.
- You could be limiting yourself to too narrow an area and not appreciating that relevant material could be just around the corner in a closely related field.
- Maybe your key search terms are not well chosen, are loosely defined or not focused enough. For example, if you type in the search term 'preceptorship and nursing' you will find a great deal of information. However, the term 'preceptorship' is used in the USA to describe the first year a nurse works in the health service after graduating, but in the UK and Australia this is used to describe clinical support of student and novice staff.
- Unfortunately, there is another possibility: that there's nothing in the literature because it's not a worthwhile area of research.

## Quality of the literature

You learn to judge, evaluate and look critically at the literature by judging, evaluating and looking critically at it. That is, you learn to do something by practising. There are some questions you could find useful and, with practice, you will develop many others:

- Is the problem clearly spelt out?
- Are the results presented new?
- Was the research influential in that others picked up the threads and pursued them?
- How large a sample was used? Was the sample size justified?
- How convincing is the argument made?
- How were the results analysed?
- What perspective are the authors coming from?
- Are the generalisations justified by the evidence on which they are made?
- What is the significance of this research?
- What are the assumptions behind the research?
- Is the methodology justified as the most appropriate to study the problem?
- Is the theoretical basis transparent?

# Critical appraisal and consideration of the level of available evidence

## Becoming familiar with the process of critical review

Critically appraising literature commonly involves using some kind of appraisal tool (see Useful websites). Such tools are designed to help you read and think about the study in a systematic manner. After working your way through the questions in the tool, you should have some idea about the worth of the article you have appraised. But this will only be achieved if you actually can 'tell' the answers to the questions posed in the tool. Frequently, novice reviewers may not easily be able to use these tools because they actually may not know whether the researchers have met the stated criteria or not. Thus they may have little more idea about the quality of the research at the end of the appraisal than at the beginning.

How then do you get the knowledge you need in order to be able to use these appraisal tools adequately? Here we outline some of the strategies you can use to become familiar with the critical review process:

1  Regularly read high-quality research papers. Commonly an article published in a **peer-reviewed journal** has been critically appraised by someone who is an expert in either content or study design used, or both. High-quality peer-reviewed journals often use three or four reviewers. In the case of quantitative studies, most high-impact journals will also use a statistician to check whether the statistical analysis was correctly conducted. What this means is that if you read journal articles published in peer-reviewed journals, you start to get a sense of how a well-written, well-reported, valid study will read. The status a journal has in the research world is its **impact factor**.

2  Practise critical appraisal. In a critical appraisal process, it really is a matter of practice makes perfect. Some ideas for getting you started are to:
    –  Practise on your own.
        •  Start small and simple.
        •  Perform a literature search in the area of your interest.
        •  Of these articles, find one that is a few pages long.
        •  Find one that has attracted some correspondence to the editor. This will help you see what others have said (for more on this see the next section).
        •  Skim-read (Schneider et al. 2013) your article through, then go and do something else for a while.
        •  Read it through more thoroughly again, this time making some notes about any questions that spring to your mind.
        •  Look up the answers to your questions in a research text or dictionary, or seek out someone with expertise to answer your questions.
        •  Complete a critical appraisal tool such as CASP (see Useful websites) for your article.
        •  Follow this process by telling a colleague or your classmate about the article, the key points, what it found that was new and the significance of these findings for clinical practice.
    –  Practise with others.
        •  A very good way of becoming familiar with critical appraisal is to join a journal club. A journal club typically meets regularly to discuss and critically appraise journal articles. Participating in such a group allows you not only to keep abreast of current literature but also gives you experience in reading and understanding research literature. If you do not have a journal club at your workplace or within your study group, then seriously consider starting one.

**Peer-reviewed journal:** A journal that publishes a paper that has been submitted to an editorial committee and passed by a process of blinded peer review before it is accepted for publication.

**Impact factor:** Calculated for each journal based on citation of articles across a year. The higher the impact factor the more widely read the journal is.

3 Read reviews done by others. There are two ways you can easily access reviews conducted by others. The first is reading reviewers' comments on a manuscript and the second is reading critical reviews posted on the internet.

## Read reviewers' comments from open-access published journals

Open-access journals offer free availability to readers and quick online publication of research articles. The review process for these journals is open and provides novice researchers and students with excellent real-world examples of critical appraisal in action.

The 'pre-publication history' of articles allows you to read the manuscript originally submitted, the reviewers' comments, the authors' response, alterations made, follow-up reviewers' comments and the final article.

This gives good insight into the review process and the kinds of comments reviewers typically make. It may be interesting for you to realise that almost invariably the reviewers require the authors to justify some aspect of their study and further refine their article before it can be published, which process improves the articles.

Examples of some open-access published journals in the discipline of nursing and midwifery are listed in Useful websites.

## Read critical reviews posted on the internet

Another way of becoming familiar with the critical review process is to read a critical review conducted by another person. One example is the Joanna Briggs Institute site, which has a range of critical reviews in its Rapid Appraisal Protocol internet database (RAPid). Many of the reviews on this site have been conducted by students. Another example is an internet site called Best BETs (Best Evidence-based Topics), developed by the Emergency Department of Manchester Royal Infirmary, UK, to provide quick and easy access to a range of critical reviews of research literature typically conducted by clinicians at this hospital. Visitors can browse 'critical appraisals' in the databases section (see BestBETS at <www.bestbets.org>).

## THINKING DEEPLY

Generally you need to read a large number of research reports in printed hard copy or on the internet. Then you come across some grey literature, conference proceedings (see also Chapter 15) and very short communications by researchers who want to report their brief research results. It is important that you develop methods that facilitate your reading and so that you gain the most from all these sources.

## Critique methods

In this section, methods for critiquing articles on **quantitative** and **qualitative research methods** will be considered. We use a case study of a cohort study to give a practical example of the application of a critical appraisal tool (CAT). We will provide links to web-based resources for the particular method you are interested in later in the chapter.

**Quantitative research methods:** Deductive research methods such as randomised control trials, quasi-experimental studies, cohort studies, observational, descriptive or exploratory designs. These methods test for cause and effect, explore relationships between variables and control variables.

**Qualitative research methods:** Inductive research methods such as grounded theory, ethnography or phenomenology, which explore human experience and 'emancipate' it—set it free from the constraints of labelling.

## Use of critical appraisal tools to critique literature

There are a number of critical appraisal tools available (see Further reading and Useful websites). While these look a little different, they all provide you with a step-by-step systematic, logical process for appraising research literature.

### Interactive critical appraisal tools

Web-based critical appraisal tools have been specifically developed for healthcare students such as nurses and midwives to help them to organise, conduct and archive summaries of evidence. These include the Critical Appraisal Tool maker (CATmaker) (Badenoch et al. 2004) and RAPid. CATmaker is a free interactive tool that enables you to store research questions, search strategies and/or complete appraisals; however, the RAPid CAT is available to JBI subscribers. In addition to CATmaker features, RAPid is designed to assist users to appraise and summarise evidence from a wide range of sources, including the results of qualitative studies. Once you have completed a RAPid appraisal you are invited to contribute it to the RAPid database. Both of these tools have drop-down boxes that allow users to logically work their way through an appraisal.

### Critical appraisal tools

**Systematic review:**
A method used to review the existing literature on a particular question, by identifying, appraising, selecting and synthesising all high-quality research evidence relevant to that question.

In a **systematic review** of CATs, Katrak and others (2004) found that there were more than 100 CATs currently in use. Such a wide choice presents the novice reviewer with a problem of which tool to use in which circumstance. They can be broadly classified into design-specific and generic. Both of these have advantages and disadvantages of use. Choosing a design-specific tool can assist you to appraise a specific study design; a generic tool is more flexible but may lack specific items to enable you to determine the quality of a certain design.

## Box 14.2

**EXAMPLE OF USE OF A CRITICAL APPRAISAL TOOL**

Article appraised: M. Lim, M. Hellard & C. Aitken (2005). The case of the disappearing teaspoons: Longitudinal cohort study of the displacement of teaspoons in an Australian research institute. *British Medical Journal* 331, 1498–500. Available online at <www.bmj.com/cgi/content/full/331/7531/1498>.

This case study will follow the CASP 12 questions to help you make sense of cohort study guidelines for critical appraisal of a quantitative research article. The CASP tool is completed using each of the CASP headings, which helps the reader decide whether the research article is credible and worthy of use within evidence-based practice. We have chosen an article that is short and fairly simple. You should also be aware that the article chosen is satirical. We are not suggesting we have completed the tool perfectly or completely, but it should give you an idea of what you need to consider when you complete a CASP tool.

This tool is completed with brackets around the answers we have chosen; our comments about the rationale for each of these choices follows.

*Q. Did the study address a clearly focused issue?*

[Yes]   Can't Tell   No

In order to answer this question you need to know what is meant by 'clearly focused'. The kinds of things that need to be considered here are listed in the appraisal tool, but simply put, this aspect of clear focus means that the researchers did not try to do too much. For example, if they were also trying to investigate missing knives and forks then this may have resulted in a much less focused study.

*Q. Did the authors use an appropriate method to answer their question?*

[Yes]　Can't Tell　No

A cohort design is used to observe a group that is linked in some way because they share common characteristics—in this case, marked teaspoons. The cohort are studied over a period of time to observe an outcome (in this case, disappearance).

The researchers' principal method was a longitudinal cohort, which was used to study the disappearance rate of a group of teaspoons. But they also used a survey of staff members. While a survey is not normally part of a cohort study, it was an appropriate addition as it adds insight to the study question—why are the teaspoons going missing?

At this point you are asked 'Is it worth continuing?' If your first two answers were anything other than yes then there is probably no point continuing because either the study is not worth reading (if you have circled 'no') or (if you have circled 'can't tell') you may not yet have the necessary skills to complete the appraisal.

The next section of the appraisal tool is all about rigour.

*Q. Was the cohort recruited in an acceptable way?*

Yes　Can't Tell　No

This asks you whether a selection bias might have occurred because if so it may imply that the ability of the researchers to generalise their findings is limited. As we read in Chapter 10, generalisability means the ability the researcher has to claim that because a certain finding has occurred in one setting the same thing will occur in another similar setting.

The tool then poses the following questions:

- Was the cohort representative of a defined population?
- Was there something special about the cohort?
- Was everybody included who should have been included?

The cohort in this study was artificially constructed and as such all sections of the cohort, such as all teaspoons, were identical and all were present at the commencement of the study. Therefore the answer to this question is not applicable to this study so you would leave this answer blank.

*Q. Was the exposure accurately measured to minimise bias?*

Yes　[Can't Tell]　No

This question is gauging measurement or classification bias and wants to know:

- Did they use subjective or objective measurements?
- Do the measures truly reflect what you want them to (have they been validated)?
- Were the subjects classified into exposure groups based on the same procedure?

*(Continued)*

*(Continued)*

Once again you are required to have some knowledge of how a measurement or classification bias may occur. Basically, this section is asking you to determine if the exposure to disappearance was accurately measured. Could something else have happened to the teaspoons? In this case it was difficult for the researchers to determine if the teaspoons had disappeared forever, or only temporarily because they were in use at the time of the count.

*Q. Was the outcome accurately measured to minimise bias?*

[Yes]   Can't Tell   No

This question has several sub-questions about reliability and validity, namely:

- Q. Did the researchers use objective measurement?
- Q. Do the measures truly reflect what you want, i.e. have they been validated?
- Q. Has a reliable system been used to detect all missing teaspoons?
- Q. Were the measurement methods similar in the different groups?
- Q. Were the subjects and/or assessors blinded to the exposure (does this matter)?

This approach seemed to be reasonably reliable and valid although the researchers don't discuss a number of issues, for example the timing of their weekly teaspoon count. If, for example, the count was conducted at lunchtime this may have resulted in more teaspoons appearing to have disappeared than if they conducted the search in the first or last part of the day.

The approach established this as a valid method of data collection by using a pilot study. For a recap on reliability and validity please see Chapters 10 and 11.

*Q. Have the authors identified all important confounding factors? List the ones you think might be important, that the authors missed.*

Yes   Can't Tell   [No]

Much of the correspondence regarding this paper discussed potential confounding factors that the authors missed including:

Teabags and forks (Woodall 2005)
The researchers themselves (Aitken 2005)
Coffee and tea drinkers (Lisse 2005)
Dishwashers (Underwood 2005)
Children (Baker 2005)
Dishes (Grantholm 2006)
Teaspoons used for other purposes (Silver 2006)
Gender of staff (Smith 2005, Cannizzaro 2006)
Attrition rates (Shadbolt 2006)
The weather (Bowler 2006)
The spoon fairy (Scholten 2006)

*Q. Was the follow-up of the subjects complete and long enough?*

Yes   Can't Tell   [No]

- Q. What are the results of this study?
- Q. How precise are the results?

There is no indication that the researchers did anything other than a cursory search; the teaspoons may have been in use when the final count occurred.

The results are reported in an unusual way for a cohort study, that is, there is no relative risk (RR) reported (see Chapter 15 for more on relative risk). However, the researchers report statistically significant findings (see Chapter 12 on statistical significance).

The 95% confidence interval (CI) is narrow (0.76—1.28), indicating that the results are likely to be precise (see Chapter 12 for information about CI).

*Q. Do you believe the results?*

[Yes]   Can't Tell   No

The results are logical and make sense.

*Q. Can the results be applied to the local population?*

[Yes]   Can't Tell   No

Even though teaspoons may differ a little from place to place the results are generalisable across many different workplaces. However, these are not generalisable to other places where teaspoons are used, such as a home.

*Q. Do the results of this study fit with other available evidence?*

[Yes]   Can't Tell   No

This is the first reported empirical study to study this phenomenon, but the results fit with anecdotal everyday observation.

## Critical appraisal of statistics

Understanding results when statistics have been used is one of the most challenging areas for many novice researchers. Probably a good approach to the critique of statistics is to consider the question 'Has the researcher provided justification for the types of statistical tests used?' Most researchers understand that their readers might not necessarily understand the subtleties of the statistical tests they have used and will usually provide an explanation about what their results mean.

A study by Zellner and others (2007) examined quantitative articles published in 13 nursing research journals during 2000. They found that the 10 most common statistics were 'mean, frequency distribution, standard deviation, range, percentiles, percentages, quartiles, t-test, ANOVA, correlation, Cronbach alpha and Chi-Square' (p. 562). These 10 statistics represented 80% of all statistics used in the 462 articles they reviewed. So if you can understand these descriptive statistics you will very likely understand most articles in the disciplines of nursing and midwifery. Thus it would be a good idea to look up and aim to understand the meaning of these statistical tests and terms. When you come across new statistical methods look these up and add them to your knowledge base for the language of statistics. An article by Beitz (2008) offers some very good information about decision-making for statistical tests in nursing research and how to problem-solve and question the statistics being used.

When making an appraisal of a qualitative study the CAT may look a little different from the CASP tool used above. The following questions are typical:

Writing style, author credibility, title and abstract

- Is the journal article well laid out with clear section headings and signposting?
- Are definitions explained and is clear language used?
- Are the researchers' qualifications and affiliations provided?
- Does the title reflect the study design, topic and findings?
- Upon reading the abstract do you have a vivid picture of the research, why it was conducted?

Aim/purpose, literature review and theoretical framework

- Is the aim or purpose of the study clearly articulated?
- Have the author(s) provided the research question(s)?
- Is the literature review extensive, contemporary and does it include key articles?
- Is the literature review critical and unbiased?
- If a literature review is not provided, have the author(s) justified this and do they relate their findings to the literature in the discussion section of the paper?
- Do the author(s) acknowledge their interest in the study and reflect on bias and conflicts of interest?
- Has a conceptual framework been identified and if so is it justified and applicable to the study?
- Has the use of a conceptual framework influenced or biased the reporting of the study findings?

Method, sampling, data analysis, philosophical integration and ethical considerations

- Have the author(s) stayed true to the method they have identified?
- Could you replicate this study from the description provided of sampling and data analysis?
- Is the sampling method adequate and is the sample size justified?
- Could other participants have added breadth of understanding of this phenomenon?
- Does the article advise that a study proposal was considered by an ethics committee and was approved?
- Have the participants been adequately informed of the study risks and has the matter of anonymity and confidentiality of data been addressed?

Rigour, presentation, links to the literature and implications for practice

- Are the findings consistent with other studies?
- Are the findings reported in a clear manner with examples of participant transcripts to support claims for themes?
- Have the aims of the study been addressed, research questions answered or considerations been made for methodological limitations that caused answers to not emerge?
- Were credibility, confirmabilty, transferability, dependability, fittingness and trust-worthiness discussed?
- Is the importance of the implications for findings discussed and appropriately considered?
- Is the citation of literature consistent with what is within the text and is it adequate and extensive?

Sources: Adapted from Cutcliffe & Ward 2006; Ryan et al. 2007

## Learning to critically appraise: Collating, describing and critiquing

Now that you have 'made sense' of the article you are ready to collate the evidence you have gathered about its worth in order to write a critical appraisal. When students are asked to write a 'critical appraisal' of literature, it is a common mistake to criticise rather than critique. What you are asked to do when you critique literature is to systematically and logically examine the article to look for:

- what was said and how well it was said
- what assumptions underlie the author's argument
- what issues were overlooked
- what implications were drawn
- what consequences for change in practice arise from the study.

The following is an example of a critical appraisal of the 'teaspoon' study and would be the type that would be used in a journal club setting. The sections in displayed quotes are all that you would actually see in an appraisal. The text provides guidance and insight into what is written.

## Introduce article to be reviewed and set in context

This section of your critical appraisal need not be long and can be quite descriptive. For example:

> This study sought to determine the rate of teaspoon disappearance from staff tearooms and whether the rate of loss was influenced by the relative value of the teaspoon. The workplace involved was a research institute.

The next section of your critique is a step-by-step critique of key elements in the article. We commence with the title and work through each of the headings as laid out in the article itself:

> The title identifies the phenomenon studied (missing teaspoons), the place the study took place (Australian research institute) and the method used (longitudinal cohort study). The title is therefore both succinct and descriptive, giving the reader a clear idea of what the study is about.
>
> The article should also provide information concerning who the researchers are, their qualifications and if they are appropriate individuals to undertake the research. While the authors' qualifications are not given, their position within the institution is cited as 'director, research assistant and research officer'. This indicates that they probably have the research skills required to have conducted this investigation effectively. Furthermore, all work within the study setting, indicating that all are aware of and interested in the issue of missing teaspoons.
>
> This article was published in the *British Medical Journal*, a respected peer-reviewed journal. The journal was no doubt chosen by the researchers because it is a journal which is used by the target reading population, namely health professionals interested in understanding the phenomenon of missing teaspoons.

## Abstract

The abstract should provide a comprehensive and clear summary of the study and should include all its major features.

> The information in the abstract is a clear and concise account of what is in the study, making this a well-structured and adequate abstract.

## Introduction

The introduction outlines the research problem, in this case that teaspoons are going missing from the researchers' workplace tearooms.

With the stated high incidence of teaspoon loss the findings of this study could have significant benefits to workers in understanding the phenomenon of teaspoon loss from workplace tearooms.

## Literature review

The literature review should cover all the current theory and research regarding the study and should contextualise the paper.

The authors state that they did not find any literature concerning the phenomenon of interest. They used three well-known search engines.

While the use of Google as a search engine in a scholarly publication should be questioned, Google Scholar and MEDLINE are suitable search engines to use. The authors' search strategy would seem a little perfunctory, but after replicating their stated strategy and adding the words 'cutlery' and 'misplaced' from the same five-year period (1999–2004) and using the same search engines, verification was achieved. There was no published research concerning the phenomenon of interest at the time the study was conducted.

## Research approach (methodology/methods)

The method section is the section of the research article where the author explains in detail exactly how they conducted the study. This section should clearly indicate how sampling occurred, information about data collection and analysis, validity, reliability and trustworthiness of the data, and ethical issues. The method section should be so clear that the reader can replicate the study methods used (Baglione 2012).

In the case of this study the method was a longitudinal cohort approach. This method is used when the researcher wishes to follow a defined group (marked teaspoons) over a period of time. It is therefore a suitable method to use to answer the research question.

## Sampling

The authors used 70 teaspoons. They gave no explanation of why this number was chosen but they did allow for other teaspoons to be added to tearooms by others because they only counted the teaspoons they had marked.

## Validity and reliability

The authors addressed reliability and validity issues by conducting a pilot study. It is difficult to determine how rigorous data collection was because the researchers don't discuss the timing of their weekly teaspoon count. If, for example, the count was conducted at lunchtime this may have resulted in more teaspoons appearing to have disappeared than if they had conducted the search during the first or last part of the day. Furthermore, while all teaspoons were counted by members from the same team, they do not discuss if or how interrater reliability was established. This leaves the reader wondering if some team members may have conducted a more thorough search for teaspoons than others.

## Ethical issues

The only ethical consideration mentioned in this paper was the statement that approval for the study was given by the 'director of the institute' (p. 4). This is problematic because this authorising person was also one of the stated researchers. In a study of this nature that involves inanimate objects there might be a prima facie case for no ethical considerations.

However, after the data collection period ended, workers were made aware of the study and asked to complete an anonymous survey. It is possible that teaspoon thieves may have felt guilty at this point in the study and non-thieves may have thought they were being accused of theft. Therefore, this study should have been reviewed by a properly formed institutional ethics committee in order to ensure that there was careful and sensitive revelation of the study and the fact that there were missing teaspoons. Anonymity of participation should have been examined by an impartial third party to ensure ethical compliance. Counselling should have been offered for traumatised staff members vicariously accused of theft. Furthermore, no details were given of what would happen to the anonymous surveys, such as how long they would be retained, where, and who would have access.

### Findings/results

The results are reported in an unusual way for a cohort study: the researchers use percentages of disappearance and there is no relative risk (RR) reported. However, the researchers report statistical significance at $p \leq 0.05$ difference between tearooms that are communal and those that are not. The 95% CI is narrow (0.76—1.28), indicating that these results are likely to be precise. Overall the results are logical and make sense.

### Conclusions/recommendations/implications for nursing

The conclusions should be clear and concise and should revisit the original objectives of the study (Baglione 2012). While the researchers do confuse the reader with talk of teaspoons 'slipping away' to another planet and spoonoid lifestyle, generally speaking the conclusions are logically presented and in keeping with the findings of the study.

Some recommendations are not made by the authors but have since been suggested by other BMJ readers including:

* chaining teaspoons to the tearoom wall via a 'strongly mounted wall bracket' or
* forcing staff to provide their own teaspoon.

Furthermore, the authors do exaggerate the implications of their findings by suggesting that they have implications for the national research agenda.

### Conclusion

The conclusion to your critique should effectively and succinctly summarise the main findings of the critique process to establish the significance of the study's findings:

This study addresses a previously unidentified gap in research literature. However, there are some shortcomings related to rigour and attention to detail which leave the reader wondering about some aspects of the study design.

## Collation and description of the literature

In practical terms, it is necessary to have an overall picture of how the thread runs through your analysis of the literature before you can get down to actually describing the literature. One strategy that many writers use as a way to begin the literature review is to proceed from the general, wider view of the research they are reviewing to the specific problem. This is not a formula but is a common pattern and may be worth trying. Maybe use a summary sheet for each paper you review or at least write notes and highlight important sections that you need to review. These notes may be attached or even written onto the paper directly so that your opinion on each section is not lost. You may use a grid-like system to make short notes of your articles and the information that is coming out of each to assist you to use and collate all the literature.

| Article | Concept 1 | Concept 2 | Concept 3 | Concept 4 |
|---|---|---|---|---|
| | How the literature defines the issue | Extent of the problem in contemporary times | Interventions and their levels of effectiveness | Attitudes of clinicians to change to practice |
| Abercrombie 2009 | Does not define | Provides extensive statistics from 3 key countries | Sample size was large across 3 locations | Not included |
| Finch 2010 | Differs from all other texts | Focus on Australia | Large cohort study | Considerations made |
| Gozzo 2008 | Similar to Myer | Focus on Australia | Large cohort study | Included in limitations section |
| Myer et al. 2008 | Similar to Gozzo | Focus on Australia | Large cohort study | Not included |

Whatever the pattern that fits your work best, you need to keep in mind that what you are doing is writing about what was done before. But you are not simply reporting on previous research. You have to write about it in terms of how well it was done and what it achieved. For example, a series of paragraphs of the kind:

'Green (1975) discovered…'

'In 1978, Black conducted experiments and discovered that…'

'Later Brown (1980) illustrated this in…'

demonstrates neither your understanding of the literature nor your ability to evaluate other people's work.

Maybe at an earlier stage, or in your first version of your literature review, you needed a summary of who did what. But in your final version, you have to show that you have thought about it, can synthesise the work and can succinctly pass judgment on the relative merits of research conducted in your field. So, to take the above example, it would be better to say something like:

'There seems to be general agreement on x (White 1987; Brown 1980; Black 1978; Green 1975), but Green (1975) sees x as a consequence of y, while Black (1978) suggests that x and y are interrelated.

While Green's work has some limitations in that it…, its main value lies in…'

Approaching your writing in this way forces you to make judgments and, furthermore, to distinguish your thoughts from assessments made by others. It is this whole process of revealing limitations or recognising the possibility of taking research further that allows you to formulate and justify your writing.

A literature review is not just a summary, but a conceptually organised synthesis of the results of your search. It must

- organise information and relate it to the argument you are developing
- synthesise results into a summary of what is and isn't known
- identify controversy when it appears in the literature
- develop questions or recommendations for further research.

Although we value 'unbiased' scientific research, the truth is that no author is free from outside influence, such as a particular theoretical framework or model (e.g. a feminist examination of gender inequity in medical research), the author's rhetorical purpose (e.g. a researcher's reasons for advocating the effectiveness of a certain drug) or an experience-based practical perspective (e.g. the belief that one approach to pain management is more effective than another). The value of your review depends not simply on how many sources you find, but also on your awareness of how these different perspectives affect the way that research on your topic is conducted, published and read.

In critically evaluating, you are looking for the strengths of certain studies and the significance and contributions made by researchers. You are also looking for limitations, flaws and weaknesses of particular studies, or of whole lines of enquiry.

Indeed, if you take this critical approach to looking at previous research in your field, your final literature review will not be a compilation of summaries but an evaluation. Then it will reflect your capacity for critical analysis.

You can then continue the process of making sense of the literature by gaining more expertise, which allows you to become more confident, and by being much more focused on your specific research. You are still reading and perhaps needing to reread some of the literature. You are thinking about it as you are analysing texts or other data. You are able to talk about it easily and discuss it. In other words, it is becoming part of you. At a deeper level than before,

- you are now not only looking at findings but are looking at how others have arrived at their findings
- you are looking at what assumptions are leading to the way something is investigated
- you are looking for genuine differences in theories as opposed to mere semantic difference
- you are gaining an understanding of why the field developed in the way it did
- you have a sense of where it might be going.

## Considering the application of evidence to practice

Using appraisal tools can help you to understand studies and their potential application to practice. Research is a word that often holds negative connotations as uninteresting. Evidence-based practice is focused on the recognition and uptake of the best available evidence to support practice. In many ways the findings of research studies can challenge clinicians and managers to consider change. There are many resources readily available, but at a local level clinicians need good critique skills to evaluate what they are reading and managers need confidence in the evidence to embark on the often difficult process of change to practice.

## Implications for evidence-based practice

The level of evidence is based on a study research design (see Table 1.1 in Chapter 1) because it indicates the rigour of the overall research process. However, research users still have to be able to critically review research reports (journal articles, conference proceedings and conference presentations) in order to identify their strengths and weaknesses. As users, clinicians then will have the confidence to apply the research evidence in their own practice.

# SUMMARY

- The critical appraisal of research is a fundamental skill to help in the uptake of contemporary evidence and facilitates practice development. You need to be able to seek information and then critically appraise it.
- There are various critical appraisal tools which can assist clinicians and readers, but the final work they must do is make sound decisions about the value of the literature. Recommendations for change or no change to practice are only as good as the reader's knowledge base.
- A journal club is an excellent way to bring novices and experienced clinicians together and improve decision-making.
- Evidence may indicate a need to change practice, but it also needs to be implemented after careful consideration of the clinical significance, that is, the impact on service users, clinical staff and the organisation's overall plan and budget. If the procedural change reduces care and active intervention or is not culturally or fiscally sound it may deliver poorer results in the long run.

## PRACTICE EXERCISE 14.1

a   Bob and his team review publications relating to chest pain. Following is a part of an article:
'Fifteen hospitals agreed to participate in the study. Of these, data were provided by ten senior nurse managers who completed questionnaires of 55 patients who presented to the hospitals with chest pain.'
What information do Bob and his team need to further explore the quality of this article? List two.
ANSWER: A few are: interrater reliability (see Chapter 11), how chest pain is measured (see Chapter 11) and how many patients were approached and how many agreed (dropout rate).
b   Ann and her team also review the literature. Following is a part of the article:
'Seven patients who presented at the hospital with chest pain were approached and invited to participate in the study. They were individually interviewed at their homes using open-ended questions. Interviews were recorded by audiotape and transcribed verbatim. Four themes were derived from the data...'
What information do Ann and her team need to further explore the quality of this article?
ANSWER: Examples are: How many interviewers were involved? What process was used to derive the themes? (see Chapter 8).

## PRACTICE EXERCISE 14.2

Think about the research topics that you are interested in. List these and consider:
1   Why have you chosen these topics?
2   What personal and professional bias do you bring to each topic?
3   Consider ways you may overcome these biases.

PRACTICE EXERCISE 14.3

- Use your library home page or favourite database to search the online databases for a topic that is of interest to you.
- Identify a research paper by looking at the abstract or the description of the paper within the indexing.
- Identify the methodological approach used. If you are not sure ask a colleague to assist you.
- Go to one of the internet web pages and choose an appropriate tool to critically appraise this article. (Hint: Check the JBI, Cochrane Collaboration and the CASP web pages. See also the CONSORT tool.)
- Note how this helps you to read and understand the article as well as be critical about the strengths and limitations presented.
- Write a brief summary of this article using your notes from the critical appraisal tool.
- What themes have come out of this paper? If you are unsure consider what key points have been presented.
- Now consider how you would use this work to critique other articles concerning this topic and compare and contrast the strengths and limitations within a paper.

## FURTHER READING

Burns, N. & Grove, S. (2009). *The Practice of Nursing Research: Appraisal, Synthesis, and Generation of Evidence*, 6th edn. St Louis, MI: Saunders.

Coughlan, M., Cronin, P. & Ryan, F. (2007). Step by step guide to critiquing research. Part 1: Quantitative research. *British Journal of Nursing* 16(11), 658–63.

Creswell, J. (2013). *Qualitative Inquiry and Research Design: Choosing among Five Approaches*, 3rd edn. Thousand Oak, CA: SAGE Publications.

Crombie, I. (1996). In *The Pocket Guide to Critical Appraisal*. London: British Medical Journal Publishing Group, pp. 23–9.

Newell, R. & Burnard, P. (2011). *Vital Notes for Nurses: Research for Evidence-Based Practice*, 2nd edn. Hoboken, NJ: Wiley-Blackwell.

Ryan, F., Coughlan, M. & Cronin, P. (2007). Step by step guide to critiquing research. Part 2: Qualitative research. *British Journal of Nursing* 16(12), 738–44.

## USEFUL WEBSITES

The following websites have useful information for critically appraising a research article.

CASP—The Critical Appraisal Skills Program:

<www.caspinternational.org/?o=1001>

The CASP International Network (CASPin) is an international collaboration which promotes the teaching and learning of critical appraisal. Once within these web pages, click on the 'Appraise' tab and you will find critical appraisal tools for various research designs. CASP offers links to additional resources and evidence-based web pages, making it a one-stop shop for critical appraisal.

Evidence Based Nursing Guides and Tools originates at McGill University in the USA and offers an extensive list of resources, downloadable critique tools and examples of critical appraisals using these tools:

<www.mcgill.ca/library/find/subjects/health/evidence>

Evidence Based Practice Checklists, available from the University of Glasgow:

<www.gla.ac.uk/researchinstitutes/healthwellbeing/research/generalpractice/ebp/checklists>

Offers several downloadable critical appraisal checklists and a useful section with key terms called a 'jargon buster'.

Some additional internet web pages are worth looking at if you are searching for grey data or systematic reviews. You will have extensive access if you locate these via your library web page and not as an individual:

Australian Digital Thesis Collection:

<http://adt.caul.edu.au>

CDBSR—Cochrane Data Base of Systematic Reviews:

<www.cochrane.org>

DARE—Data Base of Reviews of Effectiveness Centre for Reviews and Dissemination:

<www.crd.york.ac.uk/crdweb>

JBI—The Joanna Briggs Institute:

<www.joannabriggs.edu.au>

The University of Sheffield, School of Health and Related Research (ScHARR):

<www.shef.ac.uk/scharr>

## REFERENCES

ANMAC. (2006a). National competency standards for the registered nurse. <www.nursingmidwiferyboard.gov.au/Search.aspx?q=competency%20standards>.

ANMAC. (2006b). National competency standards for the midwife. <http://en-us.nielsen.com/content/nielsen/en_us/industries/media.html>.

Badenoch, D., Sackett, D., Straus, S., Ball, C. & Dawes, M. (2004). CATmaker version 1.1. <www.cebm.net>.

Baglione, L. (2012). *Writing a Research Paper in Political Sciences: A Practical Guide to Inquiry, Structure and Method*, 2nd edn. Thousand Oaks, CA: SAGE.

Beitz, J. (2008). Statistical test selection and analysis: Demystifying a 'mysterious' process. *Journal of Wound Ostomy and Continence Nursing* 35(6), 561–8.

Cheek, J., Gillham, D. & Ballantyne, A. (2005). Using education to promote research dissemination in nursing. *International Journal of Nursing Education Scholarship* 2(1), Article 31. <www.bepress.com/ijnes/vol2/iss1/art31>.

Cutcliffe, J. & Ward, M. (2006). *Critiquing Nursing Research*. Salisbury, UK: Quay Books.

Katrak, P., Bialocerkowski, A., Massy-Westropp, N., Kumar, S. & Grimmer, K. (2004). A systematic review of the content of critical appraisal tools. *BMC Medical Research Methodology* 4(22).

Lim, M., Hellard, M. & Aitken, C. (2005). The case of the disappearing teaspoons: Longitudinal cohort study of the displacement of teaspoons in an Australian research institute. *British Medical Journal* 331, 1498–500.

Ryan, F., Coughlan, M. & Cronin, P. (2007). Step by step guide to critiquing research. Part 2: Qualitative research. *British Journal of Nursing* 16(12), 738–44.

Schneider, Z., Whitehead, D., Elliot, D., LoBiondo-Wood, G. & Haber, J. (2013). *Nursing and Midwifery Research: Methods and Appraisal for Evidence-Based Practice*, 4th edn. Sydney: Mosby Elsevier.

Zellner, K., Boerst, C. & Tabb, W. (2007). Statistics used in current nursing research. *Journal of Nursing Education* 42(2), 55–9.

CHAPTER 15

# UNDERTAKING A SYSTEMATIC REVIEW

Ritin Fernandez, Maree Johnson and Rhonda Griffiths

## CHAPTER LEARNING OBJECTIVES

By the end of this chapter you will be able to:

- appreciate the importance of a systematic review as a source of evidence
- describe the importance of developing a review protocol
- understand how to formulate a focused clinical question
- explain the development of a comprehensive literature search strategy on a specific clinical question
- appreciate the importance of assessing the quality of included studies
- understand the processes of conducting a meta-analysis, meta-synthesis and narrative synthesis.

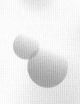

# Introduction

A systematic review is a compilation of all scientific studies on a particular topic according to predetermined criteria (Cullum et al. 2008). Systematic reviews are recognised as the highest form of evidence (NHMRC 2009) because they include all available evidence, because the conclusions are based only on research that passes a rigorous **critical appraisal** and because the methods used in the review are explicit and open to the criticism of readers. The outcome of the systematic review is the presentation of the findings in a summary format. Results of a review may validate current practice or provide evidence to change practice or identify that more research is necessary in the area (Fineout-Overholt et al. 2008). Robust and credible systematic reviews are the basis of clinical practice guideline or policy development in nursing and midwifery. In addition, they are increasingly required by funding bodies as the first step in any research proposal.

**Critical appraisal:** A term used to assess the outcomes for evidence of a research study's effectiveness.

# The process of a systematic review

Although systematic reviews are considered to be secondary research, they involve a formal process that is transparent and reproducible. The following sections will discuss various steps required to undertake a systematic review.

## Planning the review

The first step is the formation of the review team. There is no ideal number of reviewers that are required in order to complete a systematic review, but the number will be influenced by the scope of the topic and the support and resources available. Nevertheless, it is essential that the review team has extensive clinical experience in the topic under consideration, experience of the systematic review process, and an interest and commitment to developing evidence as a basis for practice (Littell et al. 2008).

## Developing the protocol

As in any scientific endeavour, a protocol should be established beforehand. A protocol for a systematic review is equivalent to a proposal for a research study. A developed protocol ensures that the *systematic review* is as rigorous as possible within practical limits.

Systematic reviews that are published in the Cochrane Library or in the JBI Database of Systematic Reviews and Implementation Reports require that the systematic review titles and protocols are registered and approved before the review is conducted (see Useful websites). This is a means of informing other researchers and clinicians of the systematic reviews currently in progress, thus avoiding duplication (Higgins & Green 2011). In addition, the peer review process for approval ensures that the systematic **review protocol** is well defined and provides explicit strategies to reduce the risk of bias and/or misuse. The steps in developing a protocol for a systematic review include:

**Review protocol:** A well-defined document that provides explicit strategies to undertake a systematic review so that bias is reduced.

- formulating a research question
- developing criteria for the inclusion of studies
- defining the search process
- identifying the methods that will be used to assess the quality of the studies
- defining the methods that will be implemented to collect/extract the data
- detailing the process for data analysis and summary of the evidence.

Figure 15.1  Steps in undertaking a systematic review

## STEP 1

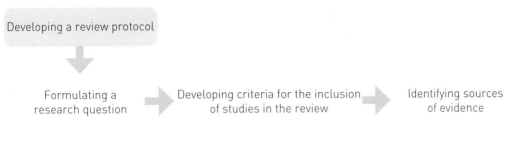

## STEP 2

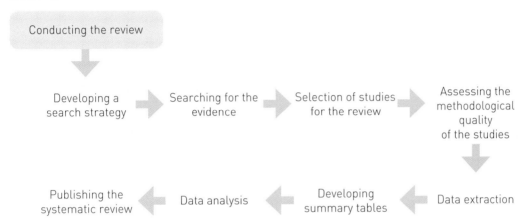

Formulating a research question

To design and execute a systematic review successfully the researcher must be very clear about what is being studied and the nature of the research question (Polit & Beck 2012). Poorly developed questions will result in a large number of citations, many of which will not be relevant to the question under investigation; or they may result in few citations and the ones that are relevant may not be identified. Well-formulated questions that are specific and focused will direct the development of a search strategy for identification of relevant studies (Aslam & Emmanuel 2010). A well-designed research question is a precise statement, based on the characteristics of the *P*atient/Population, *I*ntervention, *C*omparison and *O*utcome (PICO) (Richardson et al. 1995). Studies have shown that the use of the PICO framework improves the specificity and breakdown of clinical problems and leads to more complex search strategies and more precise search results (Boudin et al. 2010). The PICO format has also been used to develop questions for qualitative studies. In this case the *P* stands for participants, the *I* for phenomena of interest and *CO* for Context. Examples of poorly designed and well-designed questions are presented below in Tables 15.1 and 15.2.

**Table 15.1**  Examples of poorly developed clinical questions

Is tap water effective in cleansing wounds?
Does a baby's birth weight have an impact on their subsequent development?

**Table 15.2** Example of a precise clinical question for quantitative studies

| Patients or problem | Intervention | Comparison | Outcome | Patients or problem |
|---|---|---|---|---|
| Patients with chronic wounds | Cleansing with tap water | Cleansing with normal saline | Infection rate Healing rates | Patients with chronic wounds |
| Well-formulated question | What is the effect of cleansing with tap water compared to normal saline on the infection and healing rates of chronic wounds? | | | |

### Developing criteria for the inclusion of studies in the review

The criteria for the inclusion of individual studies must address questions of relevance and validity. Relevance is the ability of the selected article to answer the research question posed by the systematic review. Therefore, in order to be relevant, the eligibility criteria are based on the components of the review question. The eligibility criteria therefore consist of the participants/population, interventions, comparisons and outcomes of interest. For systematic reviews, the validity of a trial or an individual study is the extent to which its design and conduct are likely to prevent systematic errors or bias (Smith et al. 2011). Validity in systematic reviews is therefore largely dependent on the study design. For example, the most reliable research design that will provide the evidence for the effectiveness of an intervention is the randomised controlled trial.

### Types of participants/populations

The criteria for considering types of participants included in the individual studies should encompass the likely diversity of studies as well as ensure that a meaningful answer can be obtained when studies are considered in aggregate. This can be done by, first, identifying a clear definition of the disease or condition and, second, by considering the broad population and setting. Both these criteria are present in the following:

> Potable tap water may not be available in all countries or settings, therefore a recent review on water for wound cleansing included studies that used all types of water including boiled and cooled water.

As systematic reviews are carried out to provide evidence for a global audience, a reason should be given for excluding studies with specific population characteristics or settings. For example, in the systematic review on water for wound cleansing, patients with burns were excluded as the initial management of burns requires a sterile environment (Fernandez & Griffiths 2012).

### Types of interventions

The criteria for considering the interventions of interest and the comparators should be made explicit. Particular attention should be given if the interventions are being compared with an inactive control (e.g. placebo, no treatment or usual care), or with an active control (e.g. a variation of the same intervention or a different drug). Complex interventions such as behavioural or educational should have their core components clearly articulated. The mode, frequency, duration and person delivering the intervention should also be clearly stated (Higgins & Green 2011):

> The RCT on wound cleansing stated that tap water was collected from a designated faucet after letting the water run for three minutes.

### Types of outcomes

The outcomes investigated in the systematic review should be meaningful to clinicians, patients, the general public, administrators and policy-makers. The primary outcome of interest and the secondary outcomes should be clearly identified. In addition, the methods used to measure these outcomes should also be specified before commencing the review. In some cases, the reviewers might decide to include studies that have used only objective measures (e.g. wound culture results) rather than subjective methods (wound assessment criteria) for outcome measurement. Another important consideration in deciding the criteria for types of outcomes is the timing of the outcome measurement. It is important to give this considerable thought as it can influence the results of the review (Higgins & Deeks 2008).

> The results of infection rates in all wounds cleansed with either tap water or normal saline cannot be grouped together as there are different types of wounds. Individual studies could have measured outcomes for different types of wounds. Therefore a strategy could be to group the wounds into pre-specified types such as acute or chronic wounds.

It is important to include all outcomes in a review as it will identify the gaps in the primary research and provide researchers with priorities for future studies (Higgins & Green 2011).

### Types of studies

It is important to pre-specify the study designs that will be included in the review, taking into account that certain study designs are more appropriate than others for answering particular questions. For example, reviews that ask questions about the effects of healthcare interventions are best answered by including RCTs (Jadad & Enkin 2007). A rationale for why studies were included or excluded is often provided when reporting the review. For example, a study by Speirs and colleagues (2013) of interventions for homeless women excluded qualitative studies because 'the focus of the study was on effectiveness, requiring comparison groups and defined interventions that could be generalisable to communities'. Other aspects that need to be considered when deciding the types of study are matters relating to language and publication status. A rationale for excluding studies due to language or publication status should be provided.

In a systematic review on the infection control management of Methicillin-resistant Staphylococcus aureus (MRSA) in acute care studies (Halcomb et al. 2008) that were published before 1985 were excluded from the review. The rationale given for this was that the use of universal precautions only became mandatory after that year and the inclusion of studies before that would have resulted in flawed findings.

### Identifying sources of evidence

The aim of the search strategy is to undertake a comprehensive search to facilitate retrieval of all published and unpublished clinical trials (Lefebvre et al. 2008). A comprehensive literature search, which minimises the risk of bias, is another difference between a

## THINKING DEEPLY

**Deciding what to review**

Your manager has asked you as a clinical nurse specialist to review the evidence for the use of tap water compared to normal saline for cleansing wounds. You have formulated the following question:

In patients with acute or chronic wounds, what is the effect of cleansing with tap water compared to normal saline on the infection and healing rates?

What types of studies would be suited for a systematic review on the above question? Give a reason.

ANSWER: Randomised controlled trial studies, quasi-randomised trial studies, cohort studies, pre-test and post-test studies, case-control studies and qualitative studies.

systematic review and a traditional review (Crowther et al. 2010). A comprehensive and unbiased literature review incorporates both published and unpublished works and should include:

- relevant studies/reports from a variety of databases (e.g. MEDLINE, CINAHL, Cochrane Library, Cochrane Controlled Trials register, Healthstar) and the internet (Montori et al. 2005)
- a review of the reference list of the retrieved articles
- hand-searching journals that are relevant to the research question (Hopewell et al. 2007a)
- personal communication, which is a valuable source for locating grey literature such as conference papers, theses and government reports (Hopewell et al. 2007b)
- consultation with content specialists
- attempt to locate studies/reports in other languages.

## TIPS AND SKILLS

A comprehensive search is the foundation for a valid and reliable systematic review and should include both published and unpublished works where possible. Failure to identify a diversity of literature from a wide range of sources could result in a biased review (Hopewell et al. 2007a, b).

## Conducting the systematic review

### Developing a search strategy

A clearly defined search strategy is needed to direct an effective literature review and ensure efficient use of resources. The benefits arising from a search strategy include the ability for others to replicate the study, thus reducing the potential for systematic bias.

A precisely described search strategy should include identification and documentation of all steps of each phase of the search for later reference. These are:

- the date, the time period, search terms and combinations of search terms used
- the sources searched and the number of articles located

- the searcher's identity, designation and contact number, and finally
- whether assistance from the librarian for the development and implementation of the search strategy was obtained (Whitlock et al. 2009).

Retaining the computer search printouts and saving a copy for future reference is recommended.

As each database has its own unique indexing terms, individual search strategies should be developed for each database. During the development of the search strategy, consideration should also be given to the diverse terminology used and the spelling of keywords as this will influence the identification of relevant trials. Search terms can be identified from the keywords used in the individual publications. The PICO model is a good guide to devising a logical list of the search terms. This procedure is likely to result in an extensive volume of literature, which then has to be systematically filtered to identify relevant articles and reports for the study.

## Searching for the evidence

### Electronic database search

The success of an electronic search is strongly related to the skill of the searcher in using effective strategies. Electronic database searching can be performed using various methods such as searching using text words, subject headings, truncation and wildcards. Text word searching will retrieve all articles on the database that contain the relevant word in the title or abstract, so the search is likely to include a number of articles that are irrelevant to the question. However, the search can be made more sensitive by using wildcards at any point within the word. This will ensure that the search retrieves articles with all versions of the word (Cullum 2000; Cullum et al. 2008).

Most databases develop their own subject headings to enable searches to be more focused than free text searches. Articles are categorised under subject headings that are deemed to be significant topics in the article. This method provides a consistent way to retrieve information that may use different terminology for the same concepts.

Truncation is another method used to retrieve all possible suffix variations of a root word. For example, the search 'ultraso$' will retrieve the words ultrasound, ultrasonography, ultrasonogram, ultrasound, etc. However, unlimited truncation should be used with care, since documents with unwanted words will be accidentally retrieved (Pohl et al. 2010). For example, the search 'card$' would retrieve documents with the words 'cardiac', 'cardiology', 'cardiothoracic', etc., but also 'cards' and 'cardigan'.

Table 15.3 is an example of a table describing the various search terms used within a systematic review for a study assessing the effect of doll therapy for people with dementia.

**Table 15.3** Search strategy for Ovid MEDLINE

| Search ID | Search Terms | Results |
|---|---|---|
| 1 | Dementia | javascript:__ doPostBack('ctl00$ctl00$FindField$FindField$historyControl$HistoryRepeater$ctl00$linkResults','')108 726 |
| 2 | dement* OR BSPD | javascript:__doPostBack('ctl00$ctl00$FindField$FindField$historyControl$HistoryRepeater$ctl01$linkResults','')132 392 |

*(Continued)*

**Table 15.3** Search strategy for Ovid MEDLINE *(Continued)*

| Search ID | Search Terms | Results |
|---|---|---|
| 3 | Alzheimer* | javascript:__ doPostBack('ctl00$ctl00$FindField$ FindField$historyControl $HistoryRepeater$ctl02$ linkResults','')135 654 |
| 4 | creutzfeldt* OR jcd OR cjd | javascript:__ doPostBack('ctl00$ctl00$FindField$FindField$ historyControl$HistoryRepeater $ctl03$linkResults','')13 625 |
| 5 | Kohlsch* OR 'amelo-cerebro-hypohidrot*' OR *' OR aphasia* OR frontotemporal* OR Huntington* OR Kluver* N2 Bucy* OR Diffuse Neurofibrillar* N4 calcification* | 62 158 |
| 6 | Lewy* N2 bod* | javascript:__ doPostBack('ctl00$ctl00$FindField$ FindField$historyControl $HistoryRepeater$ctl05$linkResults','')11 223 |
| 7 | Pick* N2 diseas* | javascript:__ doPostBack('ctl00$ctl00$FindField$ FindField$historyControl$ HistoryRepeater$ctl06$linkResults','')6 090 |
| 8 | 1 OR 2 OR 3 OR 4 OR 5 OR 6 OR 7 | javascript:__ doPostBack('ctl00$ctl00$FindField$FindField $historyControl$HistoryRepeater $ctl07$linkResults','')271 798 |
| 9 | doll OR dolls OR dolly OR dollies | javascript:__doPostBack('ctl00$ctl00$FindField $FindField$historyControl$HistoryRepeater $ctl20$linkResults','')14 439 |
| 10 | Play Therapy | javascript:__doPostBack('ctl00$ctl00$FindField $FindField$historyControl$HistoryRepeater $ctl21$linkResults','')880 |
| 11 | Play Therap* | javascript:__doPostBack('ctl00$ctl00$FindField $FindField$historyControl $HistoryRepeater$ctl22$linkResults','')1 460 |
| 12 | 10 OR 11 | javascript:__ doPostBack('ctl00$ctl00$FindField$ FindField$historyControl $HistoryRepeater$ctl23$linkResults','')1 460 |
| 13 | 9 OR 12 | 14 521 |
| 14 | 8 AND 13 | 410 |

**Searching the literature** using wildcards such as the '#' (hash sign) and '?' (question mark) are other strategies that can be used to retrieve all relevant studies. Following the search using the key terms, the use of Boolean operators AND, OR, NOT is a way of constructing the research question, indicating the relationships between the search terms as well as limiting the search. Searching the available databases is a complex activity. Skill and specialist training is undertaken by librarians to conduct these reviews.

**Searching the literature for a systematic review:** A defined scope of literature with prior specification of eligibility criteria.

## Manual searching

It is important to be aware that not all journals are indexed by an electronic database, so manual searching may be a very important part of the search strategy. Manual searching involves searching through the reference list of articles that have been found to throw light on the clinical question. It may also involve searching the indexes of journals that are likely to publish articles relevant to the question. It is, however, labour-intensive and time-consuming (Hopewell et al. 2007a).

## Searching the grey literature

Grey literature is information that is either unpublished or has been published in non-commercial form. Publication bias is a common problem identified in systematic reviews, which arises when only published data is included. Researchers have indicated that including grey literature in systematic reviews helps to overcome the problem of publication bias (Hopewell et al. 2007b). In particular, RCTs that result in no significant difference being found are often difficult to publish in refereed journals, but are nonetheless important to include in systematic reviews. Grey literature is now freely available on many websites and is selectively indexed by numerous commercial database vendors.

Examples of grey literature include:

- government reports
- policy statements and issues papers
- conference proceedings
- pre-prints and post-prints of articles
- theses and dissertations
- market reports
- working papers
- newsletters and bulletins.

## TIPS AND SKILLS

Use the PICO table to list the search terms under the appropriate headings. If you are a student or academic it is best to find out who are the specially trained librarian staff within your local facilities who can assist you with the search.

- Consult with the librarian to identify:
  - search terms and combinations of terms
  - electronic databases to search, journals to hand-search
  - the retrieving of articles.
- Save the search strategy for future use.
- Use a reference management database such as EndNote.

Cochrane reviewers receive support with database searching from the Collaborative Review Group. Each review group has a database of all published and unpublished clinical trials that are both electronically identified and hand-searched according to their specialty. The review group librarian searches this database and provides the reviewer with a list of all eligible trials.

## Selection of studies for the review

The searching processes locate all citations that reflect the research question, and in many instances the citations may be listed in more than one database. Importing the references and abstracts identified from the search into a bibliographic software such as EndNote and removing duplicate citations will therefore prevent unnecessary waste of time (Higgins & Green 2011).

Not every study remaining after the removal of duplicates will be eligible for inclusion in the systematic review. Selection for the potential inclusion of the studies is made in a two-stage process. First, the titles and abstracts of the individual studies are verified against the inclusion and exclusion criteria and the full text obtained of relevant citations. Some citations will be rejected at this stage. If the title and abstract are inconclusive, the full text should be obtained for further assessment. The second stage is applying the inclusion and exclusion criteria to the full text of the citation. Publications that pass the relevance test are then tested for validity, which means assessing the methodological quality of the study.

## TIPS AND SKILLS

Apply the inclusion and exclusion criteria first to the title and abstract. If the title and abstract meet the criteria, obtain the article for further assessment. Have two or more investigators review each citation independently. Assessing the methodological quality of individual studies is done by two investigators independently.

- - - - - - - - - - - - - - - - - - - - - - - - - - - - - - - - - - - - - - - - - - - - - - - - - - -

### Assessing the quality of the studies

Critical appraisal helps to eliminate methodologically poor studies, so reliable and systematic methods for the assessment of the methodological quality of the studies are imperative. Numerous assessment tools and checklists have been published to assess the validity of the methodological quality of individual studies (Moher et al. 1995). Systematic reviews published in the Cochrane Library and on the JBI database require the use of their own quality assessment tools for assessing risk of bias in studies (Higgins & Green 2011). An example of the critical appraisal form used by the Joanna Briggs Institute is shown in Appendix 15.1.

The common elements of these quality assessment tools include questions to determine the extent to which the design and conduct of the study are likely to prevent the four causes of systematic errors (Table 15.4).

The assessment of the methodological quality of the studies for the review should be conducted independently by two reviewers, with disagreements or indecision being referred to a third person. The name of the author(s) and the journal source should be

**Table 15.4**  Causes of systematic error

| Level | Intervention |
|---|---|
| Selection bias | Systematic differences in comparison groups<br>Knowledge of treatment assignment |
| Performance bias | Systematic differences in care provided apart from the intervention being evaluated |
| Attrition bias | Systematic differences in withdrawals from the trial |
| Detection bias | Systematic differences in outcome assessment<br>Systematic differences in self-reported and objectively measured outcomes |

concealed from the reviewers to reduce bias. The reason for rejecting articles should be documented for future reference. In Cochrane reviews each study is weighted to reflect its design and methodology. An average weight is subsequently calculated as a guide to the quality of the studies in the review.

## Data extraction

**Data extraction** is the collection of relevant information from the publications using a data collection form to enable a standardised approach. The type of information collected is determined by the review question and so the data collection form will vary between systematic reviews (Leong 2007). A data extraction form should include information that will identify the primary study and the reviewers such as study citation, reviewer information/code, participant demographics, participant inclusion/exclusion criteria, description of the interventions, description of the outcome measures, follow-up period, and the number and reasons for withdrawals and dropouts.

Development of the data collection form is an onerous task, so enough time should be set aside for it. Caution should be exercised when developing the form to ensure that it is succinct and captures the relevant information (Higgins & Deeks 2008). The form should be pilot-tested and the information obtained should be closely examined for relevance to the question. Spreadsheets are useful tools when designing a data collection form. Appendix 15.2 shows an example of a data extraction form used by JBI.

**Data extraction:** The process of extracting the methods and results from existing research studies for further meta-analysis or presentation in summary tables within a systematic review.

## Developing summary tables

The aim of systematic reviews is to present the best available evidence in an easily understood summary form. These summaries are presented in a table built specifically from the extracted data. The summary table assists in the data analysis and provides an overview of vital information from individual studies. A range of aspects can be presented including study citation, country and year, study design, study sample size, interventions, outcome measures, overall rating of the study quality, and study findings. The tabular format is concise but comprehensive, enables comparison of the critical elements, identifies similarities and dissimilarities in the articles, and facilitates interpretation of the results by the target audience (see Table 15.5).

**Table 15.5** Example of a summary table

| Author, Year, Country | Study type/ Level of evidence | Participants | Interventions | Outcomes | Notes |
|---|---|---|---|---|---|
| Griffiths 2001 Australia | RCT/II | 35 patients with 49 chronic wounds | Group A: wounds irrigated with tap water Group B: wounds irrigated with normal saline | *Infection* Group A: No infection was found among 23 wounds Group B: 3 infections were found among 26 wounds *Healing* Group A: 8 healed among 23 wounds Group B: 16 healed among 26 wounds | Allocation performed using a list of random numbers nominated by person not entering patients into the trial. Both patients and outcome assessors were blinded to the treatment. Criteria for wound infection: Presence of pus, discolouration, friable granulation tissue, pain, tenderness, pocketing or bridging at base of the wound, abnormal smell and wound breakdown. 4 patients in each group withdrew from the study. Wounds were assessed at the end of 6 weeks. Quality of tap water reported to meet Australian National Health and Medical Research Council requirements. |

## Data analysis

Systematic reviews were started to present pooled data from RCTs reporting the results of medical research. The methods used for data analysis depend largely on the design of the studies. For quantitative studies the summary is generally presented as a meta-analysis, while evidence from qualitative studies is presented as a meta-synthesis.

## Meta-analysis: The synthesis of quantitative data

**Meta-analysis:** A statistical method used to combine the results of several studies that address a set of related research hypotheses.

A **meta-analysis** is a statistical method that synthesises the findings of several small studies as if they were one large, powerful study in order to draw conclusions about a specific research question (Gallin & Ognibene 2012). In the medical literature the terms meta-analysis and systematic review are often used interchangeably, although meta-analysis is only one component of a systematic review (Ioannidis et al. 2008). Meta-analysis can be undertaken using the Review Manager (RevMan) software from the Cochrane Collaboration or any other commercially available software.

## Carrying out a meta-analysis

Meta-analysis can only be carried out if the studies included in the review are sufficiently homogeneous. Studies are assumed to be clinically homogeneous if they are similar enough in design, population and outcomes to permit the data to be combined (Gallin & Ognibene 2012).

Studies that are clinically homogeneous can be combined in a meta-analysis to determine a summary estimate of effect. The effect is summarised in different ways with relative risks (RR) or odds ratios (OR) calculated for dichotomous data and weighted mean difference (WMD) for continuous data (Egger et al. 2008).

Relative risk is used when the outcome of interest has relatively low probability. It is used to compare the risk of developing side effects in people receiving a placebo versus people who are receiving an established (standard of care) treatment (Egger et al. 2008). The odds ratio is the ratio of the odds of an event occurring in one group to the odds of it occurring in another group. The weighted mean difference is used to combine measures for continuous variables when the mean, standard deviation and sample size in each group are known. Each study is given a weight depending on the amount of influence it has on the overall results of the meta-analysis. This method assumes that all the trials have measured the outcome on the same scale. The calculation of these and other subsequent statistics relevant to meta-analysis is undertaken using RevMan, Meta Analysis of Statistics Assessment and Review Instrument (MAStARI) or any other commercially available software.

After deciding on the effect measure, heterogeneity across the studies should be investigated to examine statistically the degree of similarity in the outcomes of the studies. Simply averaging the odds ratios from all the studies would give misleading results, due to equal weight given to all studies, although smaller studies are more subject to chance. To overcome this error, the studies included in the meta-analysis should be combined using either the fixed or random effects model. Choosing the appropriate effects model for the combination is vital. The fixed effects model answers the question whether the studies included in the meta-analysis show that the treatment or exposure produced the effect on average. On the other hand, the random effects model answers the question, on the basis of the studies that are examined, Is it possible to comment that the treatment or the exposure will produce a result? For studies that are homogeneous, combining studies using the fixed effects or random effects models will produce similar results.

Statistical homogeneity indicates that the variation in results is larger than what would have been expected by chance (Perera & Heneghan 2008). The commonly used statistical test to measure the statistical heterogeneity is the I2 test, which is independent of the number of studies included in the meta-analysis (Higgins et al. 2003). The I2 is a statistic that measures the proportion of inconsistency in individual studies that cannot be explained by chance (Higgins et al. 2003). A I2 value of less than 25% indicates that the studies are homogeneous and so can be combined using a fixed effects model, while a I2 value of more than 75% indicates that the studies are highly heterogeneous and should be combined using a random effects model (Higgins et al. 2003). Figure 15.2 shows an example of the meta-analysis graph for continuous data.

Figure 15.2   Meta-analysis graph for continuous data

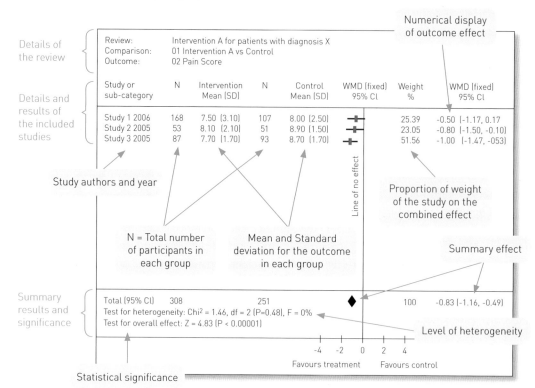

## Meta-synthesis: The synthesis of qualitative data

**Meta-synthesis:** A qualitative approach for drawing inferences from similar or related studies, identifying key features and presenting findings representative of all data.

Qualitative studies should not be disregarded, because they provide substantial evidence for clinical decision-making. **Meta-synthesis** has been developed for the same reasons as meta-analysis, that is, to overcome discrepancies associated with individual studies (Hannes & Macaitis 2012). Meta-synthesis involves examining research findings from individual qualitative studies and creating summary statements that authentically describe the meaning of these themes (Pearson et al. 2007). The Cochrane Collaboration Qualitative Research Methods Group (QRMG) provides resources and short courses to assist researchers to undertake the meta-synthesis. In addition, the Joanna Briggs Institute has developed software called Qualitative Assessment and Review Instrument (QARI) that enables researchers to carry out systematic reviews and meta-synthesis of qualitative data (see Useful websites).

### Carrying out a meta-synthesis

The process of meta-synthesis entails identifying relationships between the findings of existing studies and making interpretations across comparable studies (Barnett-Page & Thomas 2009). This has three distinct phases: identification of the key findings of each study, determining how these findings relate to those of other studies, and combining common findings into themes to generate a description of the phenomenon (Ryan et al. 2009).

### Identification of the key findings of each study

This phase involves careful reading and rereading of each primary study to search for phrases, metaphors and themes that occur repeatedly throughout the included studies

(Downe 2008). The illustrations from the text that demonstrate their origins are also recorded. This process is a form of confirming the authenticity of the association between each finding in terms of how clearly and/or directly it can be attributed to participants in the primary research (Pearson et al. 2007).

*Relating themes across studies*

Once the findings have been identified it is important to combine these using methods appropriate to the specific type and nature of data that have been extracted. The key findings from the primary studies are grouped on the basis of similarity in meanings into categories or areas of similarity. The categories are re-examined to interpret the content of each, and to identify consistencies and incongruities.

*Description of the phenomenon*

These categories are then subjected to a meta-aggregation in order to produce a single comprehensive set of synthesised findings. A synthesised finding is an overarching description of a group of categorised findings that allows for the generation of recommendations for practice (Pearson et al. 2007).

An example of a meta-synthesis is presented in Figure 15.3. This meta-synthesis was undertaken to identify the characteristics of nursing teams. A total of five findings grouped in three categories showed that nursing teams exhibit accountability for their actions, commitment to the nursing team and an enthusiastic, motivating attitude (Pearson et al. 2006).

Figure 15.3   Meta-synthesis characteristics of nursing teams

| Synthesis | Category | Finding |
|---|---|---|
| Characteristics of nursing teams<br>The function of a nursing team requires nurses to exhibit a variety of characteristics such as accountability for their actions, commitment to the nursing team and an enthusiastic, motivating attitude. | Commitment to the nursing team produces cohesiveness among the groups. | A successful, cohesive team can be produced when individuals are committed to the nursing unit. |
| | Nurses become accountable for the actions when working within a team functioning approach to care delivery. | Nurses practising with a primary care team describe a feeling of responsibility of the patient's care.<br>There is an increased awareness of accountability for nurses practising in a team of primary care. |
| | The effectiveness of a team can be improved when members are enthusiastic and motivated towards the team's goals. | Individual enthusiasm and supportive culture encourage teamwork.<br>Motivation improved among team members as a result of awareness of shared problems. |

Source: Pearson et al. 2006

*Narrative synthesis*

Summarising evidence or knowledge in the form of a meta-analysis is not always possible and in these cases the evidence is presented as a narrative synthesis. In addition, a narrative synthesis can be complementary to a meta-analysis or meta-synthesis. In narrative synthesis the findings are explained in a text format. The drawbacks of narrative

**Narrative synthesis:**
Summarising evidence in the form of a meta-analysis is not always possible and in these cases the evidence is presented in a text format as a narrative synthesis.

synthesis are that it lacks transparency and reproducibility and that currently no process is available to guide this form of analysis. The systematic review on the infection control management of MRSA in acute care (Halcomb et al. 2008) and interventions for homeless women (Speirs et al. 2013) provide excellent examples of narrative reviews in which the complete process of a systematic review was carried out. However, because of the lack of homogeneity in the studies, a **narrative synthesis** of the results was the best way to present the evidence within the systematic review.

## THINKING DEEPLY

### The dilemma of equivocal evidence

We often assume that all systematic reviews will provide a definitive answer, but sometimes this is not possible and clinicians need to consider additional issues. As a clinician you would like to decide whether the model of care you are using in your ward is the best possible way to deliver nursing care. As an evidence-based practitioner, you seek out any systematic reviews available. You locate the paper by Fernandez and associates (2012).

The conclusions of this study were that: 'There were no significant differences in nursing outcomes relating to role clarity, job satisfaction and nurse absenteeism rates between any of the models of care' (p. 324). What issues might you explore further in the various studies to inform your decision-making?

## New approaches: Overview of Reviews (umbrella reviews)

As the number of published systematic reviews increases, researchers have devised methods that would enable them to combine multiple systematic reviews in a single review of the evidence, just as journal articles are combined in a systematic review. The Cochrane Collaboration (Becker & Oxman 2008) has developed a method to complete Overviews of Reviews, also referred to as umbrella reviews. Overviews can summarise evidence from more than one systematic review for the same condition where different outcomes are addressed; different interventions for the same disorder; the same intervention applied to different problems or populations; and the adverse effects of an intervention for more than one condition.

Cochrane Overviews are arranged under the following headings: Background; Objectives (not a research question); Methods; Main Results; and Author's Conclusions. Unlike the source systematic reviews that include quality assessments of included articles, the method for completing an Overview of Reviews does not validate the quality of the original research reports used in the systematic reviews. The limitations of the source systematic reviews are assessed and meta-analysis across reviews may be included to provide direct comparisons of the effects of different interventions.

## Where to publish the completed systematic review

Once the systematic review has been completed, the findings need to be published so that they can be used in the development of guidelines to be used in clinical practice. If the initial protocol is published in the Cochrane Library or the JBI Database of

Systematic Reviews and Implementation Reports, the complete review is also published in the same database. But systematic reviews can also be published on other health databases such as MEDLINE and CINAHL. JBI and the Cochrane Collaboration have developed software that consists of a predeveloped format for the standardised reporting of systematic reviews.

## Joanna Briggs and the Cochrane Collaboration

The Joanna Briggs Institute was established in 1996 to provide an evidence base for nursing practice and to devise strategies for the effective dissemination and implementation of that information within the healthcare setting. The JBI is a growing, dynamic, international collaboration involving nursing, medical and allied health researchers, clinicians, academics and quality managers across 40 countries in every continent. The JBI has made evidence available at the point of clinical care by providing nurses with clearly presented summaries of research findings called 'Best Practice Information Sheets' <www.joannabriggs.org>.

The Cochrane Collaboration is an international not-for-profit organisation that has been established to provide up-to-date, accurate information about the effects of healthcare on the global health community. The Cochrane Collaboration is named after the British epidemiologist Archie Cochrane and was founded in 1993. The Cochrane Library consists of more than 5600 reviews on various health-related topics. The systematic reviews published in the Cochrane Library are carried out by a global network of dedicated volunteers who are supported by a small number of staff from within the Collaboration.

### Implications for evidence-based practice

Nursing practice is largely based on tradition and rituals (Porter 2010). According to various bodies (NHMRC 2009), a systematic review is considered to be the highest level of evidence because of the rigorous methods used and the unbiased results. The findings are therefore used for the development of evidence-based guidelines and policies for clinical practice. One of the most important aspects of evidence-based nursing is that patients and their families are informed about the various options available to them in relation to their treatment and care. The results of evidence searches should be shared with them so that joint decision-making can result. Information should be shared on a partnership basis, with the practitioner providing explanations so patients are able to decide what will work best for them.

In addition to giving evidence for clinical practice, systematic reviews also provide implications for further research.

Students taking higher degree courses often commence with a systematic review, identify the gaps in the literature and then complete primary research to address the gaps. Furthermore, funding bodies require evidence from systematic reviews in applications that seek grants for primary research.

The systematic review forms a crucial part of evidence-based nursing and midwifery. Results of the review are made available to health practitioners in

*(Continued)*

*(Continued)*

a briefly described document. In Australia, this document, the Best Practice Information Sheet, is prepared by JBI and is widely available through the internet. However, relevant information including the research team and the process used to develop this Best Practice Information Sheet is included in JBI's Technical Reports. The use of a Best Practice Information Sheet can also vary from one organisation to another organisation (Dobbins et al. 2010). Ongoing development to conduct systematic reviews of qualitative research will further assist nurses and midwives to apply the evidence in their care delivery.

Finally, even though evidence obtained from systematic reviews is considered to be the highest level of evidence, the systematic review needs to be critically appraised before the evidence is implemented. The evidence should also be carefully considered according to its clinical significance, impact on service users and costs.

# SUMMARY

- A robust and credible systematic review provides the basis for clinical guideline and policy development.
- Identifying and defining the clinical question for the review is an important first step in the process.
- Developing and registering a Review Protocol (a plan of your review process) will enhance the quality of a systematic review.
- Appropriate inclusion and exclusion criteria will provide formal constraints that will enhance the focus of the comparison of studies.
- Data extraction and quality assessment of the included studies are best undertaken by two independent reviewers.
- Meta-analysis of the findings of similar studies using statistical procedures will allow the researcher to combine the findings in a meaningful way.
- Narrative synthesis is used when studies are too diverse to be combined for meta-analysis.

## PRACTICE EXERCISE 15.1

Betty is a registered nurse working at a large volunteer organisation which provides health and social services to homeless people. Betty has been asked by her supervisor to find out about available evidence that the organisation can use to provide health promotion services to homeless women with or without children. Betty can gain access to more than three libraries in her local communities and uses many databases for her search.

a  What are keywords that Betty can use to begin her search? Please also use an asterisk when applicable. It is expected that Betty can discuss this task later with librarians.

b  List three databases that Betty uses for her search. It is suggested that health promotion services can be for physical health, mental health, early disease prevention or early disease detection such as screenings.

ANSWER:

a  Some keywords are homeless, NOT 'Man or men or male', female, wom?n, intervention, self exam, health behave*, intervention, crisis intervention, health care, continuum of care, primary health care, patient care, case manage*, treatment planning.

b  Examples are EBSCO, CINAHL Plus with Full Text, Academic Search Complete, Scopus, the Cochrane Collaboration, Psychinfo.

## PRACTICE EXERCISE 15.2

As a graduate nurse, you have observed an increasing use of restraints by staff in a busy nursing home. You would like to know what types of restraint can be used and their relevant guidelines. You intend to introduce changes within the organisation and would like to know potential barriers so you can discuss the issues with your supervisor.

Start your search by:

- identifying the Best Practice Information Sheet relating to the use of restraints
- searching databases to explore whether health organisations have adopted the best practice

- listing potential barriers
- analysing whether the identified barriers will be applied in your organisation or not.

Hint: Go to the JBI web page and then look for the Best Practice Information Sheet.

## PRACTICE EXERCISE 15.3

You are required to develop a search strategy to identify the relevant papers relating to wound cleansing. Which of the following databases would you search?

MEDLINE, CINAHL, EmBaSE, PsycInfo, PEDRO, Cochrane

Compile a search strategy using the search terms listed below.

Search history

| | | | |
|---|---|---|---|
| 1) Wound$ | 2) lacerat$ | 3) bruis$ | 4) Ulcer$ |
| 5) Infect$ | 6) Heal$ | 7) Solution$ | 9) Sodium Chloride |
| 10) water | 11) Clean$ | 12) Irrigat$ | 13) Swabb$ |
| 14) Scrub$ | 15) Soak$ | 16) bath$ | 17) Shower$ |

Hint: You can find answers in the article by R. Fernandez & R. Griffiths (2008). Water for wound cleansing. *Cochrane Database of Systematic Reviews* 23(1), CD003861. It is an electronic resource.

## APPENDIX 15.1
# JBI CRITICAL APPRAISAL CHECKLIST FOR EXPERIMENTAL STUDIES

Reviewer ................................................................................ Date ...............................

Author ...............................................................Year ....................... Record Number ...............................

| | Yes | No | Unclear |
|---|---|---|---|
| 1. Was the assignment to treatment groups random? | | | |
| 2. Were participants blinded to treatment allocation? | | | |
| 3. Was allocation to treatment groups concealed from the allocator? | | | |
| 4. Were the outcomes of people who withdrew described and included in the analysis? | | | |
| 5. Were those assessing outcomes blind to the treatment allocation? | | | |
| 6. Were the control and treatment groups comparable at entry? | | | |
| 7. Were groups treated identically other than for the named interventions? | | | |
| 8. Were outcomes measured in the same way for all groups? | | | |
| 9. Were outcomes measured in a reliable way? | | | |
| 10. Was there adequate follow-up (>80%)? | | | |
| 11. Was appropriate statistical analysis used? | | | |

Overall appraisal: Include Exclude Seek further info

Comments (Including reasons for exclusion)

.................................................................................................................................................
...............................
.................................................................................................................................................
...............................
.................................................................................................................................................
...............................
.................................................................................................................................................
...............................

Joanna Briggs Institute Quantitative Data Critical Appraisal Scale reproduced with
Permission of the Joanna Briggs Institute

## APPENDIX 15.2
# DATA EXTRACTION FORM (QUANTITATIVE DATA)

Author ............................................................................. Record Number.........................

Journal ...................................................................................Year ...........................

Reviewer ...............................................................................................

Method ................................................................................................

Setting ...............................................................................................

Participants............................................................................................................

..............................

....................................................................................................................................

..............................

Number of Participants ......................

Group A ..................... Group B ......................

Interventions

Intervention  A  ..............................................................................................................

....................................................................................................................................

..............................

Intervention  B  ..............................................................................................................

.......................................................................................................................... ....

..............................

**Outcome Measures**

| Outcome Description | Scale/Measure |
|---|---|
|  |  |
|  |  |
|  |  |

Results............. .............. ............. ............. ............. ............. ............. ............. ............. .............

............. ............. .

**Dichotomous Data**

| Outcome | Treatment Group Number/total number | Control Group Number/total number |
|---|---|---|
|  |  |  |
|  |  |  |

**Continuous Data**

| Outcome | Treatment Group Mean & SD (number) | Control Group Mean & SD (number) |
|---|---|---|
|  |  |  |
|  |  |  |
|  |  |  |

Authors Conclusion ...........................................................................................................................................
...........................
...........................................................................................................................................................................
...........................
...........................................................................................................................................................................
...........................
Reviewers Conclusion ......................................................................................................................................
...........................
...........................................................................................................................................................................
...........................
...........................................................................................................................................................................
...........................

Joanna Briggs Institute Quantitative Data Extraction Tool reproduced with Permission of the Joanna Briggs Institute

These tools are found within the Joanna Briggs Institute Meta Analysis of Statistics Assessment and Review Instrument (JBI MAStARI) <http://mastari.joannabriggs.edu.au>

## FURTHER READING

Craig, J. V. & Smyth, R. L. (eds) (2011). *The Evidence-Based Practice Manual for Nurses*, 3rd edn. Edinburgh: Elsevier.

Downe, S., Gyte, G. M. L. & Dahlen, H. G. (2013). Routine vaginal examinations for assessing progress of labour to improve outcomes for women and babies at term. *Cochrane Database of Systematic Reviews* 2013(7), CD010088.

Joanna Briggs Institute. (2012). *The JBI approach*. <http://joannabriggs.org/jbi-approach.html>.

Myors, K. A., Schmied, V., Johnson, M. & Cleary, M. (2013). Collaboration and integrated services for perinatal mental health: An integrative review. *Child and Adolescent Mental Health* 18(1), 1–10.

NHMRC. (2009). NHMRC additional levels of evidence and grades for recommendations for developers of guidelines: Stage 2 consultation. <www.nhmrc.gov.au/_files_nhmrc/file/publications/synopses/cp30.pdf>.

Portney, L. G. & Watkins, M. P. (2009). *Foundations of Clinical Research: Applications to Practice*, 3rd edn. New Jersey: Pearson Education.

Straus, S. E., Tetroe, J. & Graham, I. D. (2013). *Knowledge Translation in Health Care: Moving from Evidence to Practice*. West Sussex: John Wiley & Sons.

## USEFUL WEBSITES

Cochrane Collaboration: <www.cochrane.edu.au>

The Cochrane Collaboration is an international network of more than 31 000 people from over 100 countries who work together to help healthcare practitioners, policy-makers, patients, their advocates and carers make well-informed decisions about healthcare, by preparing, updating and promoting the accessibility of Cochrane Reviews.

*Evidence-Based Nursing Journal*: <http://ebn.bmj.com>

This journal publishes selected research studies and reviews that report important advances relevant to best nursing practice from the health related literature. The clinical relevance and rigour of the studies is assessed to identify research that is relevant to nursing.

The US Institutes of Health: <www.clinicaltrials.gov>

ClinicalTrials.gov is a web-based resource that provides patients, their family members, healthcare professionals, researchers and the public with easy access to information on publicly and privately supported clinical studies on a wide range of diseases and conditions. It is also a searchable database about current ongoing clinical research studies of human participants conducted around the world.

The New York Academy of Medicine–Library–Grey Literature Report

<www.nyam.org/library/pages/grey_literature_report>

The report is a bimonthly publication of the New York Academy of Medicine Library, alerting readers to new grey literature publications in health services research and selected public health topics.

<www.prisma-statement.org/statement.htm>

This website gives a template for a flow chart. A flow chart depicts the flow of information through the different phases of a systematic review.

## REFERENCES

Aslam, S. & Emmanuel, P. (2010). Formulating a researchable question: A critical step for facilitating good clinical research. *Indian Journal of Sexually Transmitted Diseases* 31(1), 47.

Barnett-Page, E. & Thomas, J. (2009). Methods for the synthesis of qualitative research: A critical review. *BMC Medical Research Methodology* 9, 59.

Becker, L. A. & Oxman, A. D. (2008). Chapter 22: Overview of reviews. In: J. P. T. Higgins & S. Green (eds), *Cochrane Handbook for Systematic Reviews of Interventions*. Version 5.0.1 [updated September 2008]. The Cochrane Collaboration, 2008. Available from <www.cochrane-handbook.org>.

Boudin, F., Nie, J., Bartlett, J. C., Grad, R., Pluye, P. & Dawes, M. (2010). Combining classifiers for robust PICO element detection. *BMC Medical Informatics and Decision Making* 10:29, doi:10.1186/1472-6947-10-29.

Crowther, M., Lim, W., & Crowther, M. A. (2010). Systematic review and meta-analysis methodology. *Blood* 116(17), 3140–6.

Cullum, N. (2000). Users' guides to the nursing literature: An introduction. *Evidence Based Nursing* 3(3), 71–2.

Cullum, N., Ciliska, D., Haynes, R. B. & Marks, S. (2008). *Evidence-based Nursing: An Introduction*: Blackwell Pub./BMJ Journals/RCN Pub.

Dobbins, M., DeCorby, K., Robeson, P., Husson, H., Tirilis, D. & Greco, L. (2010). A knowledge management tool for public health: Health-evidence. *BMC Public Health* 10(1), 496.

Downe, S. (2008). Metasynthesis: A guide to knitting smoke. *Evidence Based Midwifery* 6(1), 4–8.

Egger, M., Smith, G. D. & Altman, D. (2008). *Systematic Reviews in Health Care: Meta-analysis in Context*. London: The BMJ Publishing Group.

Fernandez, R. & Griffiths, R. (2012). Water for wound cleansing. *Cochrane Database of Systematic Reviews* (1) CD003861.

Fernandez, R., Johnson, M., Tran, D. T. & Miranda, C. (2012). Models of care in nursing: A systematic review. *International Journal of Evidence-Based Healthcare* 10, 324–37.

Fineout-Overholt, E., O'Mathúna, D. P. & Kent, B. (2008). How systematic reviews can foster evidence-based clinical decisions. *Worldviews on Evidence-Based Nursing* 5(1), 45–8.

Gallin, J. I. & Ognibene, F. P. (2012). *Principles and Practice of Clinical Research*. London: Elsevier.

Halcomb, E. J., Fernandez, R., Griffiths, R., Newton, P. J. & Hickman, L. (2008). The infection control management of MRSA in acute care. *International Journal of Evidence-Based Healthcare* 6(4), 440–67.

Hannes, K. & Macaitis, K. (2012). A move to more transparent and systematic approaches of qualitative evidence synthesis: Update of a review on published papers. *Qualitative Research* 12(4), 402–42.

Higgins, J. & Deeks, J. J. (2008). Selecting studies and collecting data. *Cochrane Handbook for Systematic Reviews of Interventions: Cochrane Book Series*, pp. 151–85.

Higgins, J. & Green, S. (2011). Cochrane handbook for systematic reviews of interventions (Vol. Version 5.1.0) [updated March 2011]: The Cochrane Collaboration.

Higgins, J. P., Thompson, S. G., Deeks, J. J. & Altman, D. G. (2003). Measuring inconsistency in meta-analyses. *British Medical Journal* 327(7414), 557–60.

Hopewell, S., Clarke, M., Lefebvre, C. & Scherer, R. (2007a). Handsearching versus electronic searching to identify reports of randomized trials. *Cochrane Database of Systematic Reviews*, 18(2), MR000001.

Hopewell, S., McDonald, S., Clarke, M. & Egger, M. (2007b). Grey literature in meta-analyses of randomized trials of health care interventions. *Cochrane Database of Systematic Reviews*, 18(2), MR000010.

Ioannidis, J. P., Patsopoulos, N. A. & Rothstein, H. R. (2008). Reasons or excuses for avoiding meta-analysis in forest plots. *British Medical Journal* 336(7658), 1413–15.

Jadad, A. & Enkin, M. (2007). *Randomized Controlled Trials: Questions, Answers and Musings*, 2nd edn. Singapore: Blackwell BMJ Books.

Lefebvre, C., Manheimer, E. & Glanville, J. (2008). Searching for studies. *Cochrane Handbook for Systematic Reviews of Interventions*. New York: Wiley, pp. 95–150.

Leong, S. T. (2007). Systematic review made simple for nurses. *Nursing* 16(2), 104–10.

Littell, J., Corcoran, J. & Pillai, V. (2008). *Systematic Reviews and Meta-analysis*. Oxford and New York: Oxford University Press.

Moher, D., Jadad, A. R., Nichol, G., Penman, M., Tugwell, P. & Walsh, S. (1995). Assessing the quality of randomized controlled trials: An annotated bibliography of scales and checklists. *Control Clinical Trials* 16(1), 62–73.

Montori, V. M., Wilczynski, N. L., Morgan, D. & Haynes, R. B. (2005). Optimal search strategies for retrieving systematic reviews from Medline: Analytical survey. *British Medical Journal* 330(7482), 68.

NHMRC (National Health and Medical Research Council) (2009). *NHMRC Levels of Evidence and Grades for Recommendations for Developers of Guidelines*. <www.nhmrc.gov.au/_files_nhmrc/file/guidelines/evidence_statement_form.pdf>.

Pearson, A., Field, J. & Jordan, Z. (2007). *Evidence-based Clinical Practice in Nursing and Healthcare: Assimilating Research, Experience and Expertise*. Adelaide: Blackwell Publishing.

Pearson, A., Porritt, K. A., Doran, D., Vincent, L., Craig, D., Tucker, D. et al. (2006). A comprehensive systematic review of evidence on the structure, process, characteristics and composition of a nursing team that fosters a healthy work environment. *International Journal of Evidence-Based Healthcare* 4(2), 118–59.

Perera, R. & Heneghan, C. (2008). Interpreting meta-analysis in systematic reviews. *Evidence Based Medicine* 13(3), 67–9.

Pohl, S., Zobel, J. & Moffat, A. (2010). Extended Boolean retrieval for systematic biomedical reviews. Paper presented at the Proceedings of the Thirty-Third Australasian Conference on Computer Science–Volume 102. Brisbane, Australia, 18–22 January 2010, Australian Computer Society.

Polit, D. & Beck, C. (2012). *Nursing Research: Generating and Assessing Evidence for Nursing Practice*. New York: J. B. Lippincott.

Porter, S. (2010). Fundamental patterns of knowing in nursing: The challenge of evidence-based practice. *Advances in Nursing Science* 33(1), 3–14.

Richardson, W. S., Wilson, M. C., Nishikawa, J. & Hayward, R. S. (1995). The well-built clinical question: A key to evidence-based decisions. *ACP Journal Club* 123(3), A12–13.

Ryan, R. E., Kaufman, C. A. & Hill, S. J. (2009). Building blocks for meta-synthesis: Data integration tables for summarising, mapping, and synthesising evidence on interventions for communicating with health consumers. *BMC Medical Research Methodology* 9(1), 16.

Smith, V., Devane, D., Begley, C. M. & Clarke, M. (2011). Methodology in conducting a systematic review of systematic reviews of healthcare interventions. *BMC Medical Research Methodology* 11(1), 15.

Speirs, V., Johnson, M. & Jirojwong, S. (2013). A systematic review of interventions for homeless women. *Journal of Clinical Nursing* 22 (7–8), 1080–93.

Whitlock, E. P., Lopez, S. A., Chang, S., Helfand, M., Eder, M. & Floyd, N. (2009). Identifying, selecting, and refining topics. In *Agency for Healthcare Research and Quality: Methods Guide for Comparative Effectiveness Reviews* [posted April 2009]. Rockville, MD. <www.ncbi.nlm.nih.gov/books/NBK47096>.

CHAPTER 16

# DISSEMINATING RESEARCH

Penny Paliadelis, Glenda Parmenter and Jackie Lea

## CHAPTER LEARNING OBJECTIVES

After reading this chapter you will be able to:

- understand research dissemination as an essential part of the research process
- recognise the importance of sharing research that contributes to the body of nursing and midwifery knowledge
- identify the core why, how and where components of preparing research findings for dissemination
- recall the different avenues available to share research findings
- identify barriers to the dissemination of nursing and midwifery research and related strategies for overcoming them
- explain how to access relevant guidelines for abstract and manuscript submissions.

### KEY TERMS

publish
conference
dissemination
abstract
scholarship
target audience
peer review
collaboration

# Introduction

The aim of this chapter is to demystify the process of disseminating nursing and midwifery knowledge. It will present a discussion of writing for publication focusing on developing your understanding of how and where to publicise research findings and professional knowledge. The importance of disseminating research findings will be discussed. The barriers to publishing will be identified and strategies for overcoming them will be provided. Some approaches will be presented that will assist in maximising opportunities to **publish** or present research findings by targeting the right journal or **conference**. In addition, strategies for developing and preparing conference posters and presentations, journal manuscripts and project reports will also be outlined. Case study examples of Australian conference papers and journal articles will be used to demonstrate the process of turning research outcomes and/or clinical innovations into publications, reports, media releases and conference papers.

# Avenues for research dissemination and how to target the right one

The **dissemination** of research findings provides and builds evidence for practice (Oermann et al. 2008), and to maximise the benefits of research, dissemination needs to occur as broadly as possible to allow access by students, other researchers and the wider community (NHMRC 2012). To increase awareness and communication of research findings so that they can be transferred to clinical practice, it is essential that research be disseminated in journals and conferences that are geared to clinicians (Oermann et al. 2008). The most common vehicles for disseminating research are conference and poster presentations, journal articles, books and book chapters, policies, guidelines, reports and media releases. This section will give you practical advice and tips on how to prepare for dissemination successfully. The first and most important step is to target the most appropriate means of dissemination for your particular project.

## Conference papers and posters

It is important to be aware of up-and-coming conferences and seminars and when the calls for **abstracts** are being made, as this will give you the opportunity to put your work forward. Most national and international conferences call for abstracts up to 12 months before the conference date. This allows plenty of time for the abstracts to be peer-reviewed and the results communicated to the author(s). Once your abstract is accepted for a presentation or poster, you need to confirm your attendance and pay conference registration fees and book travel and accommodation, if required.

However, before you can submit your abstract for consideration you must first know how to find calls for conference abstracts. One strategy for becoming aware of such calls is to look for preliminary conference notices in Australian and international nursing publications, such as the *Nursing Review*, the *Australian Journal of Nursing* or the *Journal of Nursing Scholarship*. In addition, belonging to professional nursing bodies such as the Australian College of Nursing (ACN) or an interest group such as Palliative Care Australia will assist in identifying appropriate conferences to showcase your work. Membership of professional groups will provide you with information about upcoming conferences, and national and international organisations such as the International Council of Nurses have conference alerts on their website.

**Publish:** To disseminate literature or information to others, generally in a printed format.

**Conference:** A meeting or gathering of professionals for discussion and sharing of ideas.

**Dissemination:** The circulation of a piece of research, which means publishing it or presenting it as a conference paper.

**Abstract:** A brief synopsis outlining the focus of a conference paper, article, report or poster and usually submitted for peer review.

A further strategy for finding calls for conference papers is to use a popular search engine like Google and be specific about what you are looking for. For example, if you have completed a research project that explored more effective pain assessment tools for elderly post-operative patients, you may want to search for 'pain management conferences 2014'. This strategy will give you a list of conferences both in Australia and internationally. However, if you only want to present your work locally then you may need to change your search term to something more specific such as 'nursing conferences in Queensland 2014'. Another suggestion for finding calls for conference papers is to search for conferences that target specific research methodologies. For example, there is an annual International Qualitative Health Research Conference, which is entirely devoted to the presentation and discussion of a range of qualitative methodological approaches. If you are a nursing student, discuss conference or article opportunities with academic staff in your discipline or your higher degree research supervisors.

Once you have identified a conference that is relevant to your research, you need to consider the conference themes, abstract instructions and deadlines. Each conference will have different requirements and you need to tailor your abstract to fit the guidelines (see Practice exercise 16.4 for an example of an abstract). Jackson and Sheldon (2000) provide an excellent light-hearted and easy-to-read guide to developing an abstract that you will find useful despite the age of the publication. Additionally, Weinert (2010) provides a more contemporary view of the highlights associated with preparing an abstract. If you have not attended many conferences and you are a little nervous about public speaking then maybe you could consider presenting a poster in the first instance. Information about how to present your research as a conference paper or poster is outlined in many articles. For example, Taggart and Arslanian (2000) and Keely (2004) outline the steps to the construction and formatting of a poster that will assist you in presenting an easy-to-read, informative and well-designed poster. Another strategy for delivering a successful verbal conference presentation is to rehearse your delivery with colleagues and friends. Ask for feedback on the timing of your slides, the amount of information on each slide and the pace of your presentation.

The example in Figure 16.1 shows that a poster presentation can be engaging and informative. This one was printed on fabric, making it easier to transport to an international conference in the USA in 2013. Jackson and Sheldon (2000) and Nemcek (2009) outline key elements of preparing and presenting a poster for a conference that will assist you to develop a quality poster presentation. Appendix 16.1 provides an outline of the key elements for preparing a poster. It is important to remember when preparing your poster that although oral presentations often receive the most attention, the quality of poster presentations at conferences equals and at times exceeds that of oral presentations (Dossett et al. 2012).

Another matter that needs to be considered when submitting a conference abstract is the date and location of the conference. While it might be flattering to have an abstract accepted for an international health promotion conference in Helsinki, it is important to consider whether you can find the funding to cover the costs of attending and presenting your paper or poster. In addition, you will need to discuss leave arrangements with your employer. Remember, the costs of presenting at an international conference can be prohibitive, when you take into account the prices of airfares, accommodation, conference registration, transfers and meals. If you plan ahead, grants to present at international conferences may be available from a number of sources. For example, many

**Scholarship:** The conduct of scholarly pursuits, usually within the academic world.

employers offer some conference funding. Some professional nursing organisations have competitive **scholarship** rounds, such as the Australian College of Critical Care Nurses, and others may also have competitive grants available. To secure conference funding you may be required to provide details of the conference, a copy of your accepted abstract and a detailed budget and itinerary.

**Figure 16.1    Example of a poster presentation**

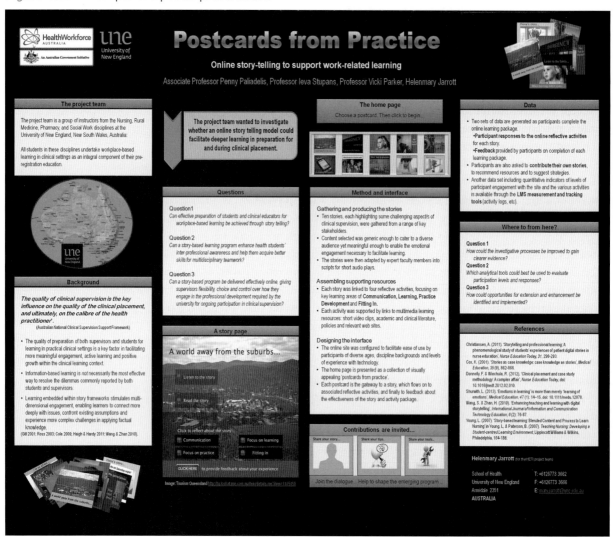

Source: P. Paliadelis, I. Stupans, V. Parker & H. Jarrott (2013). *Postcards from practice: Online story-telling to support work-related learning*. Poster presented at the International Institute for SoTL Scholars and Mentors (IISSAM) Storytelling conference, Loyola Marymount University, Los Angeles, USA.

## Preparing manuscripts for scholarly journals

If you are searching for an appropriate journal in which to publish an article about your project, one obvious place to start is your own reference list. For example, if you found that you drew on a number of articles from the *Journal of Nursing Management* to inform your project, this may be the right journal to aim at when writing your manuscript. Always have a look at the types of articles that the journal publishes, look at the focus, the content, the style and the length of published articles and consider whether you can write about your project in a similar style (Dimitroulis 2011; McIntyre et al. 2007). University or hospital librarians can also help with finding the right journal for your manuscript.

Having identified a journal that is relevant to your project and/or your **target audience**, the next step is to go to the journal website and review the author guidelines. The information provided is vital, as in order for your submission to be considered for publication you must comply with the stated word limit, formatting and referencing style, so that the editor will consider your manuscript appropriate for **peer review**. Reputable scholarly journals send manuscripts out to at least two reviewers in a double-blind process. This means that the reviewers do not know who the authors are, and the authors do not know who the reviewers are. Reviewers of manuscripts for publication are usually asked to comment on style, structure, originality, significance, interest, and scientific, methodological and technical soundness. The editor then makes the decision to accept the manuscript for publication, accept with changes, or reject the manuscript as not suitable for publication. In most cases the reviewers' feedback is sent to the authors along with the editor's decision.

The review process for most major nursing journals can take many months, and it is quite common for the reviewers' feedback to indicate that some changes are required before the paper is suitable for publication. For novice authors, this can be a long and daunting process. But it is important not to become disheartened, as all authors have had manuscripts sent back to them requiring substantial changes, while some may have had manuscripts rejected. Sometimes the journal is not the right one in which to publish your work, or maybe you do not make the significance of your project clear. Most journals now manage the entire process of submission and review online. Figure 16.2 illustrates the stages in the online submission process. Always read the reviewers' feedback carefully, use their suggestions to polish your manuscript, and most importantly, remember that this is a learning process—all successful authors were once novices!

Another important thing to consider when preparing a manuscript for publication is that journals have very strict requirements about the originality of the work under consideration. Upon submission of your manuscript, you will be asked to sign a declaration that the work has not been previously published, nor is it under consideration for publication elsewhere. This precludes you from submitting the same manuscript to several journals at once (Saver 2006b). One further possibility is to submit your manuscript to an 'Open Access' journal; this means that if it is accepted for publication, you, as the author, must pay a fee to have it published, and the article is then freely available to anyone. Many reputable publishers are now offering this option as it is usually a much faster process from submission to publication and the citation rates are usually higher.

## Books and book chapters

If you believe that you have a new project, idea or information that may be suitable to be published as a nursing or midwifery textbook, then usually the first strategy is to approach a publisher to ask how you go about submitting a book proposal. Many publishers have instructions for potential authors on their websites. Most publishing houses ask for the potential author(s) to produce a clear and compelling case for publication. This will usually include one or more sample chapters and your review of whether similar texts are available and how your text will differ. Once the publisher considers the proposal, they may conduct market research. This means that they send

**Target audience:** The primary group of people who are most interested in the content of a conference paper or journal article.

**Peer review:** The process of subjecting scholarly work, research or ideas to the scrutiny of others who are peers in the same field or discipline area.

Figure 16.2    Stages of online manuscript submission

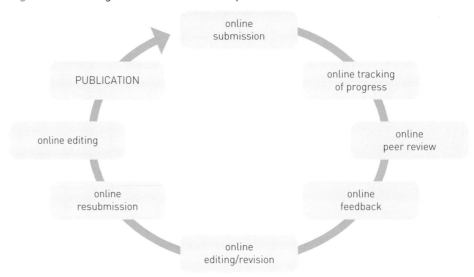

your proposal and sample chapter(s) to experts in the field, and based on the feedback, they may decline your proposal or agree to publish. If your proposal is accepted you will receive a book contract. You will then have to agree on a timeline for submission of chapters or the entire manuscript and a proposed publication date. A similar process occurs with book chapters. However, it is common for editors of the book, or those who submitted the initial proposal, to invite contributors to write specific chapters (Happell 2008). Royalty payments will be negotiated and may vary from one publisher to another.

## Policies, guidelines and reports

The requirements for writing up and disseminating research or quality projects as policies, guidelines or formal reports will vary depending on the end-user of these documents and the nature of the publication. While it is important that all policy documents are clear and well written and disseminated to all relevant stakeholders, if it is not a publicly available document, the audience for such a report may be limited. However, this type of dissemination does not generally preclude the authors from producing a manuscript about the project for publication in a relevant journal or as a conference presentation or poster.

If you have completed a funded research project, you will probably need to compile a formal report that may be published on a website or as a publicly available record of the outcomes of the project. For example, the Health Education and Training Institute of NSW Health has links to reports of research projects that have been funded by this department over the past few years. Larger research projects that have attracted significant public funding may be written up as published reports, which may then be used to inform new statewide or national health policy. Many funding bodies have strict guidelines about how such reports are presented; similarly, public and private health organisations have policy templates and may even have departments dedicated to researching and writing new policies. Policies and guidelines are also research publications that practitioners and nursing students frequently use when they are in clinical areas.

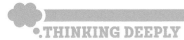

**Dissemination of quality study on a busy medical ward**

Nurses on a busy medical ward conducted a quality project that explored the number of injuries caused by pre-packaged metal closure clips that are included with many brands of bandages. The results of this study were disseminated as an internal policy document that required staff to cease using these devices and dispose of them in a sharps container. The number of injuries resulting from the use of these clips was dramatically reduced. Do you think that an article about this study would be useful if it was disseminated more widely?

## Media releases

In some situations your funding or employing organisation may ask you to prepare a media release about a project that is controversial or has popular appeal. Alternatively, a newspaper or television station may contact you for your comments on a current issue relating to your organisation or area of expertise. For example, if you have completed a project that identifies effective strategies for recruiting and retaining health professionals in rural areas, local media may wish to interview you, as this topic is of national and even global concern. The dissemination of information via media releases and reports is quite different from other forms of dissemination, as newspaper articles, news reports and radio interviews are usually short and only cover the key points. Another useful tip is to have a look at the press releases of nursing organisations, such as the Council of Deans of Nursing and Midwifery (Australia and New Zealand), which can be accessed at <www.cdnm.edu.au>, as this will give you some ideas about how to write a media release. You will also need to make yourself aware of your employer's guidelines regarding media releases before you proceed. If the research project is funded it is important to review the contract to ensure that media releases are permitted. There are a number of websites that provide valuable information about how to prepare a press release and talk to the media. An example is the following website: <www.flyingsolo.com.au/p239863654_How-to-write-a-media-release.html>.

**TIPS AND SKILLS**

Access some recent media releases from professional bodies such as the Australian Nursing and Midwifery Council or the Nursing and Midwifery Board of Australia and note the key elements/information included in the media release.

## Barriers to publishing and strategies for overcoming them

There are many avenues for disseminating and publishing research findings and these can take the form of theses, books, project reports, journal articles, conference papers and posters, policy documents, procedure manuals and media releases. However, too few nurses and midwives share their work through publication and many find the writing part of the research process daunting (Woodward et al. 2007). This is particularly evident within the clinical context where few nurses write and publish about their daily practice (Beal et al. 2008). The reason for this is that nurses and midwives encounter a number of barriers to writing and presenting their writing for publication. These barriers take four broad forms: cultural, knowledge, resource and personal barriers, and the following is a discussion of these four barriers together with some suggestions for overcoming them.

## Strategies for overcoming cultural barriers

A significant barrier to writing for publication is the culture of nursing itself. This culture has a strong tradition of favouring verbal communication over the written form (Miracle 2003). A great deal of nursing knowledge is passed on through conversations held in tearooms and at handover, and in more formal settings such as nursing conferences and seminars. In addition, there is a tendency among nurses to undervalue the role of nurse researchers and their contribution to the profession and to healthcare in general (Straker et al. 2013). Culture change happens slowly, but this change is rapidly gathering pace in nursing, with many more clinicians now becoming interested and participating in the dissemination of their clinical innovations and research findings (Kotz & Cals 2013). A significant influence on culture change is the growing number of nurses who consult the nursing literature to inform their practice. In addition, health service initiatives such as quality improvement and clinical practice development projects are creating opportunities for clinical staff to undertake local projects that are supported by health management. Such initiatives are just one way in which the culture of nursing is being transformed to become a more research-based and evidence-based one (New South Wales Nursing and Midwifery Office 2013).

## TIPS AND SKILLS

Before commencing writing make sure you have a suitable workspace, some quiet time and access to relevant resources.

## Strategies for overcoming knowledge barriers

A second barrier to publishing nursing research is a lack of knowledge about the types of papers that are suitable for publication. Many nurses believe that research and publication are the domain of academics and that the work of clinicians is not suitable for dissemination. While the research and publication work of academics is important, it is vital that clinically based nurses make local research outcomes, and the experiences that arise from them, widely known (Beal et al. 2008). These publications may take the form of research, quality assurance projects, case studies, clinical innovations or experiences, reflections on practice, or an opinion or comment on a nursing topic.

Writing can be a challenging task and not knowing where or how to begin is a powerful deterrent. Nurses often require support to enhance their writing skills and strengthen their approaches to the task of writing. However, there is usually very little in the way of support for novice writers, and finding mentors within the clinical setting can be difficult (Gough & Hampshire 2012). Nurses may also be unaware of the writing and publication process and confused about the most appropriate journal in which to present their work.

A first step to becoming a published author is to read and familiarise yourself with the range of nursing publications that are available. This will give you an insight into the journals that might be appropriate for your area of expertise or interest and the types of papers that you might develop for publication. It will also help you to prepare your own manuscript. While reading, you can note aspects of style, expression and presentation that you found particularly relevant and that give you ideas for developing your own paper. Later in this chapter some tips on how to identify appropriate journals for publication of your own papers will be provided.

Attendance and presentation at conferences, seminars and workshops is another opportunity for sharing your professional knowledge. It also raises your profile among your colleagues and allows you the opportunity to set up **collaborative** projects. While successful conference presentation does not require complex skills, the trick is to make your presentation interesting, engaging and succinct. Many nurses who attend conferences realise that they could have presented a paper themselves (Billings & Kowalski 2009b). So while attending presentations, think critically about aspects of the presentation as this will help you in preparing your own.

> **Collaboration:** A creative process where two or more people or organisations work together to achieve a common goal.

A lack of knowledge about how to approach the task of writing can be overcome in a number of ways. The first is to be aware of the steps in the writing process. These steps are set out by Hislop and associates (2008): target a journal; draft an abstract; get pre-peer review; develop a detailed outline of the paper; write drafts of all sections of the paper; and revise the draft using a revision-feedback-revision cycle. An important aspect of this approach is that it breaks the larger task into a number of smaller, more doable ones. There is a tendency for novice writers to see writing as one large and overwhelming task, the prospect of which puts them off even beginning the process (Morton 2013).

A further way to add to your writing and publishing knowledge and skills is to do a writing course, or to join or initiate a writers' support group (Stone et al. 2010). This brings together a group of like-minded people who are able to give each other the necessary support and encouragement in gaining skills in writing and publishing. Such groups also provide structure in the form of agreed timelines with collaborators and an expectation that you will continue to work on your project. This helps to sustain motivation and also provides feedback on your progress from your peers and from the more experienced members of the group (Morris et al. 2011).

## TIPS AND SKILLS

If you are a novice writer seek out an experienced author or writing support group that can mentor you in the writing process.

One strategy for gaining support and encouragement from others is to collaborate with one or more colleagues on a joint paper. This is an excellent way to share the load of writing for publication as it gives you a smaller workload and the support and encouragement of other team members. You can bounce ideas off each other and review each other's work. If possible, it is useful to have at least one member of the writing team who has experience in writing and publishing. This might be achieved by approaching a nurse academic who has an interest in your work to join the writing team as a mentor. If you do decide to collaborate on a joint paper, it is wise to discuss authorship at the outset and how and in what order authors' names will appear on the finished paper. In general, those authors have right of authorship who have contributed significantly to the conception and design of the project, the analysis and interpretation of research data, and/or drafting significant parts of the work or critically revising it so as to contribute to the interpretation (Campanelli et al. 2007; NHMRC 2007).

## •.THINKING DEEPLY

### Dissemination of research findings

Take a few moments to think about ways to foster and support colleagues in the publication and dissemination of the research.

The example below shows how a team approach to writing and publishing can work to overcome the barriers to publishing nursing research.

A small research team made up of novice and experienced researchers wanted to explore the factors that attract final-year nursing students to seek employment in rural areas. Members of the team worked together to plan the research methodology and conduct the data collection and analysis. Once the study was complete a meeting was held to discuss how the research findings would be disseminated. Tasks were shared among team members, pairing more experienced writers and presenters with novices. One researcher prepared abstracts for submission to an international evidence-based practice conference and a national nursing education conference. These abstracts were proofread for accuracy and clarity by experienced team members prior to submission. Both abstracts were accepted and conference papers were prepared. Again, more experienced team members provided critical review, support and guidance. The team then jointly submitted a manuscript for consideration to the journal *The Collegian*, and following feedback and revision, the paper was published in 2008. The article is listed in References (Lea et al. 2008).

## Strategies for addressing a lack of time and resources

A third barrier to writing and publishing for nurses and midwives is a lack of time and resources. Most clinically based staff are shift workers who are often very tired, so the energy and motivation to write may be lacking. In addition, many have family responsibilities that make further demands on their time and energy. This makes getting around to the task of writing very difficult, particularly as many nurses view writing or preparing a presentation as an extra commitment on top of their already allocated workload. Nurses may also lack a defined space in which to write and may have to share a computer with work colleagues and/or family members (Pierce 2009).

These barriers can be overcome if you use your organisational skills and assign a portion of your busy life to the task of writing. One strategy for overcoming the pressure of time is to break up the writing into a number of small tasks. It is surprising how much you can achieve in a single hour, and if you set it aside regularly this can soon add up to a considerable amount of completed work. Hislop and others (2008) refer to this strategy as 'snack' writing and suggest regular periods of 30 minutes to one hour.

It is useful if you can have a designated workspace with your work materials set out so that you can begin work easily when you have available time. It is also helpful if you have easy access to the internet as this allows you to use a huge range of nursing information that will aid you in your writing endeavours. Obtaining the latest version of a referencing tool, such as EndNote, will also save you a significant amount of time when you come to publish your work and is worth the time it takes to learn how to use the program.

Another strategy in gaining skills in an atmosphere of support is to undertake research as part of a formal course of study at a tertiary institution. This provides you with resources such as a supervision team, access to literature, computer software and sometimes a computer. It also provides a more structured environment in which timelines are set for you to achieve your writing and publishing goals.

Funding to support research, writing and publishing is also available from a number of sources. At present, the NSW Nurses and Midwives Association offers Edith Cavell Trust Scholarships that fund educational, research and conference attendance activities. The Australian College of Nursing also offers and administers a number of scholarships and grants to support education, training and research. Make yourself aware of what financial support is available to you and apply for it. Some of these funds are easily available and often do not have a large number of applicants, so your chances of success are good. A list of the web addresses of these funding bodies is presented at the end of this chapter.

## Strategies for overcoming personal barriers

Underpinning the three preceding barriers are personal barriers, such as negative thoughts and feelings, a lack of confidence in your own writing skills, and unhelpful personal work patterns or habits (Lenz & Barnard 2009). Many nurses lack confidence in their writing skills and this is compounded by a not entirely unfounded fear of rejection. A lack of mentorship and support finds many aspiring writers giving up before they have begun. Despite initial fears about writing, many beginners have overcome their fears to become successful authors. A common problem is that novice authors sit down to write before they are ready and feel frustrated when they can't think of how to start (Gough & Hampshire 2012). A wide reading of the relevant literature is the best strategy for addressing this problem as this will confirm some of your knowledge and give you clues to the gaps in the literature that your research might be filling. This will affirm that you are on the right track or give guidance about how to frame your paper.

Novice writers also need to realise that writing skills are not innate but are developed over time and with extensive practice. The more you write the better you will become. It is good practice to have patience with yourself and seek the support and guidance of more experienced mentors to keep on fine-tuning your skills. Also, don't feel that everything you write has to be perfect. It is better to begin with a very rough outline of your work and then fine-tune it in sections. Be aware that all authors write many drafts of their paper before they have produced the finished article.

## Implications for evidence-based practice

Since the early 1990s there has been an increasing need for nurses and midwives to support their professional practice with a strong research evidence base (Pierce 2009). Research is meaningless unless an account of the findings can be added to the body of nursing and midwifery knowledge and shared with others. In order to achieve this, the findings of nursing and midwifery research must be disseminated via publications and conference presentations. Publication of research activity and findings serves several functions. First, it shares nursing and midwifery knowledge, skills and experience with the wider population, allowing others to apply, critique or build on them, without unnecessary duplication. Second, it allows nurses to contribute to future nursing practice and theory by challenging traditional views and ensures that we are basing our clinical care on sound, credible and valid evidence (Hodges & Casey 2007; Saver 2006a). This allows nurses to apply the most up-to-date nursing knowledge to their clinical practice, leading to improved outcomes in patient care.

In addition to clinical practice, nurses also have a responsibility to generate and share knowledge and participate in activities of dissemination. This is because the increased demands for efficient and effective healthcare mean that nurses must be accountable for creating best practice (Billings & Kowalski 2009a, p. 152). Other professions and academic disciplines have long based their knowledge on this concept, but nursing and midwifery, as relatively new academic disciplines, are quickly catching up (Reid & Fuller 2005). Similar to many countries, nursing in Australia has emerged and matured as a profession and we need to document this emergence with a strong body of nursing literature. Therefore, it is important that we are able to gain confidence in the value of our work and our unique contribution to healthcare and to put our knowledge into writing so that evidence for practice is available to all (Keen 2007).

# SUMMARY

- It is important that nurses and midwives should disseminate their research work and thus contribute to the evidence base of the profession.
- A great sense of achievement can be derived from seeing research work developed into a published paper or conference presentation, and publication has the potential to enhance a career in nursing or midwifery.
- There are several strategies for sharing nursing knowledge within the healthcare context, and different avenues are available.
- Cultural, knowledge, resource and personal barriers to the dissemination of research can be overcome by various strategies.
- Guidelines for abstract and manuscript submissions are available and there are ways to access them.

## PRACTICE EXERCISE 16.1

Identify a journal that is relevant to your area of practice or interest. Go online to access and read the instructions for authors. Ask yourself the following questions:
Are the instructions clear?
What type of referencing style is required and are you familiar with it?
What are the format and word limit requirements for each type of manuscript?
ANSWER: For example, the *Australian Journal of Advanced Nursing* has guidelines for potential authors that can be found at <www.ajan.com.au/ajan_guidelines.html>. These guidelines described the focus and structure of the manuscript. Another example is *Nurse Education Today* author guidelines, which are at <www.elsevier.com/journals/nurse-education-today/0260-6917/guide-for-authors>.

## PRACTICE EXERCISE 16.2

Ask colleagues and peers about local or recent clinical innovations or quality projects and discover how or if they have considered disseminating the results of these projects. Then reflect on their responses.

## PRACTICE EXERCISE 16.3

If you have recently attended a lecture, workshop, training session or conference, consider the presentation and reflect on it. What worked well for you as an audience member, what was interesting, what parts were boring, irrelevant or unclear? This will assist with planning your own presentation.

## PRACTICE EXERCISE 16.4

Below is an example of an abstract submitted for presentation at an Australian Primary Health Care Conference. The conference aimed to explore opportunities for greater integration of primary healthcare within nursing and broader health services, with an increased focus on interdisciplinary care. Contributions were invited that related to the conference aim with a focus on one of the following streams: Research; Service Delivery; Education or Policy. Abstracts had a 300-word limit.

Based on these guidelines answer the following questions:

- How would you assess the suitability of the following abstract for presentation at this conference?
- Does it contain enough information?
- Which of the conference streams, if any, does it best fit?
- If you were a reviewer for the conference would you accept this paper for an oral presentation, reject it or recommend it for presentation as a poster?

**Title:** An exploration of the capacity of General Practice Nurses to improve the prevention and management of childhood obesity

Childhood obesity is a worldwide concern that poses a major threat to long-term health by increasing the risk of chronic illnesses. The 2004 NSW Schools Physical Activity and Nutrition Survey has shown that overall, 25% of boys and 23% of girls are either overweight or obese. Given the shortage of General Practitioners, it is beyond their scope to manage this issue and this is particularly so in rural areas. At the same time, the role of General Practice Nurses in Primary Health Care is expanding and has recently been recognised by the allocation of a Provider Item Number by Medicare. However, these nursing roles are relatively new and the specific role that the General Practice Nurse might play in the prevention and management of childhood obesity has not been explored.

This study explored the capacity of rural General Practice Nurses to prevent and manage obesity in children. In particular, this study investigated the existing practices, educational qualifications, organisational expectations and motivation of General Practice Nurses, General Practitioners and General Practice Managers in order to identify the potential for expanding the role of these nurses. This study employed a qualitative methodology and used focus groups conducted with the staff of general practices located in a variety of rural locations within New South Wales.

This study has identified a number of barriers to such an expanded role as well as strategies that may be employed to assist General Practice Nurses to undertake an active role in the prevention and management of childhood obesity (Paliadelis & Parmenter 2009).

## PRACTICE EXERCISE 16.5

List five potential avenues that could be used to disseminate research findings.

ANSWER: There are many examples of opportunities to disseminate research and scholarly information, for example, conference papers and posters, journal articles, policy documents, reports, textbooks and chapters in edited books.

## PRACTICE EXERCISE 16.6

There are a number of documents generated by reviewing of research systematically and used by clinicians. These documents include clinical guidelines and pathways. Based on your experiences, list specific documents you are aware of.

ANSWER: One example of evidence-based practice guidelines can be found at the Joanna Briggs Institute. The Best Practice Guidelines can be found on their website, <joannabriggs. org>.

# APPENDIX 16.1

# KEY ELEMENTS/GUIDELINES FOR DEVELOPING AN EFFECTIVE CONFERENCE POSTER TO DISSEMINATE RESEARCH

The key elements and guidelines for developing an effective conference poster presentation, adapted from Nemcek (2009) and Jackson and Sheldon (2000, p. 70), can be used as a checklist to ensure that your poster is a *storyboard of information* that communicates research outcomes and adds to the evidence base of the discipline of nursing.

## LAYOUT

- Investigate the size and type of poster required before developing: that is, check the conference organiser specifications for word count, size, headings, learning objectives, materials required for display of the poster and requirements for presentation, length and allocation of the poster presentation session times.
- The poster should be graphic, focused and organised and contain a clear message that is *showing not telling* (Jackson & Sheldon 2000, p. 70).
- Display should be eyecatching, so be careful how much text is used. A general rule for layout is 20% text, 40% charts graphs and pictures and 40% white space or background.
- Use PowerPoint for poster layout; many examples and templates for poster layouts are available on the web.

## CONTENT

- The poster should provide an overview of the study, the purpose and outcome.

**Table 1**  Suggested headings for research posters:

| Quantitative Studies | Qualitative Studies |
|---|---|
| • Conceptual model or theory<br>• Research design<br>• Sampling information<br>• Methods or procedures followed,<br>  e.g. instruments used<br>• Data analysis<br>• Key findings<br>• Clinical implications/relevance of the study | • Research question<br>• Qualitative design<br>• Sampling procedures<br>• Data collection and methods of analysis<br>• Key findings<br>• Clinical implications/relevance of the study |

- The poster should have a concise and clear title (short and snappy) in large letters that adequately describes its content. Also include under the title a clear indication of the authors.
- When organising the content, place the most important elements at eye level, avoid use of unfamiliar acronyms and use visual enhancements to draw attention and keep viewers interested.
- Choose neutral background colours and limit the colour scheme to two or three related colours.
- Use charts and graphs but make sure they are *clean of* excess lines; avoid keys and detailed legends; clearly delineate breaks with darker lines.
- Use vertical columns rather than horizontal to organise content.
- Use section headings and number sub-elements.
- Allow time for proofreading/editing the poster for typographical and spelling errors.

## DISPLAYING THE POSTER

- Arrive early on the day to set up the poster.
- You can add pockets to the poster with handouts or business cards for contact information.
- Stay with the poster for the allocated time.
- Know the information in the poster so that you can communicate appropriately with interested viewers.
- Dress professionally.

## FURTHER READING

Lester, J. D. (2011). *Writing Research Papers: A Complete Guide*, 13th edn. New York: Pearson.

Rolfe, G. (2009). Writing-up and writing-as: Rediscovering nursing scholarship. *Nurse Education Today* 29(8), 816–20.

Zemach, D. E., Broudy, D. & Valvona, C. (2011). *Writing Research Papers: From Essay to Research Paper*. Oxford: Macmillan.

## USEFUL WEBSITES

<www.acn.edu.au/scholarships>

The Australian College of Nursing is a professional nursing organisation that provides scholarships for study and professional development activities for all nurses at every stage of their career and in all settings; this includes student nurses entering the profession. The Australian College of Nursing Scholarship information can be found at the website above.

<www.health.nsw.gov.au/nursing/scholarship/Pages/default.aspx>

This NSW Health Nursing and Midwifery Scholarship site has information on undergraduate study scholarships but also gives information on scholarships for registered nurses to undertake a study tour to observe and learn about innovative and best practice in nursing and/or midwifery.

<www.nswnma.asn.au/the-lions-nurses-scholarship-information>

The NSW Nurses and Midwives Association has scholarships for its members to attend and present at conferences. For example, information on the Lions Nurses Scholarship can be found at the website above.

## REFERENCES

Beal, J. A., Riley, J. M. & Lancaster, D. R. (2008). Essential elements of an optimal clinical practice environment. *Journal of Nursing Administration* 38(11), 488–93.

Billings, D. & Kowalski, K. (2009a). Lessons learnt when writing a manuscript. *Journal of Continuing Education in Nursing* 40(2), 55–6.

Billings, D. & Kowalski, K. (2009b). Strategies for making oral presentations about clinical issues: Part 1. At the workplace. *Journal of Continuing Education in Nursing* 40(4), 152–3.

Campanelli, P. C., Feferman, R., Keane, C., Lieberman, H. J. & Roberon, D. (2007). An advanced practice psychiatric nurse's guide to professional writing. *Perspectives in Psychiatric Care* 43(4), 163–73.

Dimitroulis, G. (2011). Getting published in peer reviewed journals. *International Journal of Oral and Maxillofacial Surgery* 40(12), 1342–5.

Dossett, L. A., Fox, E. E., del Junco, D. J., Zaydfudim, V., Kauffmann, R., Shelton, J., Wang, W., Cioffi, W. G., Holcomb, J. B. and Cotton, B. A. (2012). Don't forget the posters! Quality and content variables associated with accepted abstracts at a national trauma meeting. *Journal of Trauma and Acute Care Surgery* 72(5), 1429–34.

Gough, S. & Hampshire, C. (2012). The first sentence is hardest: Writing for publication. *Journal of Operating Department Practice* 3(2), 6–9.

Happell, B. (2008). Writing for publication: A practical guide. *Nursing Standard* 22(28), 35–40.

Hislop, J., Murray, R. & Newton, M. (2008). Writing for publication: A case study. *Practice Development in Health Care* 7(3), 156–63.

Hodges, B. & Casey, A. (2007). Writing for publication: A personal view. *Paediatric Nursing* 19(2), 35.

Jackson, K. & Sheldon, L. (2000). Demystifying the academic aura: Preparing a poster. *Nurse Researcher* 7(3), 70–3.

Keely, B. (2004). Planning and creating effective scientific posters. *Journal of Continuing Education in Nursing* 35(4), 182–5.

Keen, A. (2007). Writing for publication: Pressures, barriers and support strategies. *Nurse Education Today* 27, 382–8.

Kotz, D. & Cals, J. W. L. (2013). Effective writing and publishing scientific papers, part IV: Methods. *Journal of Clinical Epidemiology* 66(8), 817.

Lea, J., Cruickshank, M., Paliadelis, P., Parmenter, G., Sanderson, H. & Thornberry, P. (2008). The lure of the bush: Do rural placements influence student nurses to seek employment in rural settings? *Collegian* 15(3), 77–82.

Lenz, B. & Barnard, P. (2009). Advancing evidence-based practice in rural nursing. *Journal for Nurses in Staff Development* 25(1), 14–19.

McIntyre, E., Eckermann, S., Keane, M., Magarey, A. & Roeger, L. (2007). Publishing in peer review journals: Criteria for success. *Australian Family Physician* 36(7), 561–2.

Miracle, V. A. (2003). Writing for publication: You can do it! *Dimensions of Critical Care Nursing* 22(1), 31–4.

Morris, C. T., Hatton, R. C. & Kimberlin, C. L. (2011). Factors associated with the publication of scholarly articles by pharmacists. *American Journal of Health-System Pharmacy* 68(17), 1640–5.

Morton, P. G. (2013). Publishing in professional journals, Part I: Getting started. *AACN Advanced Critical Care* 24(2), 162–8.

NHMRC (National Health and Medical Research Council). (2007). *Australian Code for the Responsible Conduct of Research*. Canberra: Australian Government Publishing Service.

NHMRC. (2012). *Dissemination of Research Findings*. Canberra: Australian Government Publishing Service.

Nemcek, M. (2009). Poster presentations in the primary care setting. *Primary Health Care* 19(4), 34–8.

New South Wales Nursing and Midwifery Office (2013). *Models of Care*. Accessed 20 January 2014, from http://www.health.nsw.gov.au/nursing/projects/Pages/models-care.aspx/.

Oermann, M. H., Nordstrom, C. K., Wilmes, N. A., Denison, D., Webb S. A., Featherstone, D. E., Bednarz, H., Striz, P., Blair, D. A. & Kowaleewski, K. (2008). Dissemination of research in clinical nursing journals. *Journal of Clinical Nursing* 17, 149–56.

Paliadelis, P. & Parmenter, G. (2009). An exploration of the capacity of general practice nurses to improve the prevention and management of childhood obesity. Royal College of Nursing Primary Health Care Conference, November, Adelaide, Australia.

Paliadelis, P., Stupans, I., Parker, V. & Jarrott, H. (2013). Postcards from practice: Online story-telling to support work-related learning. Poster presented at the International Institute for SoTL Scholars and Mentors (IISSAM) Storytelling Conference, Loyola Marymount University, Los Angeles, USA.

Pierce, L. L. (2009). Writing for publication: You can do it! *Rehabilitation Nursing* 34(1), 3–8.

Reid, K. & Fuller, J. (2005). Building a culture of research dissemination in primary health care: The South Australian experience of supporting the novice researcher. *Australian Health Review* 29(1), 6–11.

Saver, C. (2006a). Reap the benefits of writing for publication. *AORN Journal* 83(3), 603–6.

Saver, C. (2006b). Tables and figures: Adding vitality to your article. *AORN Journal* 84(6), 945–50.

Stone, T., Levett-Jones, T., Harris, M. & Sinclair, P. M. (2010). The genesis of 'the Neophytes': A writing support group for clinical nurses. *Nurse Education Today* 30(7), 657–61.

Straker, K. L., Brandt, P. B. & Brytus, J. (2013). Creating a culture of evidence-based practice and nursing research in a paediatric hospital. *Journal of Pediatric Nursing* 28(4), 1–4.

Taggart, H. & Arslanian, C. (2000). Creating an effective poster presentation. *Orthopaedic Nursing* 19(3), 47–9.

Weinert, C. (2010). Are all abstracts created equal? *Applied Nursing Research* 23, 106–9.

Woodward, V., Webb, C. & Prowse, M. (2007). The perceptions and experiences of nurses undertaking research in the clinical setting. *Journal of Research in Nursing* 12, 227–44.

# GLOSSARY

**Abstract**
A brief synopsis outlining the focus of a conference paper, article, report or poster and usually submitted for peer review.

**Accessible population**
The collection of all possible observation units that might have been chosen in a sample; the population from which the sample was taken.

**Action research**
A method of enquiry in which an individual or group actively engage as researchers in a process of change to address actual or emergent problems in their specific area of practice.

**Alpha error**
One of the two types of potential errors when conducting a statistical hypothesis test. It implies that one falsely assumes a significant difference between groups, when in reality there is none.

**Anonymity**
Lack of personal identifiable information; the state of having no name.

**Archie Cochrane**
A pioneer and advocate of evidence-based practice.

**Audit trail**
A decision trail that documents each step of the data analysis process. An audit is a process of observing and recording events or scrutinising pre-existing records for subsequent comparison to standards.

**Autoethnography**
The study of oneself within the context of the culture in which one lives.

**Beneficence**
A term referring to someone who is 'doing good'.

**Beta error**
This implies that a statistical test does not detect an existing difference between groups when in reality there is one.

**Bias**
Any influence that produces distortion in the results of the study.

**Bracketing**
The process of bringing to awareness, acknowledging and setting aside the researcher's assumptions and biases about the phenomenon being studied.

**Bricolage**
A research method that creatively amalgamates or synthesises a range of methodologies and strategies deemed appropriate by the researcher in pursuit of the most robust and accurate explication of findings.

**Case control study**

A study that compares a group of well individuals with a group of individuals who have the illness or health condition of interest. The two groups are compared with respect to past exposure to risk factors.

**Case-study sampling**

The selection of cases that are most appropriate to the subject under investigation.

**Causality**

A relationship of cause and effect. It has a minimum of three conditions: a strong relationship between the proposed cause and effect; the proposed cause must precede the effect in time; and the proposed cause must be present whenever the effect occurs.

**Clinical guidelines**

Recommendations for practice based on the best available evidence.

**Closed-ended question**

A question that limits responses to predetermined categories. A closed-ended question will normally be answered using a simple 'yes/no', or 'strongly agreed/agreed/strongly not agreed/not agreed'.

**Cluster random sampling**

A method where a random selection of a subset of usually geographically dispersed components of the population is made and forms the sample.

**Code**

A name given to data that have been separated into component parts.

**Cohort study**

A study in which a group free of illness is observed for exposure to risk factors that are hypothesised to increase or decrease the chance of getting the illness. The study group will be followed up through time in order to compare the frequency of the illness of groups who have different levels of exposure.

**Collaboration**

A creative process where two or more people or organisations work together to achieve a common goal.

**Concept**

A mental idea based on observations of behaviours or characteristics, for example pain and stress.

**Concurrent mixed methods design**

A design where the quantitative and qualitative data collection and data analysis are carried out within the same timeframe.

**Conference**

A meeting or gathering of professionals for discussion and sharing of ideas.

**Confidence interval**

A statement about the target population based on values derived from a sample. It tells us where the true value from the target population is likely to be.

**Confidentiality**

This is when the researcher promises to protect the identity of the participant by allocating either a code number or a pseudonym to the participant.

**Confounding variable**
An independent variable that varies systematically with the hypothetical causal variable under study. When uncontrolled, the effects of a confounding variable cannot be distinguished from those of the study variable.

**Constant comparison**
The process whereby the data and the concepts created from analysis are compared to ensure that they are a good fit and re-evaluated if they are not.

**Construct validity**
The extent to which a scale measures the underlying construct.

**Content validity**
The extent to which items on a scale reflect the concept being measured.

**Convenience sampling**
The selection of participants easily accessible to the researcher.

**Criterion validity**
Used to evaluate whether or not a scale measures what it is supposed to measure by comparing it with another measure known to be valid.

**Critical appraisal**
A term used to assess the outcomes for evidence of a research study's effectiveness.

**Critical social theory**
A theory or an intellectual form that has criticism at the centre of its knowledge production. A broad range of ideas and frameworks are used to help people question, deconstruct and then reconstruct knowledge to uncover issues of power and social inequality.

**Critique**
To critique is to read and examine the strengths and limitations of a published study.

**Crossover study**
A study that administers more than one treatment sequentially to each participant so that comparison can be made of the effects of different treatments on a dependent variable for the same participant.

**Cross-sectional study**
A study based on observation of a phenomenon at a single time for the purpose of inferring trends over time.

**Data extraction**
The process of extracting the methods and results from existing research studies for further meta-analysis or presentation in summary tables within a systematic review.

**Deductive approach**
A method of moving from the general to the specific: from the macro to the micro.

**Dependent variable**
The outcome variable that is thought to depend on or be caused by another variable, the independent variable.

**Descriptive study**

This aims to accurately describe characteristics of persons, places, situations or groups, and the frequency with which certain phenomena occur.

**Dissemination**

The circulation of a piece of research, which means publishing it or presenting it as a conference paper.

**Double-blind strategy**

A method of studying a drug or a procedure in which both the participants and researchers are kept unaware of who is actually getting which specific procedure.

**Emphasis dimension**

This considers the status of the qualitative and quantitative elements in a mixed methods study. See **time dimension**.

**Epidemiology**

A discipline that describes, quantifies and postulates causal mechanisms for health phenomena in populations.

**Equivalence or interrater reliability**

This means comparing the degree to which two raters measuring the same event obtain the same results.

**Ethnography**

A qualitative research method designed to explore cultural patterns of behaviour—social interactions and associated meanings—for individuals, groups and communities.

**Ethnonursing**

A research method used to explore and describe care patterns in cultures.

**Evidence-based practice**

A process that requires the practitioner to identify knowledge gaps, find research evidence to address knowledge gaps, and determine the relevance of the evidence to a particular client's situation.

**Experimental research design**

A research design used to test cause-and-effect relationships between variables. Research participants are randomly assigned to either an intervention group or a control group. The independent variable is manipulated for the intervention group but not for the control group. Both groups' outcomes are measured on the same dependent variable.

**External validity of research design**

The extent to which the results of a study can be generalised to other situations and to other people.

**Extraneous variable**

A variable that confounds the relationship between the independent and the dependent variables and that needs to be controlled either in the research design or through statistical procedures.

**Familiarisation**

The process of becoming familiar with the data. The process often begins by transcribing the data, reading and rereading the transcript and continuing on through the process of analysis.

**Feminism**

Feminism refers to a range of feminist thought and approaches to enquiry concerned with the social structures and processes that lead to gender inequality and oppression with the aim of achieving emancipation and equality.

**Focus group**

A form of qualitative research in which a group of people are asked about their perceptions, opinions, beliefs and attitudes towards a study topic. Questions are asked in an interactive group setting where participants are free to talk with other group members.

**Generalisation**

The extent to which findings are applicable to another similar sample or population.

**Grey literature**

Unpublished literature in the form of theses, government reports or conference proceedings.

**Grounded theory**

A systematic process of enquiry in which the researcher engages in a process of constant comparative analysis of data at each stage of the research process in order to generate theories about the phenomenon of concern.

**Hawthorne effect**

A phenomenon in which participants improve or modify their behaviour as a result of being part of an experiment or research study.

**Hermeneutics**

The interpretation of information or data.

**Heuristics**

A process of internal search with the aim of exploring and discovering personal insights and understanding of a phenomenon of intense interest to the researcher.

**Homogeneity or internal consistency**

The extent (strength of association) to which all items in the scale measure the same concept or construct. The most commonly used test of consistency is the Cronbach's alpha coefficient.

**Human research ethics committees**

HRECs are established to approve human research ethics applications.

**Human rights**

In research this applies to the participant being fully informed about the research as well as being able to withdraw from participating at any stage.

**Hypothesis**

A statement about the relationship between two variables (factors or characteristics in a study).

**Impact factor**

Calculated for each journal based on citation of articles across a year. The higher the impact factor the more widely read the journal is.

**Incompatibility thesis**

The assumption that accommodation between paradigms is not feasible.

**Independent variable**
The variable expected to cause or influence the dependent variable. In an experimental study, researchers manipulate this independent variable.

**Inductive approach**
A method of moving from the specific to the general: from empirical data to theory generation.

**Inferential statistics**
Applied during the study design to estimate the appropriate sample size according to the specified research hypothesis and during the analysis to confirm or reject the research hypothesis.

**Internal validity of research design**
A property of research design that reflects the extent to which a causal conclusion based on a study is warranted, or that can exclude other factors as alternative explanations of the observed association between the variables under investigation.

**Interrater reliability:** *see* **Equivalence**

**Likert scale**
Used to measure attitudes and beliefs. The degree of agreement or disagreement to a statement of a question is assigned a numerical value.

**Measures of central tendency**
A summary phrase in descriptive statistics for numerical data that describe the centre of the distribution. The most frequently used measures of central tendency are the arithmetic mean and the median.

**Meta-analysis**
A statistical method used to combine the results of several studies that address a set of related research hypotheses.

**Meta-synthesis**
A qualitative approach for drawing inferences from similar or related studies, identifying key features and presenting findings representative of all data.

**Method**
The prescribed systematic procedures and protocols involved in carrying out a research project.

**Methodology**
The theoretical or philosophical framework that underpins and guides the research process throughout the study; the principles that embody a research approach and guide the researcher in the application of methods. The longer word is often used to mean just 'method', and the student needs to be aware of possible confusion here.

**Mixed methods research**
Research that systematically combines the collection and analysis of both qualitative and quantitative data in the same study.

**Model**
A structure or framework designed to symbolise a concept or phenomenon.

**Multivariable procedures**
Methods, most widely used in the health sciences, that enable the simultaneous assessment of the effects of several study factors on the outcome as well as adjustment for confounding.

**Narrative synthesis**
Summarising evidence or knowledge in the form of a meta-analysis is not always possible, and in these cases the evidence is presented in a text format as a narrative synthesis.

**Naturalist paradigm**
The exploration of phenomena as they occur in their natural setting.

**Networking**
Involves the researcher either knowing or recruiting participants by asking colleagues or associates.

**Non-experimental research design**
Research in which researchers collect data without introducing any manipulation or change.

**Non-maleficence**
A term referring to someone who is 'doing no harm'.

**Non-participant observation (overt)**
Observation of participants (with their full knowledge) by a researcher who does not take an active part in the situation.

**Non-participant observation (covert)**
Observation of participants where they are not aware of being observed.

**Non-probability sampling**
Occurs where the researcher cannot ensure that each case in the population has been represented in the sample, so that they cannot claim representativeness of the sample. In addition, non-probability samples may contain bias not known or recognised by the researcher.

**Notation system**
A systematic way of describing how a mixed methods study is conducted.

**Open-ended question**
A form of question that requires the participant to answer in their own words. It allows a spontaneous, unstructured response and is sometimes called a subjective question.

**Opportunistic sampling**
On-the-spot decisions about sampling to take advantage of opportunities during actual data collection.

**Paradigm**
In the research context, paradigm has come to mean the commitments, beliefs and values, methods and outlooks shared across a research discipline.

**Parameter**
The number or data that describe a population.

**Participant observation**
A method of qualitative research in which the researcher understands the contextual meanings of an event or events through participating and observing as a subject in the research. The degree of sharing in activities between the researcher and the participant ranges from full participation to onlooker.

**Peer review**
The process of subjecting scholarly work, research or ideas to the scrutiny of others who are peers in the same field or discipline area.

**Peer-reviewed journal**
A journal that publishes a paper that has been submitted to an editorial committee and passed by a process of blinded peer review before it is accepted for publication.

**Phenomenology**
A philosophical movement and a mode of enquiry that aims to understand the essential structures or essence of phenomena of individuals' everyday experiences.

**Phenomenon**
Any observable thing or occurrence that is worth noting; plural, phenomena.

**Placebo effect**
The reported response or change in the dependent variable by an individual who does not receive an intervention or receives an inert intervention.

**Population**
A clearly defined grouping of people, animals or objects that can be identified by specific characteristics or properties useful to research.

**Positivist**
Someone who believes in the concepts of an objective reality and the notion of determinism.

**Pragmatism**
A worldview which accepts multiple realities that reflect both biased and unbiased perspectives and supports practicality when addressing the research question. It has been proposed as a paradigm that best fits mixed methods research.

**Probability sampling**
A sampling approach that allows for all participants to have an equal chance of being selected.

**Probing question**
A question aimed to help the participant think more deeply about the study issue. It is used to search in-depth information or to make a thorough examination of the study topic.

**Problem statement**
A problem statement describes what the situation is that requires changing or understanding and how the study will address this situation or problem.

**Psychometric scale**
A set of written questions or statements designed to measure a particular concept such as anxiety or stress.

**Publish**
To disseminate literature or information to others, generally in a printed format.

**Purposive sampling**
Used where the researcher recruits participants to the study based on some attribute that the researcher feels is appropriate.

## P-value

The p-value gives the probability of obtaining in a sample a difference as large as the actually observed one if in reality there is no such difference. Thus the p-value is the probability that an observed difference is attributable to chance alone.

## Qualitative research methods

Inductive research methods such as grounded theory, ethnography or phenomenology, which explore human experience and 'emancipate' it—set it free from the constraints of labelling.

## Quantitative data

These can be either categorical or numerical; statistical methods are directly linked to the type of data investigated.

## Quantitative research

A systematic investigation with a rigorous and controlled design, using precise measurements and obtaining quantifiable information to answer a research question.

## Quantitative research methods

Deductive research methods such as randomised control trials, quasi-experimental studies, cohort studies, observational, descriptive or exploratory designs. These methods test for cause and effect, explore relationships between variables and control variables.

## Quasi-experimental research design

Research in which the researchers manipulate an independent variable in order to evaluate the change of a dependent variable. However, not all of the following conditions are met in such a study: random allocation of treatment condition to participants, and a comparison group of participants to those who receive the manipulation. There is some control to increase the internal validity of the results.

## Random selection

A sampling method in which every case has the same opportunity to be selected for the study.

## Randomised controlled trial

A study in which similar people are randomly allocated to two (or more) groups to test a specific treatment. The experimental group receives the treatment to be tested. Another group, the comparison or control group, receives an alternative treatment, a dummy treatment (placebo) or no treatment at all.

## Reliability

The degree of consistency or dependability with which an instrument measures the attribute it is intended to measure.

## Research design

The overall plan for answering a research question, including an appropriate detailed plan for enhancing the integrity of the study.

## Research hypothesis

A precise statement about the research question the study will be designed to answer. It must be plausible and falsifiable.

## Research question

The question being asked by the research—the issue it sets out to explore.

**Review protocol (for systematic review)**
A well-defined document that provides explicit strategies to undertake a systematic review so that bias is reduced.

**Risk**
The level of either emotional or physical discomfort a potential participant may experience when being involved in research.

**Sample**
A subset of persons or units that carry the same characteristics as the overarching population.

**Sampling bias**
Any influence that produces systematic distortion in the sample, where increasing the sample will increase the bias effect.

**Sampling error**
Error resulting from taking a sample instead of measuring every unit in the population.

**Sampling frame**
A list (e.g. map or other specification) of all the elements in the population from which a sample is to be selected.

**Scholarship**
The conduct of scholarly pursuits, usually within the academic world.

**Searching the literature for a systematic review**
A defined scope of literature with prior specification of eligibility criteria.

**Semantic differential scale**
Scale designed to ask respondents their position or attitude to a concept using two adjectives at opposite ends of a continuum.

**Semistructured interview**
A flexible set of questions which allow new questions to be brought up during the interview as a result of what the participant says. The interviewer in a semi-structured interview generally has a framework of the topic to be explored.

**Sequential mixed methods design**
A design where the quantitative and qualitative data collection are in separate timeframes and in two distinct phases.

**Snowballing or chain sampling**
Involves starting with one or two participants and then relying on them to identify and refer to the researcher other potential participants who meet the inclusion criteria for the study.

**Stability or test-retest reliability**
The ability of a scale to produce the same or similar results with the same group of participants on two (or more) occasions.

**Statistic**
The number or data that describe a sample.

**Statistical hypothesis tests**
Procedures that allow the calculation of the likelihood of an observed difference between two or more groups that are compared.

**Stratified random selection**
A sampling method where a similar proportion of cases to the population are selected in each stratum.

**Structured interview**
A formalised set of questions used to collect quantitative research data when the order in which questions are asked of survey respondents is standardised. It is also known as a standardised interview or a researcher-administered survey.

**Systematic review**
A method used to review the existing literature on a particular question, by identifying, appraising, selecting and synthesising all high-quality research evidence relevant to that question.

**Systematic sampling**
A method where every $n$th case (set interval) is selected from the list.

**Target audience**
The primary group of people who are most interested in the content of a conference paper or journal article.

**Target population**
The entire group the researcher is interested in and to whom the study results are to be generalised.

**Theme**
A theme is generated when similar ideas from participants expressed in the data are brought together. The theme may be labelled using a word or expression taken directly from the data or else named by the researcher to best characterise the collection of data.

**Theoretical sampling**
A process where findings from a small number of cases determine theoretically important aspects that direct subsequent sample or case selection.

**Theoretical saturation**
The point at which no further data collection or coding is required because no new instances are to be found in the data.

**Theory**
A set of interrelated assumptions put forward to describe or explain a given phenomenon.

**Time dimension**
This relates to when the phases of a mixed methods study are carried out. See **emphasis dimension**.

**Triangulation**
The process of integrating the results from multiple sources of data or research methods in the same study. The word is a metaphor from engineering surveying, where readings are taken from several viewpoints.

**Type I error**
An error where the null hypothesis is rejected when it is in fact true. Also **alpha error**.

**Type II error**

The failure to reject the null hypothesis when the null hypothesis is false. Also **beta error**.

**Unstructured interview**

A method of interview where questions can be changed or adapted to meet the participant's understanding or belief. Questions can be influenced by each individual person's responses.

**Validity**

The degree to which a measurement instrument measures what it is intended to measure.

**Variable**

A characteristic or factor that will vary within a study (e.g. age, blood pressure, depression scores).

**Visual analogue scale**

A straight line, 100 mm in length, with anchors representing the extremes of the particular concept being measured.

**Vulnerable people**

Individuals who are marginalised and discriminated against in society because of their social situation—class, ethnicity, gender, age, illness, disability or sexual preference. They are often difficult to reach and require special consideration when they are involved in research. The term is also used to refer to people who are difficult to access in societies.

# INDEX